Vitreoretinal Surgery

Principles and Techniques

Vitreoretinal Surgery

Principles and Techniques

Nabin Kumar Pattnaik MD
Director and Chief Eye Surgeon
Dr. Pattnaik's Laser Eye Institute
and Referral Retina Center
M-1, Lajpat Nager-3
New Delhi-110024
(India)

Illustrations by
Mrunmayee Pattnaik MSc (Optometry)

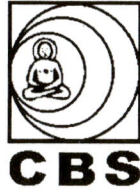

CBS

CBS Publishers & Distributors
4596/1-A, 11 Darya Ganj, New Delhi-110 002 (India)
e-mail: cbspubs@del3.vsnl.net.in   website: http://www.cbspd.com

Vitreoretinal Surgery

First Edition : 2003

ISBN : 81-239-0956-X

Production Director : Vinod K. Jain

Published by :
Satish Kumar Jain for CBS Publishers & Distributors,
4596/1-A, 11 Darya Ganj, New Delhi - 110 002 (India)
E-mail : cbspubs@del3.vsnl.net.in
Website : http://www.cbspd.com

Branch Office :
Seema House, 2975, 17th Cross, K.R. Road,
Bansankari 2nd Stage, Bangalore - 560070
Fax : 080-6771680 • E-mail : cbsbng@vsnl.net

Printed at :
Meenakshi Printers, Delhi-11 0006

Foreword

The arrival of the new millennium coincides with the remarkable and highly innovative development of vitreoretinal surgery. The future of vitreoretinal surgery looks still brighter. Dazzling biotechnological discoveries and technological marvels raise the expectations of vireoretinal surgeons. In this book an attempt has been made to provide reasonably complete and up-to-date material, which is written primarily keeping in mind the requirements of the postgraduate students and young ophthalmologists who wish to take up vitreoretinal speciality as a career.

The text has been organized in such a way that the students can easily understand, retain, and reproduce the facts and the principles. Brief introduction has been given in the beginning of each chapter to provide a clear outline of the topics discussed. The book has been well illustrated through computer-generated colour graphics and a significant number of photographs depicting operative steps of the surgical techniques have been liberally incorporated. This book simplifies and succinctly explains the surgical techniques both for the the postgraduate student who is planning to choose vitreoretinal surgery as a specialty as well as the beginner vitreoretinal surgeon who still has to understand and learn the fine nuances of the surgery which is based on modern hi-tech equipment.

It gives me a great pleasure in writing the Foreword to this book.

Dr. Nabin K. Pattnaik needs to be highly complimented for fully utilizing his talent and providing an academic insight into the different aspects of vitreoretinal surgery. All retinal surgeons will find sufficient food for thought and several practical pearls while going through this book. The text also takes one along the horizons by discussing recent advances and future directions of vitreoretinal surgery. I congratulate Dr. Pattnaik, one of my former students at Dr. Rajendra Prasad Centre for Ophthalmic Sciences, for the outstanding work done in bringing out this publication in its present form. My blessings and good wishes are always with him.

Prof. H. K. Tiwari MD
Head of Vitreoretina Unit and
Chief, Dr. Rajendra Prasad Centre for Ophthalmic Sciences,
All India Institute of Medical Sciences,
New Delhi.

Foreword

It is a pleasure to note that Dr. Nabin Kumar Pattnaik MD has written this book based on his experience around retinovitreous diseases and their management, which is understood by the majority of us. He deserves to be congratulated and commended for the effort. The two chapters that I have read are crisp and straightforward in their approach and make it easy reading. Computer-generated illustrations are great.

I am sure the book will prove very useful to postgraduates in ophthalmology and all those who decide to pursue this subspecialty as their career.

I appreciate his desire to share his experience with others and wish him good luck.

Dr. P. N. Nagpal
Eye Research Centre and Retina Foundation
Ahmedabad-380004

Preface

Two decades ago, modern vitreous surgery was a dream. Today it is the most effective tool for treating posterior segment diseases. Significant technical and technological advances have taken place in further refinement of the vitreous surgery. These advances have also helped one to understand the pathophysiological abnormalities of many common diseases. Some of the brilliant and innovative surgeons have added entirely new dimensions to treat surgically a variety of vitreoretinal diseases. Vitreous surgery has a long way to go.

This book is intended mainly for the postgraduate students and trainee ophthalmologists who are keen to take up vitreoretinal surgery as a specialty. The text should also prove useful to those wishing to update their knowledge in this rapidly advancing branch of medicine. The main emphasis has been laid on the basic as well as most advanced clinical interpretation; step-by-step surgical procedures, techniques and complications of the more commonly performed procedures have been included. The bibliography provides the reader key references for pursuing particular topics in depth to review the significant advances made in vitreoretinal surgery during the last few years. It has been necessary to keep abreast of the latest and innovative procedures and techniques to upgrade the reader.

There is no doubt that scleral buckling is the gold standard for the retinal detachment surgery till today. New instruments have given us the ability to solve problems that were previously not treatable through surgical efforts.

The first chapter is a description of basic surgical anatomy and its importance in vitreoretinal surgery. Setting up of vitreoretinal units and importance of operating microscope and wide-angle fundus observation system has been discussed in a vivid form for the understanding of the beginner. Chapters 5 and 6 deal with patient preparation and basics of pars plana vitrectomy.

A wide variety of computer-generated graphics representing the artist's view of the anatomy and surgical procedures is presented throughout the text. Three-dimensional diagrams depicting the interiors of the eye and side-views have been liberally included in all the chapters for better understanding.

Limited selection of references at the end of each chapter provides a guide for additional study. Vitreoretinal surgery is highly technical and each chapter has been developed to facilitate communication among fellow surgeons. Diabetic vitrectomy, surgery for proliferative vitreoretinopathy, macular surface disorders, ocular trauma and prematurity of retinopathy need special guide to therapeutic studies. The roles of vitrectomy in endophthalmitis and the operative complication have been given special consideration at the end. CBS Publishers & Distributors, the publishers of this book, have been patient and helpful in guiding me through the long process of the preparing the manuscript and illustrative material for publication.

Dr. Nabin Kumar Pattnaik MD

Acknowledgements

This book would not have been possible without the help and encouragement of numerous individuals from home and abroad.

I am extremely grateful to Mrunmayee Pattnaik and Jayant Bhalla for taking time and care to review the manuscript and for making computer-generated artwork. I would wish to place on record my sincere appreciation to my teachers and friends Prof. H. K. Tewari, Prof. P.N. Nagpal, Prof. R. V. Azad, Prof. Namperumalsamy, Prof. Amod Gupta, Prof. A. K. Paul of Eye Institute, Sitapur, Dr. T. P. Das, Dr. S. Natarajan, Dr. Atul Kumar, Dr. Mangat R. Dogra, Dr. Cyrus Shroff, Dr. R. P. Singh, Dr. Vinay Garodia, Dr. C. S. Chauhan and Dr. Gopal Verma for their constant encouragement. Dr. A. K. Singh, one of my dear friends, needs special thanks for his constant encouragements to write this book.

My special thanks to Dr. C. Claes, head of Vitreoretina, Department of Opthalmology, A.Z. Middelheim, Antwerp, Belgium, for support and encouragement.

I would like to thank Prof. L. P. Agarwal, former chief of Dr. Rajendra Prasad Center for Ophthalmic Sciences and former Director of All India Institute of Medical Sciences, New Delhi, for introducing me to the word of ophthalmology.

Last but not least, I would like to convey my gratitude to Mr. Y.N. Arjuna, Publishing Director of CBS Publishers, for reviewing and editing the manuscript and for making many helpful suggestions.

Finally, I would like to thank my son Dr. Abhiyan Kumar and my family members for supporting me and understanding the loss of some special moments during this task.

Dr. Nabin Kumar Pattnaik MD

Contents

Foreword by Prof H.K. Tiwari   *v*

Foreword by Dr. P.N. Nagpal   *vi*

Preface   *vii*

CHAPTER **1**
Surgical Anatomy and its Importance in Vitreoretinal Surgery   **1**

Introduction   1
Vitreous Anatomy   2
    The vitreous humour   2
    Cortical vitreous   2
    The main vitreous body   3
Important Surgical Landmarks   4

CHAPTER **2**
Setting Up the Vitreoretinal Unit   **9**

Introduction   9
Infrastructure   10
Fluorescein Angiography Unit   11
Ultrasonography Unit   11
Laser Photocoagulation Unit   12
Operating Room   12
Vitreoretinal Tray   13
Vitrectomy Accessories   13
Consumable Items   14
Duty of Responsible Staff   14
Sterilization   14
Surgeon and Trained Assistant   15
Standby Anaesthesiologist   15
Supportive Service   15
Operating Room Assistants   16

CHAPTER **3**
Operating Microscope and Wide Angle Fundus Observation System   **17**

Introduction   17
Objective Lens Assembly   18
Zoom Device   18
Beam Splitter and Eyepiece Head   18
Illumination   19

Coaxial Zoom Illumination   19
Coaxial and Oblique Zoom Illumination   19
Filter and Protection for Eyes   19
Checking of Operating Microscope after Surgery   20
Care, Sterilization and Maintenance of Microscope   20
Trouble-Shooting and Remedies of Microscope   21
Foot Switch   21
An Overview of Switching Functions of the Foot Switch   22
Fundus Contact Lenses for Vitreoretinal Surgery   23
Wide Angle Fundus Observation System   23
Binocular Indirect Ophthalmo Microscope (BIOM)   24
Erected Image Binocular Ophthalmoscopic System (EIBOS)   24
  Advantages of EIBOS   24
Diagramatic Representation of Different Parts of EBIOS   25
Description of Functions   26
How to Use   26
Cleaning and Sterilization   26

CHAPTER **4**
Basic Working Principle of Vitrectomy Equipment   **27**

Introduction   27
Foot Switch Functions   28
Back-Flush Features   29
Preparing the Vitrectomy Unit for Use   30
  Preoperating procedure   30
  Dual illumination module   31
  Diathermy module   31
  Air-module   32
  Vitrectomy/VFI module   33
  Irrigation/aspiration (I/A) and viscus fluid extraction module   34
  Compressed air inlet   34
  Irrigation   35
  Aspiration   35
Cleaning and Sterilizing Instruction for Accessories   35
  Recommendation guidelines for ethylene oxide sterilization parameters   35
  Recommendation guidelines for steam sterilization   35
  Cleaning instructions   36

CHAPTER **5**
Patient Preparation for Vitreous Surgery and Care of Instruments   **37**

Introduction   37
Patient Preparation   37
  Dilatation of Pupils   38
  Preparation of Eye   38
  Preparation for Surgery   38
  Anaesthesia   39
  Check-List of Instruments in OT   39
    Check lists for vitrectomy and fragmatome units   39

    Checking the microscope   39
    Checking the microsurgical equipment   39
   Preparation   42
   Irrigation Fluid   42
Care of Instruments   43
   Cleaning   43
   Storage   43
   Instruments Sets   43
   Disinfections and Sterilisation   43

CHAPTER **6**

Pars Plana Vitrectomy: Basic Technique   **45**

Introduction   45
Patient Preparation   45
   Mydriasis   45
   Preparation of the surgical field   46
   Irrigation fluids   46
   Conjunctival incisions   47
   Making the entry sites   47
The Infusion Cannula   49
Instrument Handling   51
Pars Plana Lensectomy   53
Steps for Removal of Lens   53
Management of Small Pupil   54
   Non-surgical treatment of small pupils   54
   Surgical treatment of small pupil   54
     Sphincterotomy or pupilloplasty   55
     Mid-peripheral iridectomy   55
     Radial iridectomy for miotic pupil   55
     Multiple sphincterotomies   55
Steps of Vitrectomy in Simple Vitreous Haemorrhage   55
   Vitreous haemorrhage flow chart   59
   Vacuum technique   61
Fluid–Air Exchange   62
   Fluid–air exchange associated with drainage of subretinal fluid   68
   Fluid–air exchange combined with drainage of subretinal fluid though a posterior
     dehiscence   68
   Fluid–air exchange after retinal reapplication using a liquid perfluorocarbon   68
   IR–PFCL exchange   68
Laser Photocoagulation   69
Closure   70

CHAPTER **7**

Retained Lens Fragments and Intraocular Lens Dislocation   **73**

Introduction   73
Identification of Rsk Factors   73
Time of Removal of Retained Lens Fragments and Dislocated Lens   74
Emphasized During Cataract Surgery   74
Loss of Lens Fragments into the Vitreous   74

CHAPTER **8**
Surgical Treatment of Macular Surface Disorder   **81**

Macular Hole   81
  Introduction   81
  Clinical features   81
  Diagnosis   83
Macular Hole Surgery   83
  When to perform surgery in macular hole   84
  Surgical technique   84
  Removal of ILM   88
Macular Pucker (Macular Distortion)   90
Subretinal Neovascularization   93
  Introduction   93
  Subfoveal choroidal neovascularization   93
  Instrumentation   94
  Surgical technique   95
  Complications   97
  Postoperative management   97

CHAPTER **9**
Diabetic Vitrectomy   **99**

Introduction   99
Anatomic Considerations   99
Indication of Diabetic Vitrectomy   103
Surgical Objectives   104
Basic Diabetic Vitrectomy   104
Segmentation on Fibrovascular Proliferation   107
Delamination of Diabetic Membrane   107
En Bloc Techniques in Diabetic Membrane   111
Diabetic Membrane Delamination: Bimanual Dissection Technique   113
Anterior Hyaloidal Proliferation   115
Intraoperative Complications of Diabetic Membrane Dissection   116

CHAPTER **10**
Surgery for Proliferative Vitreoretinopathy   **119**

Introduction   119
Classification   119
Anatomic Presentation in Proliferative Vitreoretinopathy   120
Principles of Treatment of Proliferative Vitreoretinopathy to Close All Retinal Breaks   122
Optimal Time for Operation in Proliferative Vitreoretinopathy   122
Vitrectomy Technique in Proliferative Vitreoretinopathy   122
Membrane Removal in Proliferative Vitreoretinopathy   123
Membrane Removal with Perflurocarbon Technique in Proliferative Vitreoretinopathy   128

CHAPTER **11**
**Management of Ocular Trauma and Retained
  Intraocular Foreign Bodies**   **131**

Introduction   131
Wound Closure   132

Timing of Surgery   132
The Role of Infection in Timing of Surgery   132
Risk of Imtraoperative Haemorrhage   133
Vitrectomy Endolaser Silicone Oil Tamponade   133
Removal of Foreign Bodies   133
The Role of Vitrectomy   133
Techniques of Intraocular Foreign Body Removal   134
Large Retinal Intraocular Foreign Body   138
Encapsulated RIOFB   138
Retained IOFB in the Vitreous Cavity   138
Subretinal Intraocular Foreign Body   138
Glass and Other Foreign Bodies   139
Repair of Scleral Laceration, Ruptures and Prognosis   139
Locations and Extent of Penetrating Injuries Related to Prognosis   139
Proliferative Vitreoretinopathy (PVR) in Ocular Trauma   140
Surgery of PVR in Penetrating Trauma   140

CHAPTER **12**
Retinopathy of Prematurty (ROP)   141

Introduction   141
Pathogenesis   141
Classification   141
Staging   142
  Stage 1: Demarcation line   142
  Stage 2: Ridge   143
  Stage 3: Ridge with extraretinal fibrovascular proliferation   144
  Stage 4: Partial retinal development   144
  Stage 5: Total retinal detachment   145
Plus Disease   145
Threshold Disease   145
Screening   145
Laser/Cryo Treatment in Retinopathy of Prematurity   146
Surgical Management of Retinopathy of Prematurity   146
Management of Pupil   147
Surgical Options   148
Posterior Tractional Problems   148
Peripheral Traction Problems   149
Complications   150

CHAPTER **13**
Rhegmatogenous Retinal Detachment   151

Introduction   151
Diagnosis   151
Surgical Anatomy of Conjunctiva, Tenon's Capsule and Muscles Isolation   152
Localisation and Treatment of Retinal Breaks   154
Basic Surgical Technique   155
Basic Requirement of Retinal Detachment Surgery   156
Methods of Buckling   156

Securing the Ends of the Band   159
Management of Subretinal Fluid Drainage   159
Drainage of Subretinal Fluid   160
Buckle Position, Suture Finalisation and Adjustments   161
Custodis Technique   167
Intraoperative Complications of Scleral Buckling   168
    Corneal clouding   168
    Scleral perforations   168
    Miosis   168
    Drainage complications   168
Postoperative Complication   169
    Glaucoma   169
    Anterior segment ischemia   170
    Extrusions and buckle infection   170
    Choroidal detachment   170
    Cystoid macular oedema   171
    Macular pucker   171
    Postoperative diplopia   171
    Changes in refractive error after scleral buckling   171
Main Cause of Failure of Retina Detachment (RD) Surgery   172
Failure of Primary Retinal Detachment—Pitfalls   172
Precaution with Cryotherapy   173
Precaution with Scleral Buckling   173
Preventive Steps to Avoid Primary Failure   173
Pneumatic Retinopexy   174
    Introduction   174
    Preoperative evaluation   174
    Procedure   175

CHAPTER **14**
Role of Vireous Surgery in Primary Rhegmatogenous Retinal Detachment   **179**

Introduction   179
Indication for Vitrectomy in Rhegmatogenous Retinal Detachment   180
Pars Plana Vitrectomy for Retinal Detachments   181
Primary Vitrectomy in Retinal Detachment Caused by Macular Hole   182
Primary Vitrectomy in Retinal Detachment Caused by Posterior Breaks   183
Primary Vitrectomy in Retinal Detachment Caused by Peripheral Breaks   185

CHAPTER **15**
Management of Giant Retinal Tear   **187**

Introduction   187
Diagnosis and Preoperative Evaluation   187
Location of Giant Retinal Tear   188
Mobility of Posterior Retinal Flap   188
Extent of Proliferative Vitreoretinopathy (PVR)   189
Procedure (Surgical Technique)   190
Silicone Oil Technique in Giant Retinal Tear   193

Silicone Oil Removal   199
Liquid Perfluorocarbon in Giant Retinal Tear   199
Treatment of Giant Tear   202
Postoperative Complications   203
Management of Fellow Eye   205

CHAPTER **16**
Role of Vitrectomy in Endophthalmitis   **207**

Introduction   207
Diagnosis of Endophthalmitis   207
Intravitreal Injection of Antibiotics   207
Techniques of Intravitreal Injection   208
Role of Vitrectomy in Endophthalmitis   209
Removal of the Lens Capsule   210
Tips for Vitrectomy in Endophthalmitis   210
Surgical Technique   210

CHAPTER **17**
Complications of Operative Vitreous Surgery   **213**

Introduction   213
Complications Following Sclerotomy   213
Corneal Complications   215
Retinal Complications   215
Choroidal Haemorrhage   216
Vitreous Haemorrhage   216
Lens Complication   216
Miosis During Vitreous Surgery   216
Complications of Silicone Oil   217
    Emulsification   217
    Keratopathy   217
    Cataract   217
    Pupillary block   217
    Hypotony   217
    Peri silicone proliferative macular pucker   217
    Recurrent retinal detachments   217
Glaucoma in Vitreous Surgery   218
    Pupillary block glaucoma   218
    Silicone oil glaucoma   218
    Erythroclastic glaucoma   218
    Neovascular glaucoma   218
    Steroid glaucoma   218
    Open angle glaucoma   218
Retinal Burn   218
Endophthalmitis   219

Index   **221**

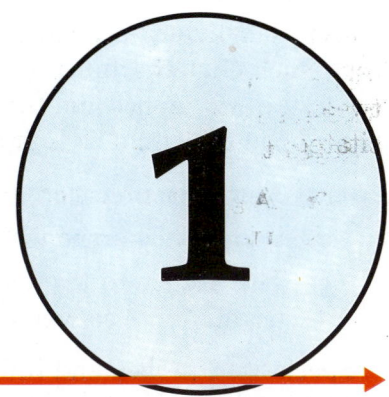

Surgical Anatomy and its Importance in Vitreoretinal Surgery

Introduction

Shafer in **1950** pioneered to initiate the surgical approach to the vitreous with his method of vitreous transplantation. This delicate and sophisticated branch was elaborated by Cibis in 1962 with his introduction of intravitreal silicone oil injection.

In **1971**, Machemer developed, the vitreous infusion suction cutter (VISC). Norton introduced the use of intravitreal sulphur hexafluoride gas, which is an adjuvant in the management of retinal detachment surgery.

Though early attempts at understanding the importance of vitreous in retinal detachment (RD) case made by **Von Graefe**, **Deutschman**, **Von Hippel**, **Rosengren** and others, the role of vitreous in the pathogenesis and surgical outcomes of retinal detachment (RD) largely buried under the success of **Gonin's** principles of retinal detachment surgery. It was **David Kasner** who in the late sixties demonstrated and introduced the concept of open sky vitrectomy in the management of patients with severe anterior segment trauma. Inspired by his work, Robert Machemer, father of modern vitreous surgery developed a mechanical device to aid **Kasner** in his open sky vitrectomy. Very soon this device was modified and used through parsplana route and this paved the way for the modern day closed parsplana vitrectomy. This device incorporated all the components of the modern day surgery in a single device was making it bulky in use. This instrument was extremely popular for a few years till O'Malley introduced the concept of "divided-system instrumentation whereby changes in the design of the probe were done such that the functions of suction, cutter, aspiration and illumination was divided between the two probes and the infusion provided through a separate sclerotomy site. This necessitated the bimanual technique by the surgeon, and the advantages are as follows:

a. A greater precision and control in stabilization of globe rotation.
b. Use of the surgeon's better hand for delicate maneuvers.
c. The ability to transform instrument position such that tissues could be approached from a more convenient direction.

Specialized probes and illumination probes could be exchanged and introduced through either port, the technique of fluid air exchange; silicone oil injection through separate cannula is now possible. Now, the vitreous surgery is refinement of microsurgical and endosurgical techniques utilized for the posterior segment.

VITREOUS ANATOMY

The vitreous humour is an inert, avascular, transparent jelly-like structure, which serves only optical functions. It consists of a delicate framework of collagen and hyaluronic acid. It is a hydrophilic gel, which becomes "fluid" when its protein basis is coagulated due to advancing senile age, degeneration and also due to chemical and mechanical trauma. The vitreous body can be divided into two parts, the cortex and the nucleus, the main vitreous body (Fig. 1.1).

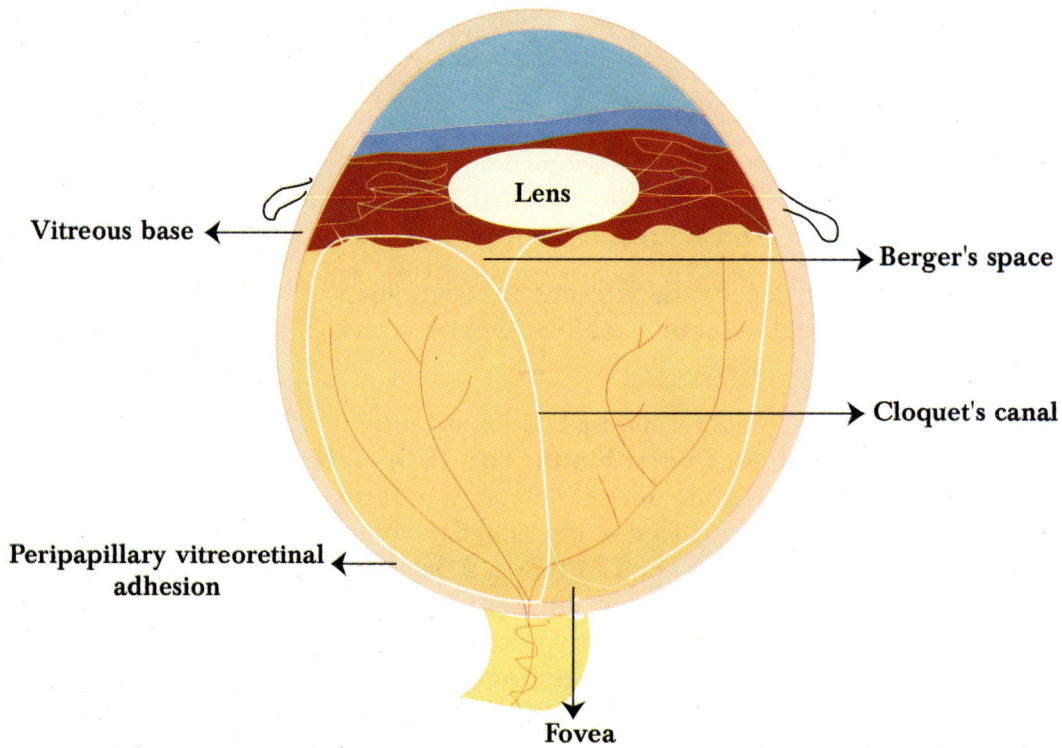

Fig. 1.1 Cross-sectional view of the eye

Cortical vitreous: It lies adjacent to the retina and is formed of cells and dense collagen fibrils. Its outer part is condensed to form the hyaloid membrane; which is loosely attached to the internal limiting membrane of the retina posteriorly as posterior hyaloid phase and firmly attached to lens anterioly as anterior hyaloid phase.

The main vitreous body (nucleus) has less dense fibrillar structure and is a true biological gel. It consists of a delicate framework (reticulum) of fine collagen fibrils interspersed with a hydrophilic mucopolysaccharide and hyaluronic acid. Microscopically the vitreous body is homogeneous, but exhibits wavy lines as of watered silk in the slit-lamp beam.

In normal adult eye, the vitreous adheres firmly to the retina at the vitreous base, which is attached 3 to 4 mm wide, and straddles around the ora serrata.

It is also attached of course less firmly to the retina around optic disc and surrounding macula. Many areas of vitreo retinal attachment are found along the retina vessels.

In early life the vitreous body is a homogenous gel consisting of a network of collagen fibrils separated from one another by macromolecules of hyaluronic acid. The density of fibrils is relatively higher near the retina and highest at the vitreous base.

With ageing the vitreous body undergoes loculation, depolymerization and precipitation of hyaluronic acid which produces liquification, as a result, the vitreous detached from the disc, it may pull loose a glial annulus, which the patient may see as a prominent ring (Vogt's ring) near the visual axis.

The macular region has a unique anatomy of the vitreoretinal junction, and is known to have increased vitreoretinal adherence, compared to the equatorial retina. This strong vitreoretinal adhesion in the macular region is not focal but is diffusely distributed throughout the posterior pole just behind the temporal vascular arcades. This increased adherence of the vitreous to the macula may predispose eyes to develop a dehiscence of the posterior vitreous cortex around the macula during spontaneous posterior vitreous detachment.

The optic nerve head or disc is the most prominent feature of the fundus. Foveola is the most functional center of the fundus. It is located in the center of the fovea, which has a diameter of about 5°. The macula is centered on the fovea and has a diameter of about 17°.

The multiple branches of the central retinal artery are readily identified by their bright red colour and relatively narrow caliber. The multiple tributaries of the central vein are recognised by their dark red colour and relatively wider caliber.

The horizontal meridians are usually identified by their radially oriented, long posterior ciliary artery accompanies the nerve. The nerve is relatively broad and has a yellow colour and the artery is usually inferior to the nerve temporally and superior to it nasally.

The ora serrata is the anterior limit of the sensory retina. The nasal ora-serrata is prominent and points anterioly but the pattern of serration is not present temporally where the ora-teeth are small or absent. Occasionally a white line is evident on the retina just posterior to the ora serrata representing the posterior limit of the vitreous base. A similar circumferential white line representing the anterior limit of the vitreous base is occasionally visible in the middle of the pars plana.

The normal fusion of the sensory retina and retinal pigment epithelium along the ora-serrata is referred to the retina choroidal adhesion. This zone is three or four mm wide in the temporal periphery but less than one mm wide in the nasal periphery. The equator is an important landmark. The distance from the ora to the equator is approximately four-disc (6–7 mm) diameter and the equator is just slightly anterior to the vortex ampullae.

IMPORTANT SURGICAL LANDMARKS

A comprehensive knowledge of surgical anatomy of the eye is essential for vitreoretinal surgery. The average anterior posterior diameter of the globe is 24 mm. In high myopia the anterior posterior diameter may be as great as 30 mm. The average circumference is 72 mm. The average horizontal diameter (23.5 mm) is slightly longer that the average vertical diameter 23 mm. The rectus muscles, superior rectus (SR), lateral rectus (LR), medial rectus (MR), arise from the posterior orbital walls, course forward through Tenon's capsule and insert into the sclera. The superior oblique (SO) arises from the apex of the orbit from the superior and the medical aspect of the optic foramen. It passes through a tendon and under the superior rectus before inserting in the sclera.

The external insertion of the muscles roughly corresponds to the anterior termination of the retina at the oraserrata internally, represented by the scalloped line.

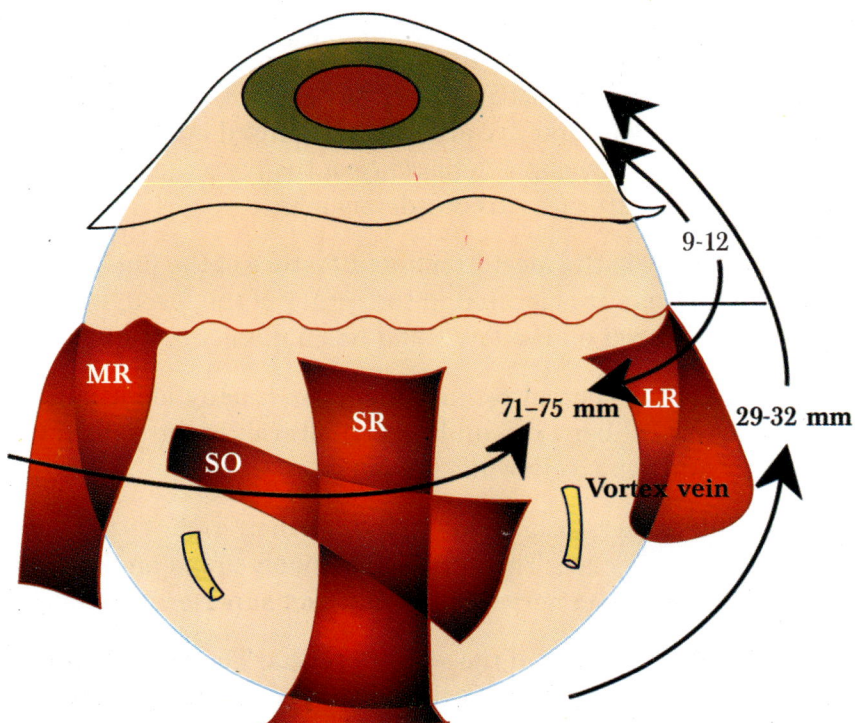

Fig. 1.2 Superior view of the external globe

The distance from the oraserrata measures on average from 5.7 mm nasally to 6.5 mm temporally. The distance from the limbus to the equator ranges from 9 to 12 mm and the distance from limbus to the posterior pole is 28 to 30 mm. Normal scleral thickness is approximately 1mm at the equator and posterior pole and 0.8 mm near the limbus. Under the rectus muscle insertion the sclera thin to 0.3 mm caution is necessary when working in this area (Fig. 1.2).

The cornea average 10 to 11 mm in width. The muscle insertion varies from 5.5 mm posterior to the limbus for the medial rectus to approximately 7.5 mm posterior to the limbus for the superior rectus. The superior rectus is the broadest insertion (10.6 to 11 mm); the medial rectus is the narrowest (9.2 to 9.7 mm) (Fig. 1.3).

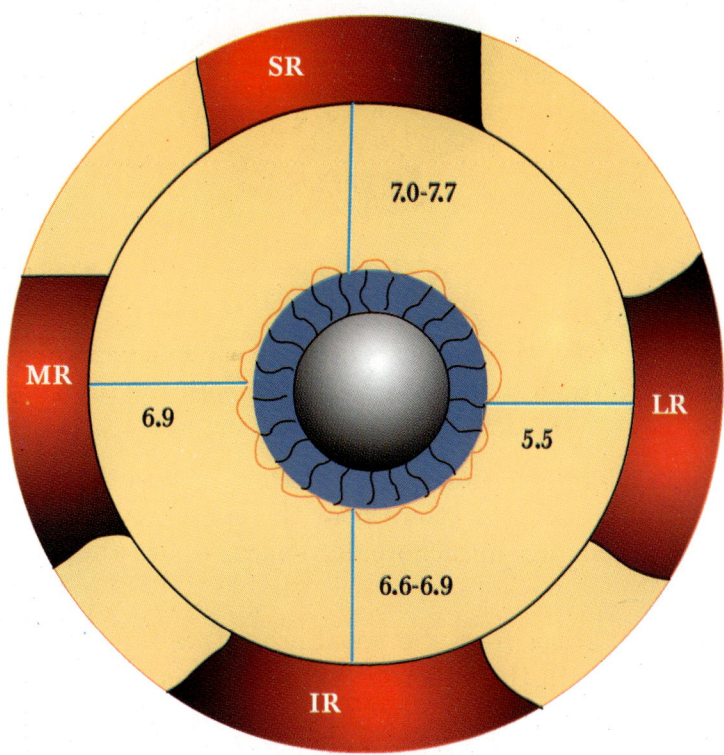

Fig. 1.3 *Muscle insertion posterior to the limbus*

The short anterior ciliary arteries course through the central part of the muscle to exit anterioly and form the greater circle of the iris. There are two arteries in each muscle expect the LR (lateral rectus); which has only one.

The choroidal circulation drains into ampullae in the choroid that give rise to the vortex vein. In most eyes the vortex vein travel posteriorly through short intrascleral course and exit approximately 14 to 18 mm posterior to the limbus and 10 to 14 mm posterior to the ora serrata (Fig. 1.4).

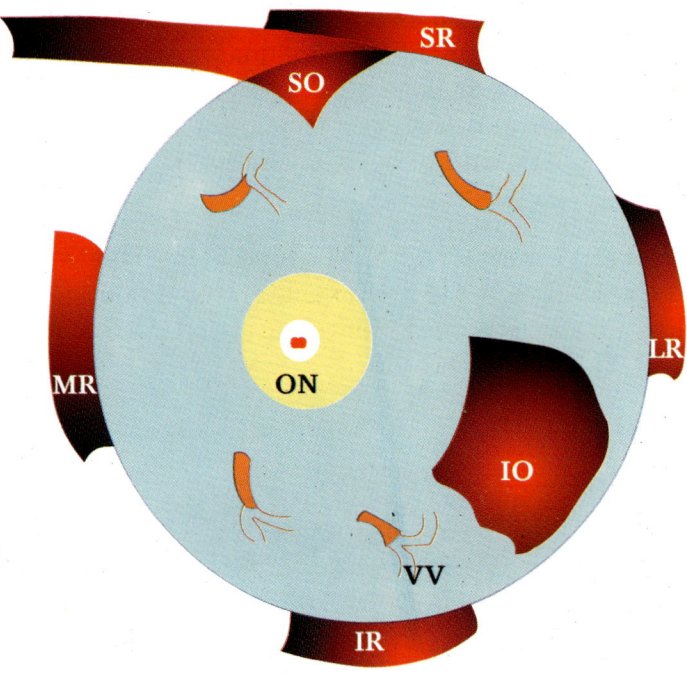

Fig. 1.4 *Posterior view of the globe showing the vortex vein*

There are approximately 5 to 7 vortex veins per eye, each vein has a variable location within the quadrants, although a vortex vein usually found beneath the insertion of the superior oblique muscle.

10 to 20 short posterior ciliary arteries enter the sclera posteriorly feeding the choroid. The long posterior ciliary arteries enter the sclera near the optic nerve and coarse anteriorly at 3 O'clock and 9 O'clock positions in suprachoroidal space, where they are often identified by indirect ophthalmoscopy.

The superior oblique (SO) arises from the nasal orbital wall, passes through a pulley as a tendon, and then passes beneath the superior rectus to insert into the sclera. The anterior border of the insertion is 12 to 14 mm posterior to the limbus and extends 7 to 18 mm posteriorly. The inferior oblique (IO) arises from the anterior-nasal aspect of the orbital wall, passes beneath the inferior rectus muscle (IR), and inserts in the inferotemporal quadrant. The anterior border of the insertion nearly parallels the inferior margin of the lateral rectus (LR), but the insertion extends posteriorly to the center of the globe. Thus falling in port over the macula.

The optic nerve exits nasal to the posterior center of the globe and is 3 mm in width (including its sheath); the diameter of the optic nerve when viewed internally is 1.5 to 1.75 mm.

The anterior chamber, which has an average volume of 0.25 ml, is defined by the cornea, the iris, and the anterior lens as its boundaries. The lens has an average anterior to posterior diameter of 3.5 mm and an approximate horizontal diameter of 9 mm. It is suspended by ligaments that insert into the ciliary processes of the pars plicata. The volume of the interior of globe is approximately 5.5 ml where the vitreous gel occupies around 4 ml in a normal adult eye.

Anteriorly, the regions of the pars plicata and pars plana are important landmarks for the vitreous surgeon. The pars plicata is occupied by a series of 70 to 80 elevated ridges (ciliary processes) that stretch posteriorly and internally for 2.5 mm from the limbus; the zonules suspending the lens are attached to these ridges (Fig. 1.5).

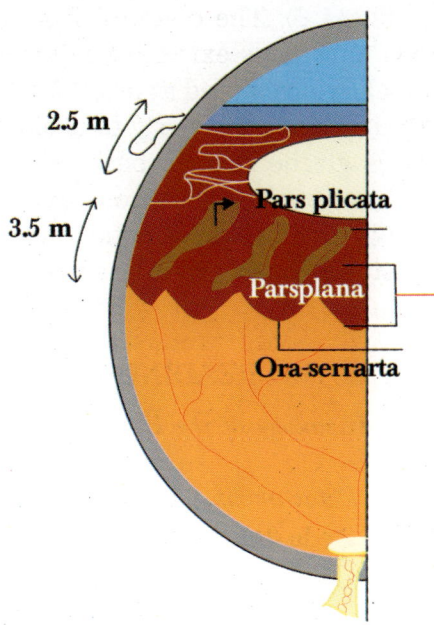

Fig. 1.5 *Diagrammatic representation of pars plana and ora serrata*

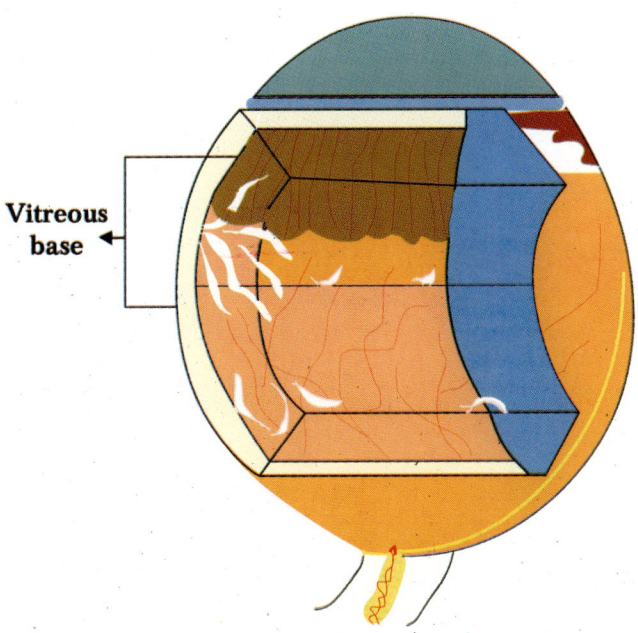

Fig. 1.6 *Vitreous base as on important landmark for the vitreous surgeon*

The pars plana is approximately 3 mm wide nasally and 5 mm temporally. It extends posteriorly from the pars plicata and is bounded posteriorly at the margin of the ciliary epithelium by the anterior retina, a scalloped border called the ora serrata. The average distance from the ora to the limbus is 5 mm nasally and 7 mm temporally. The pars plana may be wider in significantly myopic eyes. The vitreous base is 2 to 6 mm wide and straddles the oraserrata, extending 2 to 3 mm posterior to it (Fig. 1.6). The distance from the limbus to the anterior vitreous base is 5 mm, so the vitreous base thus extends farther anteriorly temporally than nasally. Incision into vitreous cavity nasally are placed at lest 2.5 mm posterior to the limbus to avoid the pars-plicata but not more than 5 mm posteriorly to avoid vitreous base. Blunt-ended instruments introduced into the eye through the vitreous base may therefore exert traction and gives rise to a peripheral retinal tear. As a result of the strong adhesion of the cortical vitreous at the vitreous base, in an eye with a posterior vitreous detachment (PVD), the posterior hyaloid surface remain attached to the posterior boarder of the vitreous base.

SUGGESTED READINGS

1. Hogan MJ, Alvarado JA, Weddell JE: *Histology of the Human Eye*, Philadelphia, WB Saunders, 1971.
2. Wilkinson CP, Rice TA: *Michels Retinal Detachment*, 2 edn, St. Louis, Mosby Year Book, 1997.
3. Jack J Kanski: *Clinical Ophthalmology*, 2 edn 341, 1988.

Setting Up
the Vitreoretinal Unit

Introduction

Modern vitreous surgery has paved the way for revolutionary developments in the field of ophthalmology. The latest apparatus no doubt is costly and rather difficult to maintain, but in the field of ophthalmic surgery a retina surgeon will be helpless without the aid of these recent wonderful well-equipped vitrectomy units.

As we know, removal of the vitreous does not compromise the functioning of the eye. Earlier use of multifunctional probes such as the standard 20 gauge instruments have been replaced by vitreous infusion suction cutter (VISC) and vitreophage. Important advances have also occurred in the system for visualization during surgery. Development of operating microscope with X-Y movements, erected image binocular ophthalmoscopic system (EIBOS) attachment, etc. have aided with all its advantages. Bimanual surgery thus becomes possible. Now one can use three ports: one for infusion, endo-illumination and other the active instrument for cutter, have become standard procedure.

The benefit and indications of vitrectomy surgery are gradually increasing day-by-day. Disease, which was considered to be incurable, has become relatively easy to manage by these new technical advances. There are numerous indications and day-by-day new indications are aided to the list of vitreous surgery. Managements of certain anterior segment disorders have also improved with the availability of vitrectomy techniques.

The growth of this specialty has been made possible by the development of new instrumentation and improved techniques. Vitreoretinal surgery as a specialty has spread rapidly to the most of the major ophthalmic institutions around the world.

INFRASTRUCTURE

To start a vitreoretinal unit, the following setup should be kept in mind.

Outpatient wing: In outpatient wing presurgical and postoperative vitreoretinal patients are examined, which should have the following.

    a. Binocular indirect ophthalmoscope (Fig 2.1).

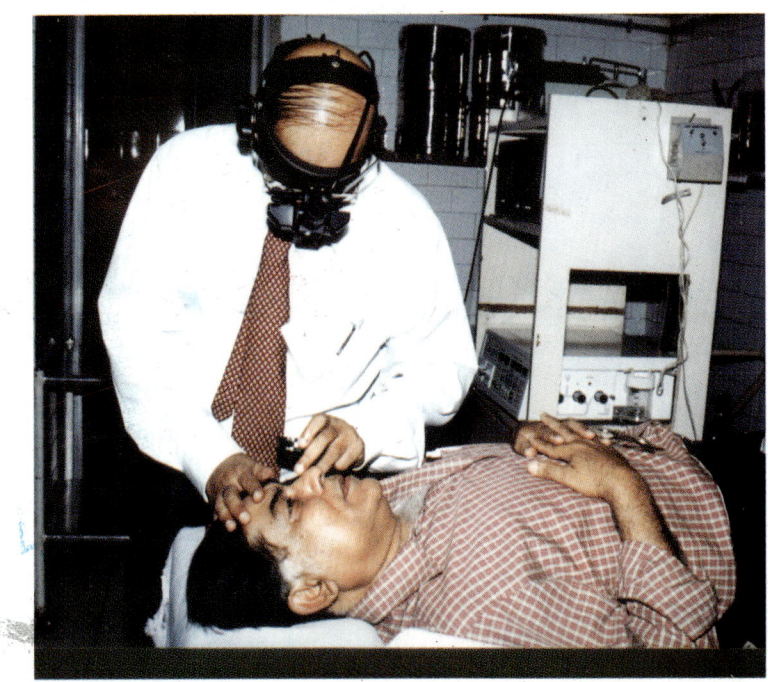

Fig. 2.1 *Indirect ophthalmoscopy*

    b. Refraction trial set and direct ophthalmoscope
    c. +20 D condensing lens
    d. Slit lamp
    e. Applanation tonometer
    f. Reclining chair
    g. Emergency drugs
    h. Oxygen apparatus

The outpatient wing should also have a fluorescein angiography unit and ultra sonography unit and also if possible electro diagnostic work-up services. Laser photocoagulation is the commonest mode of treatment of vitreoretinal diseases. Portable dido-laser, having slit lamp delivery, indirect ophthalmoscopic delivery, and endo-laser delivery system can be utilized both in out-door as well as in operation room. It should be side by side so that the laser machine can be utilized both in out door patients as well as in operation theatre.

FLUORESCEIN ANGIOGRAPHY UNIT

The fluorescein angiography unit should have the following equipment:

    a. Fundus camera for fluorescein angiography (Fig. 2.2)

    b. Sterile sodium fluorescein vials

    c. Scalp vein set (23 size) and disposable syringes.

    d. Emergency tray having all emergency drugs.

    e. Oxygen and ambu bag.

Depending upon the patient volume, fluorescein angiography can be performed either by an ophthalmologist or by the trained technician (Fig. 2.3).

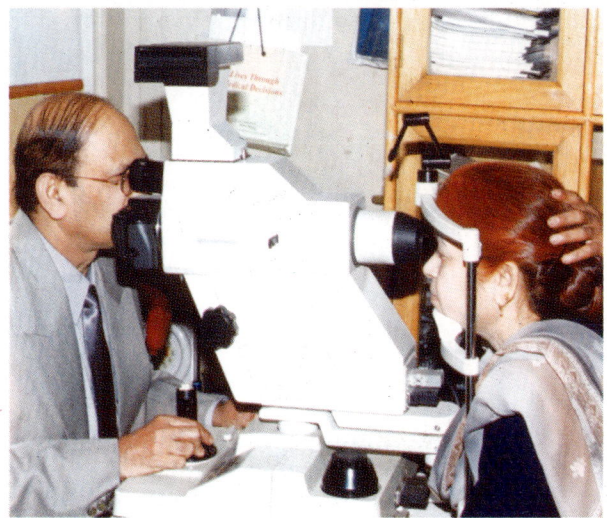 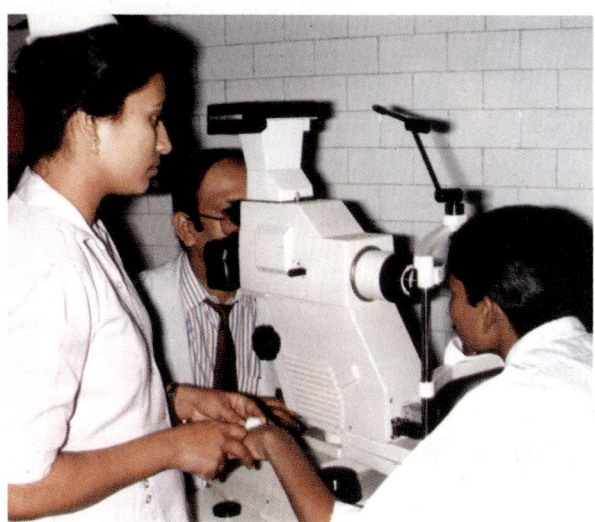

Fig. 2.2 *Fluorescein angiography unit.*   **Fig. 2.3** *Fluorescein angiography procedure.*

ULTRASONOGRAPHY UNIT

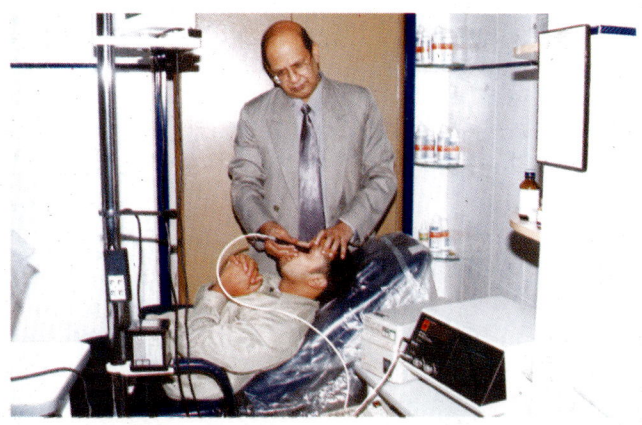

Fig. 2.4 *Ultrasound unit*

An ultrasonography unit should have the following equipment

    a. Ultrasonography equipment having A-and B-scan probes (Fig. 2.4).

    b. Reclining chair/ couch.

    c. Camera for documentation.

    d. Printer.

LASER PHOTOCOAGULATION UNIT

Laser photocoagulation is the commonest mode of treatment employed in the treatment of vitreoretinal diseases. In an institute-based unit, it is best to have separate laser machines for outpatient department and intraoperative use.

    Should be in separate room and it should be preferable close to operation theatre. Which should have:

    a. Laser machine with all its accessories.

    b. Chair and stool for the surgeon and patient.

    c. Lenses: Goldmann-3 mirror, Mainster lens, etc.

    d. Methyl cellulose/X-Y jelly

    e. Indirect ophthalmoscope with + 20 D lens

OPERATING ROOM

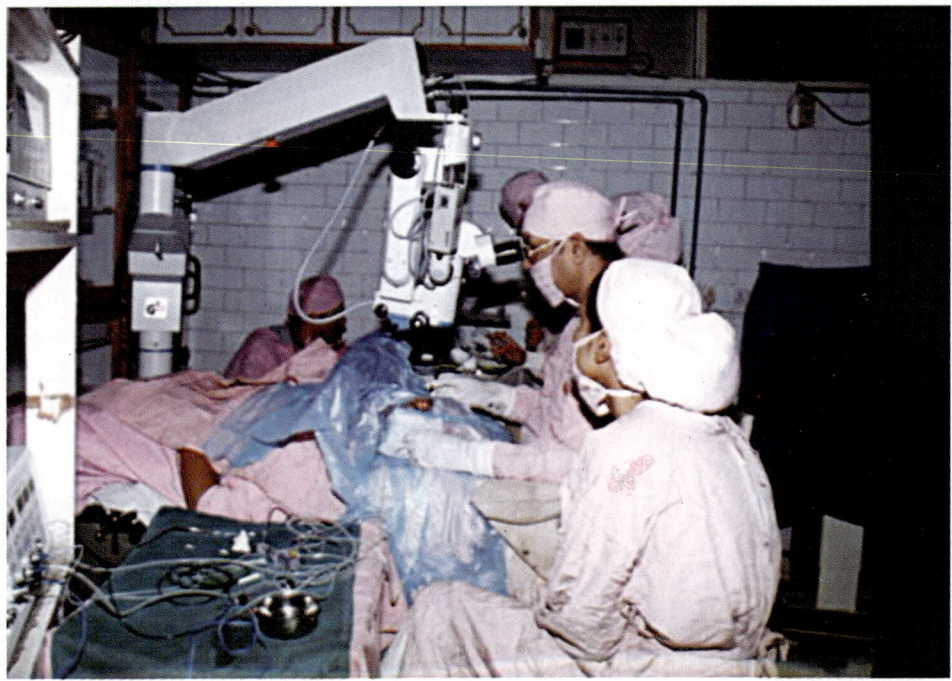

Fig. 2.5 Operation theatre

The operating room should be spacious where all machines and instruments can be placed and handled smoothly (Fig 2.5). It is preferable to have a standby vitrectomy console, which may be necessary in an emergency.

Essential major instruments required are:

1. Boyle's apparatus.
2. Vitrectomy units having endoilluminator, diathermy units, etc. in one console.
3. Good quality operating microscope having X-Y coupling, focus and zoom facility which can be controlled by foot switch.
4. Suction apparatus.
5. Laser both endo- and indirect ophthalmoscopic delivery system.
6. Air-compressor units.

VITREORETINAL TRAY

The vitreoretinal tray should have the following

a. Stainless steel cup for storing irrigating fluid.
b. Needle holder
c. Eye speculum
d. Curved and straight scissor
e. Muscle hook
f. Tying forceps

VITRECTOMY ACCESSORIES

a. Infusion cannula (6 mm, 4 mm)
b. Scleral plug with scleral forceps
c. Fragmatome needle
d. Wrench to fix fragmatome needle
e. Flute needle
f. Vitrectomy cutter
g. 3-way stopcock
h. Millipore filter
i. Vitreous forceps — end gripping
j. Vitreous scissors — 1. Horizontal
                         2. Vertical
k. Membrane peeling instruments: pick, spatula
l. Foreign body forceps
m. Intraocular magnet

n. Endolaser probes

o. Back-flush needle, etc.

p. Light pipes.

CONSUMABLE ITEMS

1. Irrigating solution: Ringer lactate or BSS plus
2. Sutures: 6.0 vicryl
   4.0/ 0.5 – dacron
   10.0 – nylon
3. Scleral buckling materials
4. Silicone oil
5. Perfluorocarbon liquid (PFCL)
6. Gloves/plastic adhesive drapes.

DUTY OF RESPONSIBLE STAFF

Vitreous instruments such as forceps, scissors, etc. should be handled with the utmost care. The tip should be cleaned immediately after use to prevent blood and debris from clogging the lever mechanism. The tips must be protected with safety guard. At the end of the surgery all the instruments should be cleaned by distilled water (not saline). Reusable vitreous cutter should be cleaned immediately after surgery with distilled water. Fiber optic cables should not be allowed to bend or get kinked. Responsible operating staff should handle the expensive and delicate instruments for packing and sterilization. It should be double-packed individually and sterilized in ethylene oxide.

STERILIZATION

Maintenance of absolute asepsis is very important in vitreoretinal set up. The surgeon and operation staff should be alert for the possibility of contamination. The following points may helpful in preventing contamination:

1. Surgical gloves are absolute prerequisite.
2. Plastic adhesive with drainage system.
3. The cutter, fiber optic cables and endolaser probe.
4. Sterilised plastic or cloth to adjust the head of indirect ophthalmoscopy.
5. Silicone oil (pre-sterilized pack)
6. Gases (SF_6 or C_3F_8) – presterilized pack
7. Prepacked sterilized PFCL (perfluorocarbon liquid)

An ultrasonic cleaner in needed to clean instruments such as vitreous scissors, forceps, etc. High-speed autoclave unit should be close to the operation room.

SURGEON AND TRAINED ASSISTANT

The vitreoretinal surgeon must be well trained at an advanced center in all aspect of vitreoretinal problems. The surgeon should have special interest in this branch and he or she should have certain qualities to be acquired for the successful practice of vitreoretinal surgery. In view of the relatively long-duration and unpredictable intraoperative course of each surgery patience is a basic prerequisite for the surgeon. If one is impatient, and too time conscious, there will be a tendency to compromise on the quality of surgery. Unlike in cataract surgery, vitreoretinal surgery is expected to be successful in only a modest percentage of cases.

The trained assistant is highly desirable to assist in these surgical procedures. He should be trained to perform the following:

1. Should assist in all vitreoretinal cases.

2. To be able to assemble and dismantle the instruments such as vitrectomy cutter, vitreous scissors, etc.

3. Should be knowledgeable in cleaning and packing these delicate instruments.

4. Should know how to load the expansive gases (SF_6 and C_3F_8) in the syringe and prepare the exact concentration for its mixture with air needed for flushing the eye.

5. Should have working knowledge of the scleral buckling material and able to identify them.

STANDBY ANAESTHESIOLOGIST

Patient undergoing vitreoretinal surgeries are also likely to suffer from diabetes, hypertension and other systemic problems. Hence, standby anaesthesiologist is necessary even for case done under local anesthesia. For emergency intravenous line with veflon is mandatory. Oxygen should be given throughout operation to prevent suffocation. Pulse oxymeter, cardiac monitor and suction apparatus should be available in good working condition. An intensive care unit to take care of the immediate postoperative period is highly desirable to face any situation among vitreoretinal patients.

SUPPORTIVE SERVICE

It is a good practice to have every patient scheduled for surgery to go through physician's examination in addition to routine laboratory tests for fitness. As vitreoretinal set up having all sophisticated instruments, service back up is necessary for day-to-day running the machines. Adequate stocks of spare bulbs for operating microscope, endo-illuminator fuses for vitrectomy console are necessary to save valuable time and in case of emergency.

The vitreoretinal surgeon needs to be trained in a good institution before setting of the unit. It requires full time involvements for successful practice. In view of relatively long duration and unpredictable long course of each surgery, lot of patience is required for a good vitreoretinal surgeon. As rightly said earlier, a good vitreoretinal surgeon should have lady's fingers, lion's heart, camel's belly, a horse's legs and eagle's eyes.

For a successful outcome of the vitreoretinal cases, co-operation of assistant, scrub nurse, operating room assistants, anaesthetist, physician and above all the surgeon who plays the master role, needs attention to the patients. All this makes it necessary for the surgeon to be prepared for experience that may be frustrating at times. Recurrences of problems are not uncommon requiring additional surgical procedures. The visual results are also not gratifying as in cataract surgery. However, the growth of this specialty has been made possible interesting, although time-consuming.

OPERATING ROOM ASSISTANTS

The operating room assistants not only look after the surgeon's need but also assist the anesthetist during intubations and extubation. He may assist in preparing the anesthetic for local anesthesia. He should also know all vitreoretinal instruments, and how to put on the indirect ophthalmoscope on the surgeon's head during surgery. Connection of endolaser, the assistant should know cryo machine and he should have a working knowledge of the vitrectomy console, so that minor faults could be rectified without the need to call an engineer.

Operating Microscope and Wide Angle Fundus Observation System

Introduction

The operating microscope is very essential tool for an eye surgeon. Understanding the components and their functions are mandatory for day-to-day microsurgery. Surgery can only be performed safely with the aid of a good operating microscope with a zoom and the fine focus capability, as well as X-Y coupling that enables the surgeon to move the microscope in horizontal plane (Fig 3.1). The optical principles provide unique binocularity magnification and illumination of the viewed object. The components of the microscope constitute the following.

1. Objective lens assembly.
2. The microscope body.
3. Binocular tube system.
4. Zoom device.
5. Microscope suspension with:
   a. Tilting device
   b. Inclination device
   c. Focusing device

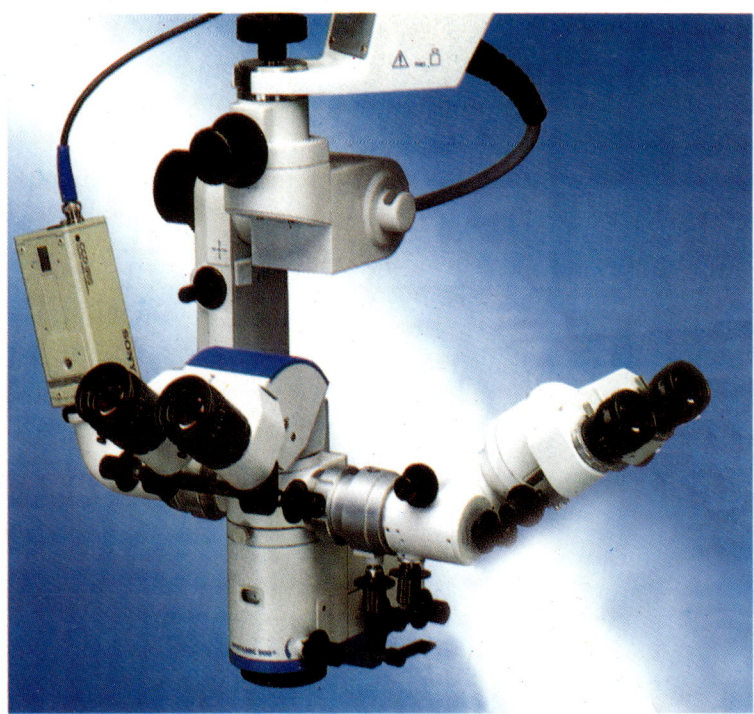

Fig. 3.1 *Operating microscope with X-Y coupling*

OBJECTIVE LENS ASSEMBLY

The objective lens with fix focal length (standard f = 175 mm) projects the object in "infinity" and at the same time provides parallel beam path of the illumination, where the illuminating spot which illuminates the object. The illuminating mirror is part of the objective lens assembly and is adjusted to the objective axis to provide attachment of different illumination modules.

ZOOM DEVICE

This zoom device continuously adjusted electromotively via zoom, which is connected, to the floor stand or ceiling unit.

BEAM SPLITTER AND EYEPIECE HEAD

For stereoscopic viewing through the operating microscope, two beam paths of the parallel beams between zoom and microscope eyepiece head are used.

The microscope eyepiece head corresponds to a binocular telescope with two ocular lenses (10 ×20b). Diopter setting may be performed from +5DSP to–8 DSP via each ocular lens provided with a setting ring with movable soft robber edges for spectacle wearers. The inclination angle of the eyepiece head may be changed in the range of 0 to 75 degree. The pupil distance (PD) is adjustable by knobs is the range of 50 to 75 mm via spindle with scale. The adjustable knobs of the spindle may be covered with sterilizable caps at both sides.

ILLUMINATION

The illuminating system originally used was an incandescent coaxial but by 1980 had been replaced by glass fiber optical illumination. The advantages of glass fiber illumination are to reduce heat production; easier bulb changing, increased field size, and increased intensity.

In a good operating microscope the following three cold light illumination systems are available which are incorporated in floor stand or the ceiling unit like.

1. Zoom illumination coaxial
2. Zoom illumination coaxial and oblique
3. Operating slit-lamp

A red reflex enhancer may be used if coaxial illumination is selected.

COAXIAL ZOOM ILLUMINATION

The illumination module forms an illuminating spot in the object plane by the light coming from fiber optic cable through lens system via a mirror in the objective group and through microscope objective lens. The illuminating spot is coupled if microscope zoom is changed and concentrates a more intensive luminous density on smaller area in cases of large magnification. The diameter of the illuminating spot is coupled to microscope magnification such that it always will be larger than the visual field. If turning knob is positioned to spot, the illuminating spot may be set to its smallest diameter and its most extensive brightness. The automatic coupling to the zoom is only performed after knob is turned back. The microscope should have a protective filter (UV yellow) and blue filter may be swiveled in to the beam path.

COAXIAL AND OBLIQUE ZOOM ILLUMINATION

The zoom illumination assembly coaxial and oblique is extended by a mirror swivable right and left by lever in an oblique illumination mount. This mirror deflects the beam path from the coaxial course and directs it through the illumination objective lens on the object field by an angle of 20 degree.

Microscope accessories are necessary and the most important is the observer scope, which may be mounted on to the beam splitter of the microscope. The magnification and visual field in the observer scope correspond to those of main eyepiece head of the microscope. The assisted enjoy the same illumination and depth of the visual field through the observer scope. The facility of a TV camera and 35 mm camera should be available for recording and still photography during the operation.

FILTER AND PROTECTION FOR EYES

The filter and protection for eyes are essential during ophthalmic surgery. Blue filter is used for stimulation of fluorescence. The ultraviolet protection is normally used which is usually the wavelength below 470 mm. Due to absorption of UV light and the blue portion of visible light, a high protection effect is achieved against photochemical damage of the eye. It is highly recommended to use filter during long-lasting surgery. In ophthalmology, only illumination system with incandescent or halogen lamps should be used. Gas discharge lamps like xenon or metal halogen as the highlight portion in the blue spectral range may cause photochemical damage to the eye.

When operating macula area, oblique illumination is ideal, as light hazard of macula will be reduced.

CHECKING OF OPERATING MICROSCOPE AFTER SURGERY

After longer break of work, the system should be checked where all electrometric functions of the suspension would be set back to the value set in the factory (Fig 3.2).

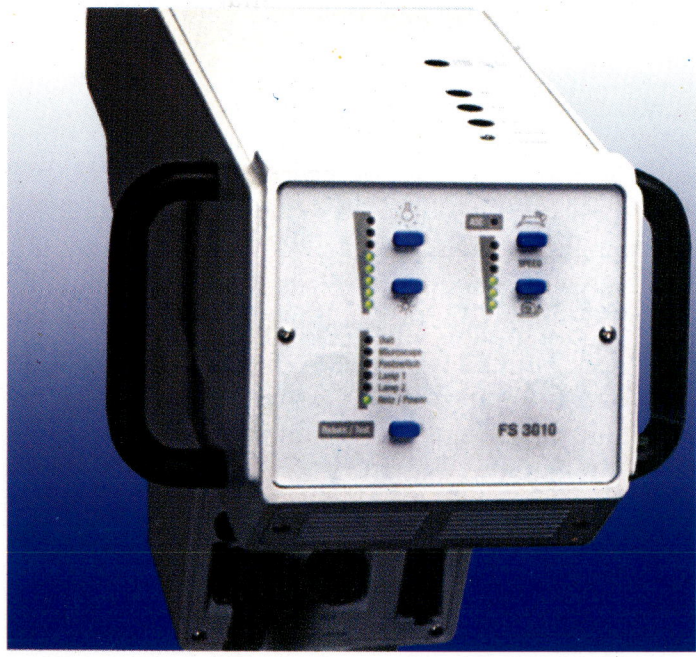

Fig. 3.2 *Error indicators*

To focus the magnification to start the work one should set small magnification and the object is set by manually moving the microscope.

The microscope can be adjusted to set largest magnification and one should later set the working magnification by depressing the foot switch. After performing this adjustment the image will remain sharp despite any change of magnification. The depth of field will be increased in case of smaller magnifications.

CARE, STERILIZATION AND MAINTENANCE OF MICROSCOPE

The clearing of the microscope may be cleaned with dry dust cloth or dust brush. Optical surface (lenses) should be cleaned with a clean linen cloth free from detergents. Over longer intervals the painted surfaces should be cleaned with damp cloth. For this purpose a watery solution of a common cleaning agent should be used. One should be sure that no water penetrates inside the microscope.

Sterilization of caps and handles may be performed in an autoclave up to max. 143° C or in hot vapor up to 165° C. If there is visible damage exchange of caps and handle may be done. The microscope is an essential part of the entire microsurgical procedure and it is the life-long investment.

TROUBLE-SHOOTING AND REMEDIES OF MICROSCOPE

One should be aware of the trouble-shooting of the microscope and its remedies. When there is no illumination, one should check the power from the main switch; look for defective fuses, halogen lamps, and also fibre-optic connection. Some time the protective cap blocks the light, which needs to be removed for illumination.

The motorized movement (X-Y) could be defective if the foot switch connection is not proper.

FOOT SWITCH

The foot switch is an important component of the microscope. It provides 12 different switching functions (Figs 3.3 or 3.4).

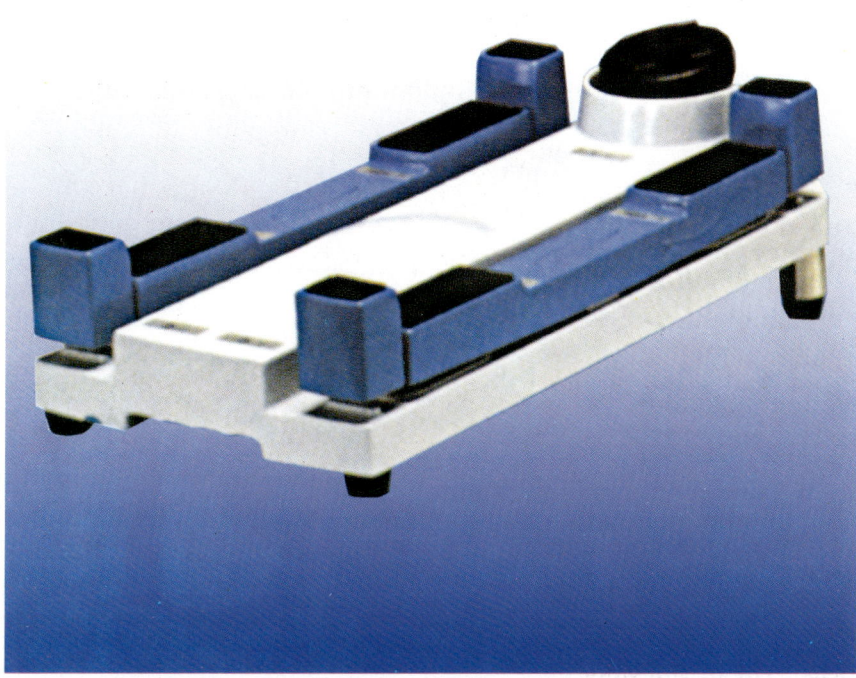

Fig 3.3 *Foot switch of operating microscope*

AN OVERVIEW OF SWITCHING FUNCTIONS OF THE FOOT SWITCH

The foot switch acts in different function by pressing different switches (Fig. 3.4).

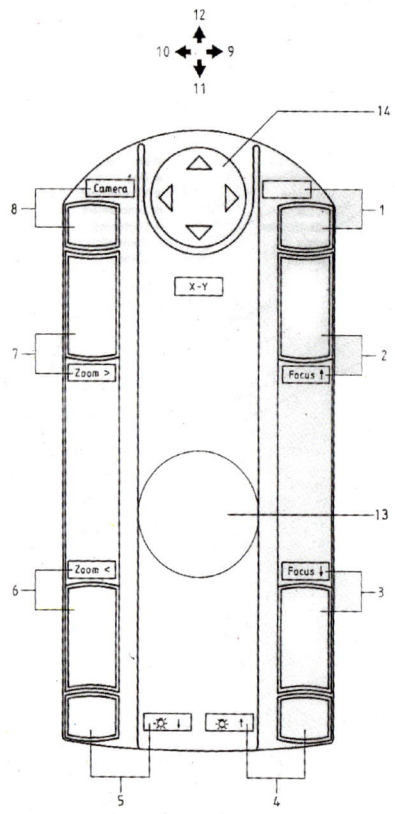

Fig 3.4 *Diagrammatic representation of foot switch*

1. Reserve
2. Focus – upward
3. Focus – downward
4. Illumination – on
5. Illumination – off
6. Magnification – smaller
7. Magnification – larger
8. Camera – release at max illumination

Position of knob by moving the knob:

9. To right side – tilt to right side
10. To left side – tilt to left side
11. Backwards – tilt in the rear
12. Forwards – tilt in front

The microscope functions can be controlled through a separate foot switch or surgeon's chair, which is electrically connected to a floor stand through cable, which can provide all the functions.

FUNDUS CONTACT LENSES FOR VITREORETINAL SURGERY

The contact lenses provide better view of ocular structures of the posterior segment. These contact lenses have lesser magnification, which is compensated by adjusting the microscope to greater magnification. Various types of contact lenses are available and they are used on the basis of the convenience of the vitreous surgeon. The contact lenses provide a wide field and also stereopsis. These are:

- Small contact lens resting on cornea, approximately 9.8 mm in diameter, which does not dislodge easily from its site during surgery. The lens stays in place due to capillary action. Since this lens is light in weight, there is no need to hold it. It is easily sterilizable by steam autoclave or ethylene oxide.

- The second type of contact lenses is those which are sewn on lenses. The contact lens is put over a metallic ring, which is sewn on lenses. The contact lens is put over a metallic ring, which is sewn at the limbus with the sclera. Within this ring the contact lens is put which just fits into it. This lens does not require an assistant's help and keeps the area to be viewed in focus with movements of the eye, but sometimes poses difficulty when blood or a bubble enters between the cornea and the lens. Another advantages of this system is that the various types of lenses can be changed for the visualization of center, mid-periphery and extreme periphery as per surgeon's choice and requirements. This lens cum ring system has also A + 78D lens for visualization on the retina is an air filled phakic eye.

- Hand-held contact lenses: In this system there is irrigation facility whereby debris and blood are constantly washed away during surgery. These lenses are cheaper and collection of fluid, blood or air bubbles does not occur between the cornea and the contact lens, and the view is clear and very widely used in developing countries.

WIDE ANGLE FUNDUS OBSERVATION SYSTEM

The wide-angle fundus observation system is the latest technologic development in which has lead to elimination of contact lens altogether and incorporation of this facility with the operating microscope itself.

Fundus visualization in vitreous retinal surgery is essential in allowing a detailed view of the entire retina, both posterior pole and periphery. Ideally it should be less dependent on assistance and surgery can be performed in air-filled phakic or pseudophakic eye. For this purpose wide-angle non-contact fundus observation systems are ideal. Some of available systems like irrigating contact lenses, wide-angle contact lens system AVI, ROLS, VPFS, OCU-LAR are available in the market. Their popularity is comparatively low as non-contact wide-angle systems like BIOM or EIBOS are available.

BINOCULAR INDIRECT OPHTHALMO MICROSCOPE (BIOM)

It was first invented by Prof. Spitnaz. This special type of non-contact BIOM has larger field of view (90°–110°). One can even visualize in small pupil and hazy media right up to the ora serrata. A detailed examination with good quality photography is possible if magnification is stepped up. It requires learning curve.

ERECTED IMAGE BINOCULAR OPHTHALMOSCOPIC SYSTEM (EIBOS)

Vitreoretinal surgery is more easy and convenient by the using wide-angle fundus observation system (Fig 3.5).

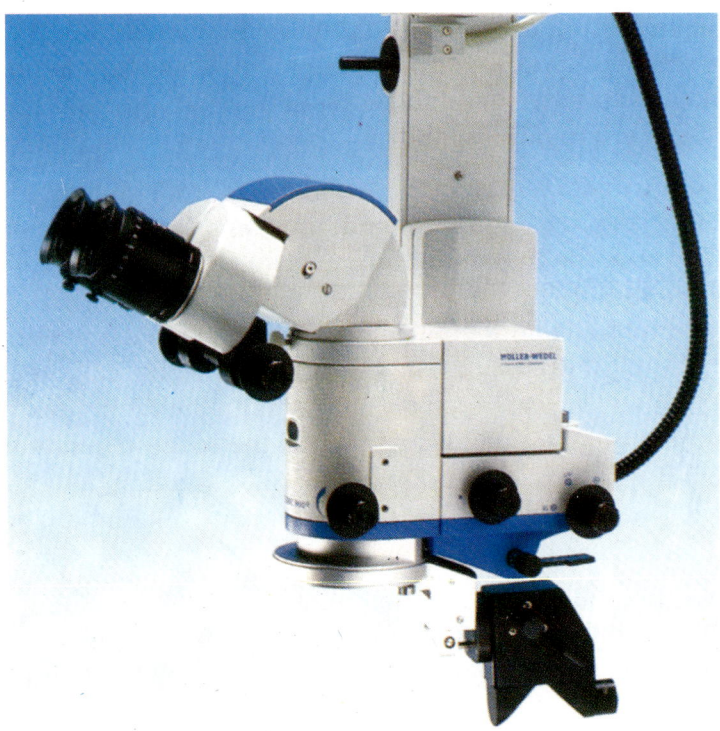

Fig. 3.5 *EIBOS attached with operating microscope*

The erected image binocular ophthalmoscopic system (EIBOS), in conjunction with the appropriate operating microscope, is designed for use in vireoretinal surgery. In fact, EIBOS is better than BIOM. It must be used only with front lens f =175 mm. The erected image binocular ophthalmoscopic system is a part of a microsurgical operating system. One should not use shorter focal length because there may be injury to the patient's eyes.

ADVANTAGES OF EIBOS

- Non-contact use in vitreoretinal surgery, approximately 100° field of view (Fig. 3.6).

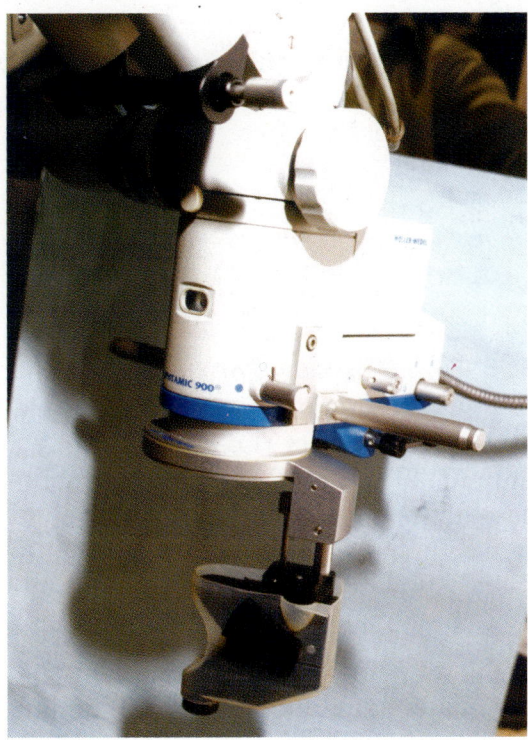

Fig. 3.6 *EIBOS Non-contact lens vitreoretinal surgery, covers approx. 100 degree field of view.*

- Simultaneous observation of fundus and incision area is possible.
- Integrated reversing optics for left–right correction.
- Safe for patient's eye by spring-loaded suspension.
- Internal focus ranging from retina to upper vitreous body.
- Ideal for quick inspection of posterior segment.
- Swing-away position without interfering with cataract and glaucoma surgery.

DIAGRAMATIC REPRESENTATION OF DIFFERENT PARTS OF EBIOS

1. EBIOS fitted at the bottom of microscope
2. Adaptor ring
3. Screw which is fitted with the microscope
4. Mount of the adaptor ring
5. Screw
6. Guide pins
7. EBIOS
8. Axle
9. Focusing lever
10. Ophthalmoscopic lens

DESCRIPTION OF FUNCTIONS

In this system an ophthalmic lens is fitted at the bottom part of the erected image binocular ophthalmoscopic system (EBIOS), which is projected into the fundus of the eye. With the help of the prism the image of the fundus is put upright. The surgeon adjusts focussing to his choice by using the lever.

A large magnification, the image of the fundus of the projected via lens and the prism system fills up the entire visual field of the microscope. When the magnification is reduced, the outer part of the iris becomes visible in the visual field. The instruments are seen non-reversed outside as well as inside the eye.

Whenever the surgeon has not used or does not intend to use the equipment during the surgery, it may be swirled backwards. It is done easily due to the rotateable adapter ring and the swiveling system. The parking position of the erected image binocular ophthalmoscopic system may be selected as required. To protect the patient's eye, the middle part of the erected image binocular ophthalmoscopic system is freely movable in range of approx. 30 mm. One can use a sterile drape covers around the bottom part of the erected image binocular ophthalmoscopic system (EBIOS) from which sterile lens protrudes.

To illuminate the retina, it is recommended to use endolight source via fiber optic cable or the operating slit lamp with slit setting to avoid reflections. One should not use coaxial or oblique illumination due to heavy reflections at the time of operation, the red reflex enhanced should be switched off.

HOW TO USE

EBIOS is used with any microscope with front lens f = 175 mm. To start the operation, the microscope is focused on to the iris of the patient's eye. The erected image binocular ophthalmoscopic system (EBIOS) is now swirled into working position. By moving the focusing lever, which is located at the right side; the fundus can be focused according to the desired position. When the focusing lever is in horizontal position, focus is deeper, i.e. on retina, and if the lever in vertical position, the focus is higher, i.e. inside the vitreous body.

CLEANING AND STERILIZATION

The erected image binocular ophthalmoscopic system (EBIOS) may be cleaned with a damp soft cloth. The glass surface can be cleaned with a cloth for optical cleaning. The component containing the prism of erected image binocular ophthalmoscopic system erected image binocular ophthalmoscopic system (EBIOS) must not be sterilized; therefore it should be covered by the sterilizable drape. The focusing lever and drape are sterilized in an autoclave up to 134° C or in hot air up to 165° C. The sterilizable drape for erected image binocular ophthalmoscopic system (EBIOS), focusing lever and ophthalmic lens can be used for sterilization.

REFERENCE

1. Horenz P: The operating microscope I. *J. Microsurgery*, 1980; 1: 364
2. Horenz P: The operating microscope II *J. Microsurgery*, 1980; 2: 22
3. Zeiss Inc: *Carl Zeiss for Ophthalmology*, Medical Division, Carl Zeiss, Inc.

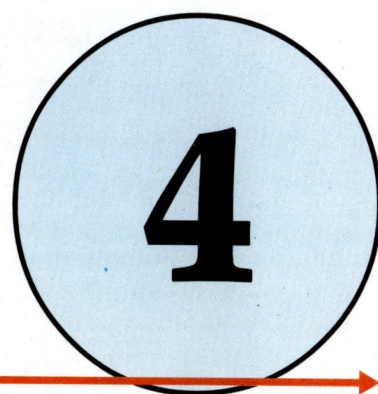

Basic Working Principle of Vitrectomy Equipment

Introduction

Every vitreous machine has several components and the functioning of each of these should be evaluated thoroughly. The most important component of any modern vitreous machine is there following:

1. Dual illumination module.

2. High frequency diathermy module.

3. Air module.

4. Vitrectomy module with viscous fluid injection (VFI).

5. Fragmentation module.

6. Irrigation/Aspiration modulated also viscous fluid extraction (VFE).

These modules may be used together or in combination as desired by the surgeon. The functioning of the modules should be interactive and a footswitch provides a convenient way of controlling several modules at once (Fig. 4.1).

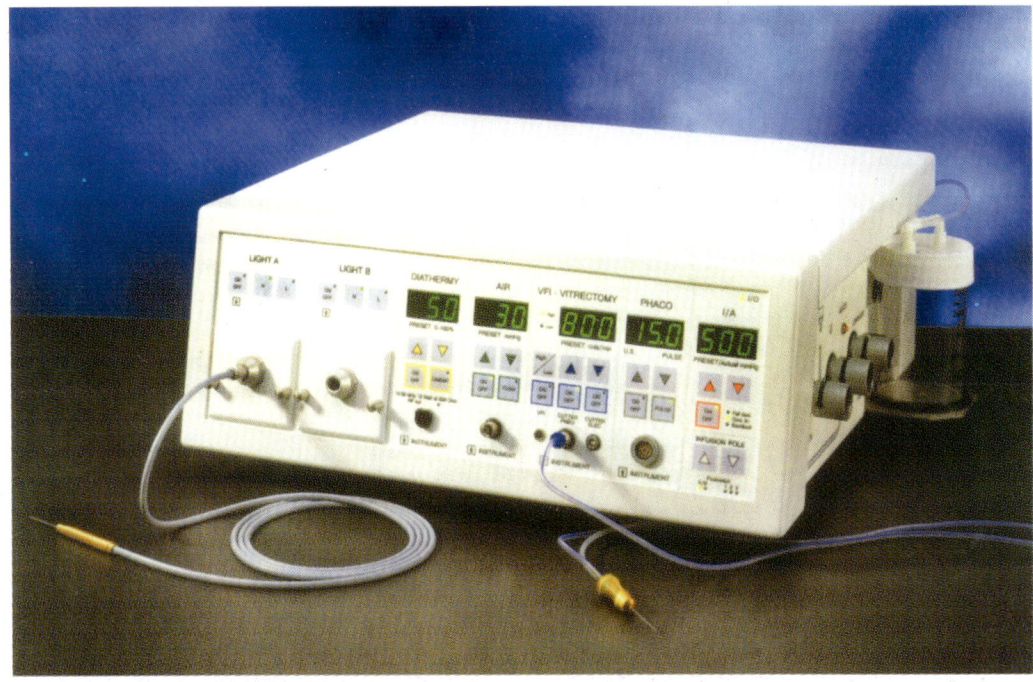

Fig. 4.1 *Vitrectomy modules*

FOOT SWITCH FUNCTIONS

The foot switch function allows the surgeon to control many different functions (Fig. 4.2).

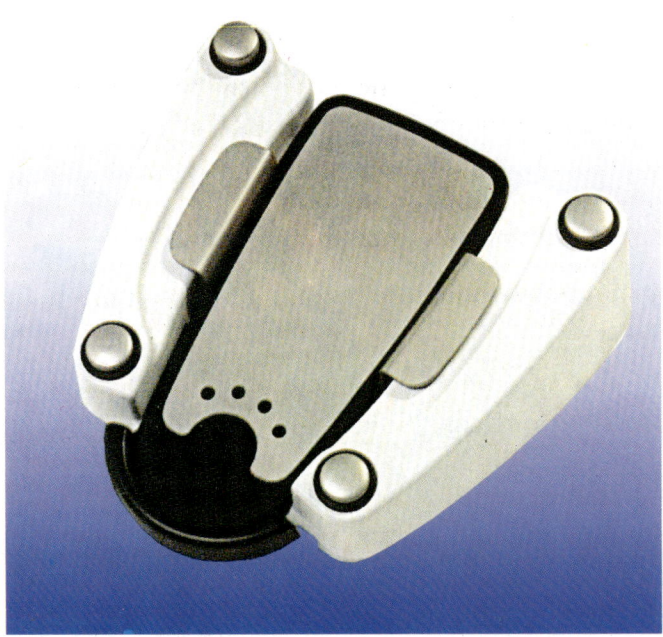

Fig. 4.2 *Multifunctional foot switch top view*

Key	Foot Switch Functions
1	Raised the infusion bottle-used with optional electric infusion pole.
2	Lowering the infusion-used with optional electrical infusion pole.
3 Program-A	1st step — Irrigation. 2nd step — Linear control of vitrectomy. 3rd step — Linear control of aspiration.
4 Program-B	1st step — Irrigation. 2nd step — Linear control of aspiration. 3rd step — Linear control of vitrectomy.
5	Continuous irrigation or viscous fluid injection.
6	Diathermy — Linear control by pressing switch 6.
7	By pressing switch 7 down active back-flush on/off.
8	By pressing switch 8 to the right scissors hold position and scissors single cut.

Audible tones: The vitrectomy unit should have audible tones in several different patterns, depending on the functions in use at the time. Using volume adjustment on the rear of the unit can control the volume. The vitrectomy unit produces audible tone, which changes in frequency to match the switch position and output power.

The tubing set when first installed must be primed to remove any air bubble. Once the automatic switch is pressed, the unit will produce a set of tones in group of three.

BACK-FLUSH FEATURES

When the irrigation/aspiration module is in use, there may be occasions where it is necessary to back-flush the accessory being used. During back flush, the infusion fluid flows in the opposite of the normal function. This back-flush feature can be used by pressing the back-flush switch, which is usually situated at the rear of the vitrectomy unit (Fig. 4 .3).

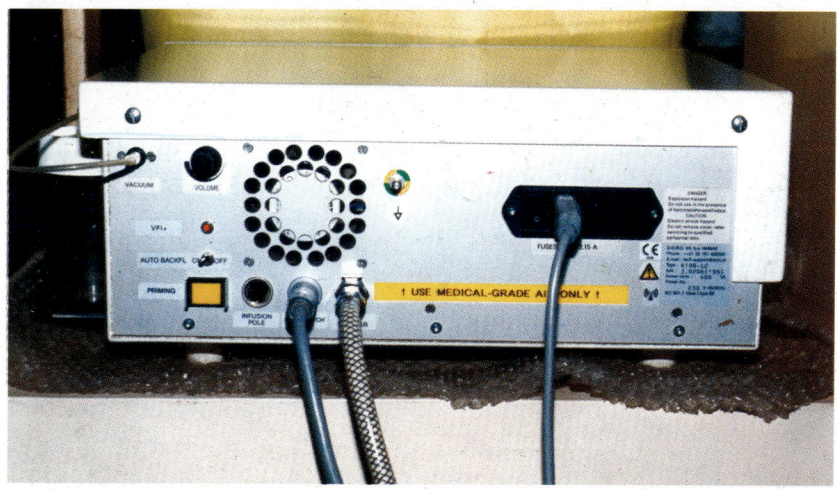

Fig. 4.3 *Vitrectomy console rear view*

Once the switch is turned on, automatic back-flush cycle will be preformed whenever the aspiration feature is stopped.

The vacuum inside the collection bottle and aspiration tubing is released immediately. The collection container is automatically vented to the outside air through the console. The aspiration tubing set is liquid-vented to the infusion bottle. This prevents residual aspiration and or tissue incarceration. During this procedure, aspiration irrigation pinch valve unit closes and the back flush pinch valve opens. This provides positive fluid pressure to the aspiration side of the tubing set. The two actions work together to stop any aspiration action very quickly.

PREPARAING THE VITRECTOMY UNIT FOR USE

The vitrectomy unit is set to use the proper voltage provided by the power-outlet. During surgery, back up of U.P.S should be installed so as to avoid operating complications and time may be saved. The unit should be placed on a firm, smooth surface. Allow at least 8 inches (20 cm) of clearance on all size of the unit. It is especially importance to allow a clear space near the fan on the rear of the unit. Like any other electrical machine, it should allow 8" (20 cm) of clearance on all sides of the unit. It is especially important to allow a clear space near the fan on the rear of the unit.

Pre-Operating Procedure

After switching on the power unit, one should connect the source of compressed air to the inlet part on the back of the vitrectomy unit. The regulator for the compressed air source should be set for 5 to 6 bar (75 –90 psi) (Fig. 4.4).

After proper connection of the tubing set, the system must be primed, so that there is no air bubble in the tubing.

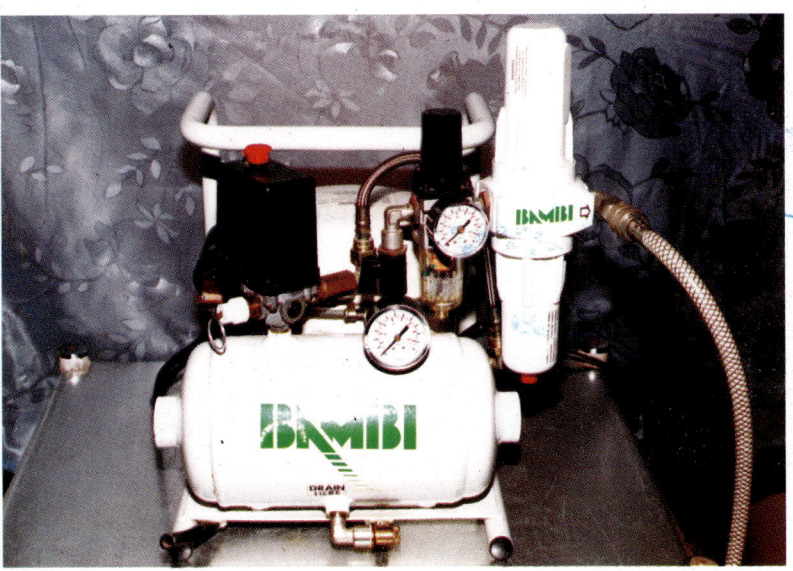

Fig. 4.4 *Air compressor unit*

Dual Illumination Module

The illumination module is intended to provide intraocular illumination during vitreoretinal surgery (Fig. 4 .5).

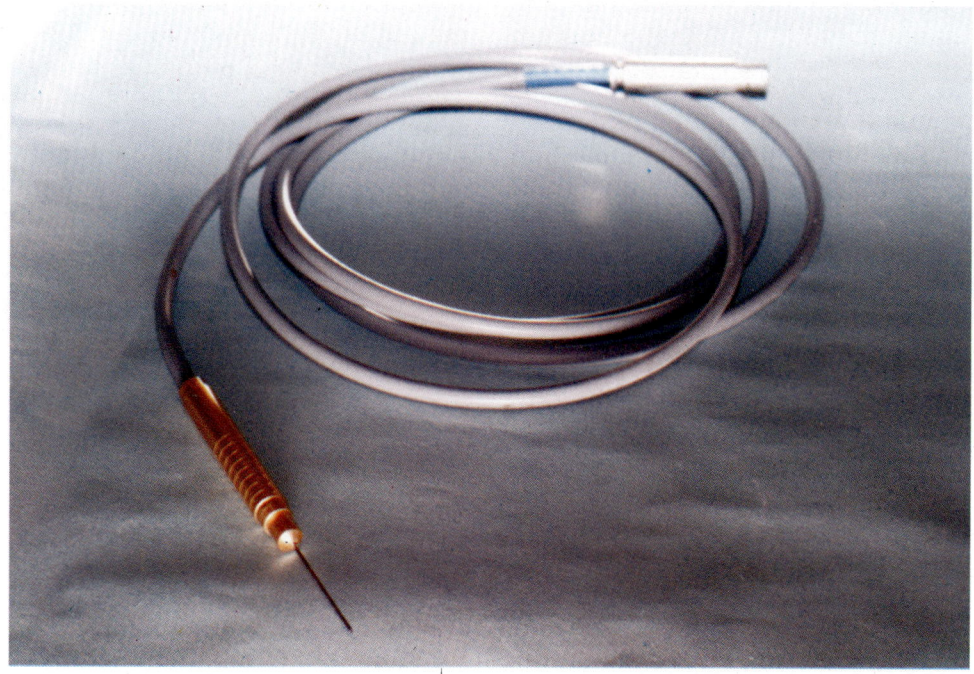

Fig. 4.5 *Endo illumination probe, 20 gauge (0.9 mm)*

Dual illumination facilities should be there once one bulb is fused; the other should work to facilitate the surgery. In typical situation if necessary both the illumination can be used at a time, one with endo-illuminator probe and the other with the fiber-optic micro forceps/scissor. The intensity of the illumination can be decreased or increased during surgery, according to the surgeon's choice. Normally halogen bulbs are used. In case the bulb is fused, before changing the bulb, shut off the vitrectomy unit and allow at least 5 minutes for the bulb to cool down. Never touch a hot bulb with bare fingers. Be very careful not to touch the surface of the bulb with finger.

Diathermy Module

The diathermy module provides high-frequency diathermy for highly selective burn placement for anterior and posterior segment surgery (Fig. 4.6). A crystal controlled solid-state oscillator at a frequency of 13.56 MH produces the RF energy.

The energy intensity delivered to the electrode can be varied continuously from 0.2 watts to approximately 12 watts. The output is regulated so that the RF energy remains constant at the reselected value. The output of the diathermy can be adjusted using the foot-switch, up to a limit, which is preset by the surgeon.

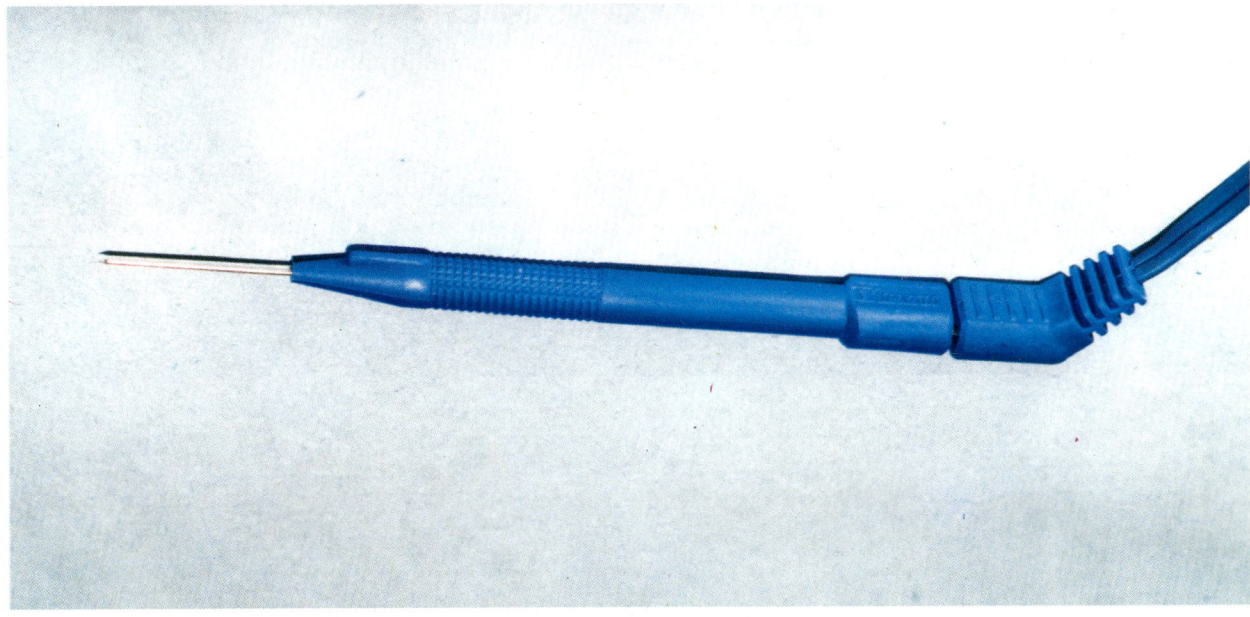

Fig. 4.6 Endodiathermy probes with tapered tip

Air-Module

The air-module provides an automatic air-infusion system. The air is delivered to the tubing set through a 0.22 mm filter to assure sterility (Fig. 4.7).

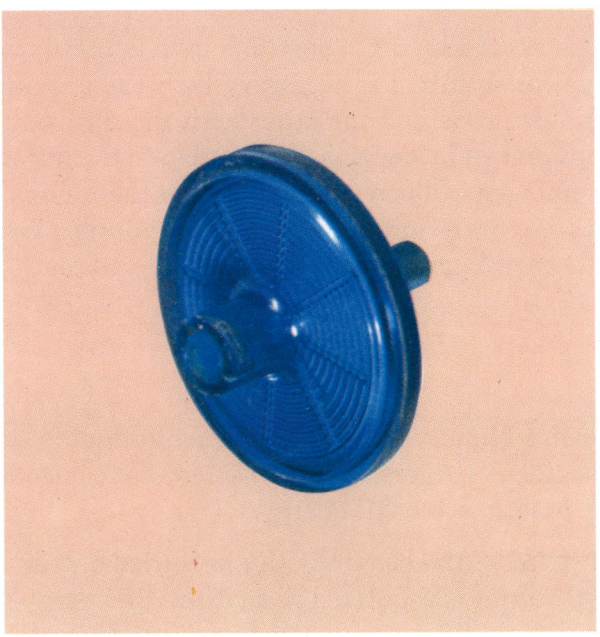

Fig. 4.7 *Millipore filter*

During operation on the posterior segment of the eye, which requires fluid–gas exchange, the air-module provides an automatic injection of sterile air at the preset pressure.

Vitrectomy/VFI Module

Vitrectomy/VFI module has three separate functions. Two of these provide outputs for electric and pneumatic vitrectomies (Figs. 4.8 and 4.9). For vitreous base surgery, vitreous shaver (Fig. 4.10) is excellent to remove the vitreous without damaging the retina. Each of these out-puts can produce a maximum frequency of 1500 cuts per minute. The upper limit of the frequency, for both the outputs, can be set using the preset controls on the front panel.

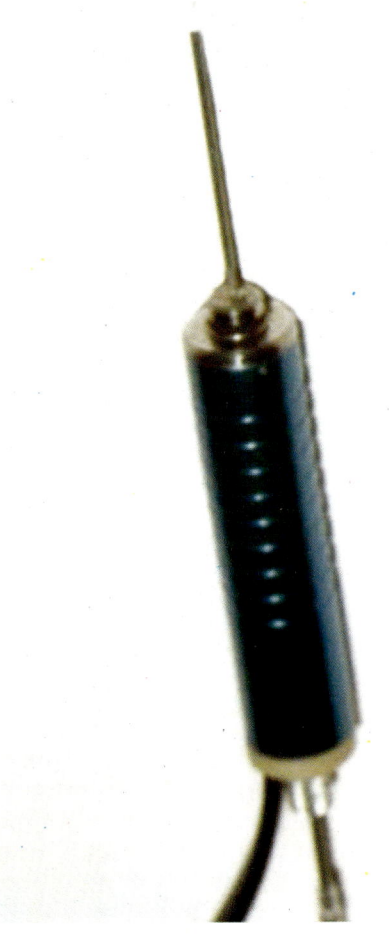

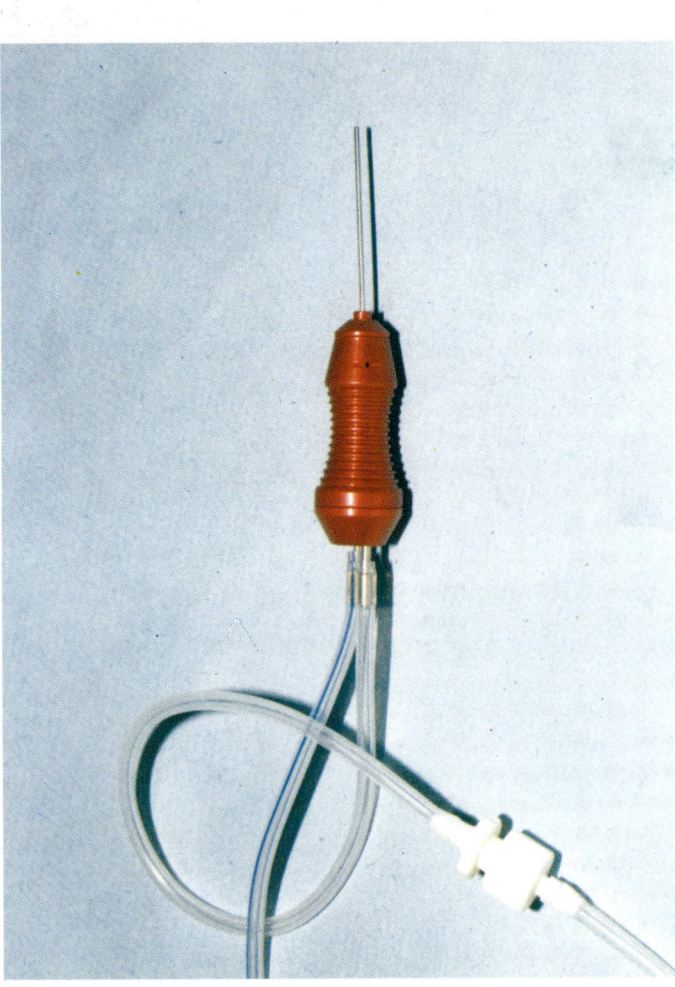

Fig. 4.8 Vitrectomy electric cutter   *Fig. 4.9 Vitrectomy pneumatic cutter*

The third function of the vitrectomy module is used with the VFI (viscous fluid injection) accessory. This provides a way of injecting viscous fluid in a controlled, automated manner. In some of the vitrectomy units the system can inject viscous fluids with a high viscosity up to 5000 centistokes or 1000 centistokes (low viscosity).

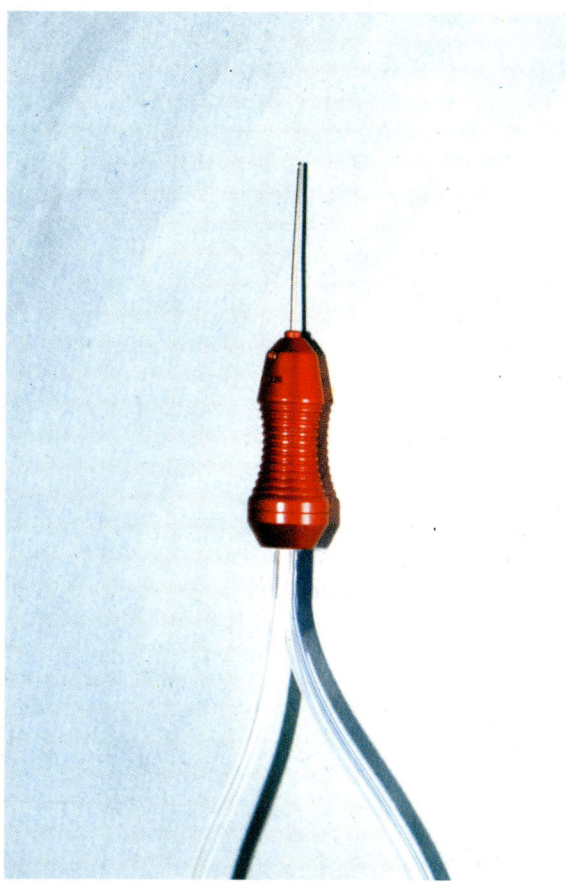

Fig. 4.10 *Vitreous shaver*

Irrigation/Aspiration (I/A) and Viscus Fluid Extraction Module

The I/A module generates a vacuum, which provides aspiration. The module include three pinch valves which control both irrigation and aspiration functions. The aspiration sounds can produce a maximum vacuum of 500 mm hg. The units should have automatic back-flush feature. When automatic back-flush feature is enabled and the footswitch is released, the vacuum inside the collection bottle to the outside air through the console. The aspiration tubing set is liquid vented to the infusion bottle. This prevents residual aspiration and tissue incarceration. The system is so accurate that when back-flush pinch valve opens, the irrigation/aspiration pinch valve of the unit closes. The two actions, taken together work to stop any aspiration action very quickly.

Compressed Air Inlet

The I/A module, a Venturi device uses compressed air to provide the vacuum used for aspiration. This system requires an air supply with a pressure of 5 to 6 Bar (75 to 90 psi). The air source must provide medical-grade quality air. This means that the air supply must be 100% free of water and oil, and should not contain particles larger than 0.3 μm.

Irrigation

The height of the irrigation above the patient's eye determines the pressure inside the eye. Each surgical procedure requires that the intra ocular pressure be set by adjusting the irrigation bottle to the required height.

Aspiration

A device based on the Venturi principal creates the vacuum used to provide aspiration. The Venturi has an inlet for compressed air, and uses the energy from the air to produce a vacuum. The orifice of Venturi is connected to the vacuum part on the rear of the unit. A short section of tubing runs to a collection container and an aspiration tubing set. When the surgeon calls for aspiration, a vacuum is created inside the collection bottle.

The aspiration function is used in vitrectomy to provide linear control of the vacuum level. To remove the viscous fluid extraction, one female side at the VFE tubing is fitted directly to the top of the collection bottle. The foot-switch provides linear control of the vacuum and thereby removes the viscous fluid (silicone oil).

CLEANING AND STERILIZING INSTRUCTION FOR ACCESSORIES

The accessories must be sterilized prior to use. It requires decontamination and re-sterilization between patient procedures. The accessories may be sterilized using either ethylene oxide (ETO) or stem. The sterilization effectiveness depends on the complete reprocessing of instrumentation (adequate cleaning, process control, and maintenance of sterility from the paint of processing to the surgical fields).

Recommendation Guidelines for Ethylene Oxide Sterilization Parameters

1. 100% ETO cycles.
2. Concentration of ETO 850 I 50 mg/l.
3. Temperature 99 F to117 F (37° to 47°C).
4. Exposure time 3 to 4 hrs.
5. Relation humidity 70%.

Recommendation Guidelines for Steam Sterilization

I. Never sterilize the accessories using dry air sterilization.
II. Handle the accessories gently; they are precision instruments.
III. During the sterilization process do not allow any of the accessories to touch any other items.
IV. Use only demineralised water for sterilization.

Cleaning Instructions

1. For device with an internal lumen, flush enzymatic cleaner through the lumen using a cleaning syringe.

2. Submerge and soak the devices in the enzymatic detergent solution for a minimum of two minutes.

3. Ringer under distilled running water to remove surface suspended particles.

4. Flush the lumen with distilled water.

5. Perform a final rinse with distilled water.

6. Dry the outside of the devices and purge the lumen with compressed air. Drying may also be accomplished by rinsing or flushing with 70% alcohol.

7. Inspect the instrument for cleanliness and damage.

Patient Preparation for Vitreous Surgery and Care of Instruments

Introduction

Vitreous surgery is a specialized, complicated and time-consuming procedure. Therefore, an idea about its setup, operation theatre arrangements, mediation and instrument backup is very important. Proper planning and preparation of patient operation theatre and surgeon himself is very essential. The surgical procedure itself is the most important event that happens to a patient. Proper management of the critical act requires teamwork. Each member of the team has a key role to play in the overall success of the surgery. The surgeon must explain to the patients and their relations about the outcome of surgery so that the patient and relations are mentally prepared to undertake smooth surgery and its outcome.

PATIENT PREPARATION

Each case has its own problems and prognosis. No two cases are similar. It is, therefore, mandatory to discuss with the patient prior to surgery. An informed consent based on the discussion with the patient is essential before surgery. Details follow-up, hospital stay and condition of the fellow eye should be explained to the patient.

The patients undergoing vitreous surgery generally have systemic problems like diabetes mellitus, cardiovascular problem, hypertension or neurological problems. Therefore, thorough laboratory tests, viz. blood sugar, oxylated hemoglobin HbA1C level, urea, creatine ECG, x-ray chest are essential for the high-risk patients. Physician and as well as anaesthetic consultation is a must for smooth running during operation and as well as in postoperative periods. However, due to associated systemic problems, local anesthesia is considered preferable over general anesthesia and it is better to have an anesthetist, around, while the surgery is on premeditation one hour before operation ensures a smooth surgical progress. All patients should have an intravenous line ready with ringer lactate or 5% dextrose adjusted according to the patient's requirements.

Dilatation of Pupils

Pupillary dilatation is highly desirable because the whole surgery is dependent upon the proper visibility of the posterior segment. Dilatation is carried out 60 minutes prior to surgery so that full dilation is achieved at the operation table. Homatropine (2%), Tropicamide or Tropicacyl are not only mydritrics but also cycloplegic which is desirable during operation.

However, certain points with regard to this should be taken care.

1. Due to the presence of preservative, these drops may be toxic to epithelium and endothelium of cornea and cause hazy media more so in diabetic patients where cornea epithelium is already in a compromised state.

2. Rigidity of the pupils often noticed due to frequent dilatation of pupils prior to surgery.

3. Phenylephrine instillation may develop high blood pressure; care should be taken for hypertensive patients.

4. Cyclopentolate has occasionally been known to produce hallucination-like symptoms.

Preparation of Eye

Local antibiotic drops in the eye should be instilled for two days prior to surgery. Eyelashes are a potential source of infection; these should be cut either on the day of operation or one day prior to surgery. Local antiseptic povidone iodine (Betadine) should be applied over the eye to be operated before sending the patient to operation theatre. In the operating room, placement of equipment utilization patterns material handling depends on the effluence of the entire surgical procedure.[1]

Preparation for Surgery

The most important aspect of vitreous surgery is to look-after the following items in operation theatre (Fig. 5.1)

1. Placement of microscope, vitrectomy machine, cryo- and endolaser.

2. Position of foot-pedal for microscope and vitrectomy units.

3. Check the working condition of suctions apparatus, pulse-oxymeter and oxygen apparatus.

4. Placements of microsurgical instruments and video arrangements.

5. Accessories like diathermy, fluid/air exchange and vitrectomy instruments should be kept ready and in order.

Anaesthesia

General anesthesia is preferred over local due to patient comfort, immobilization and better ventilation and perfusion. Since patient undergoing vitreous surgery generally have systemic ailment, a thorough history taking and medical and evaluation is a must. Proper control of the blood sugar, blood pressure and cardiac evaluation should be done prior to surgery. During general anesthesia one should take special care while using nitrous oxide. Since nitrous oxide is the mainstay in general anaesthesia: during sulphur hexafluoride (SF_6) in air fluid exchange, the nitrous oxide should be turned off at least 5 to 7 minutes before starting the procedure. While applying diathermy the anesthesist must be informed since it is inflammable and may create problem for the patient.

Local anesthesia is preferable by the ophthalmologist. As risk of the patient minimal and recovery time is quick. Peribulbar block into extraconal space with equal volumes of xylocaine and Bupivacaine with hyaluronidase using one-inch needle is very effective and provide adequate local ocular akinesia. Sub-tenon xylocaine and bupivacaine with a cannula may be continued in between if necessary.

Check-List of Instruments in OT

Prior to surgery, the following instruments should be checked for efficient and smooth functioning.

Check lists for vitrectomy and fragmatome units

  i. Vitrectomy probe—to ensure that suction and cutting are working properly.

 ii. Proper tubing and priming and checking the probe suction.

iii. Checking the illumination and its intensity.

 iv. Check the fragmatome units and its accessories.

Checking the microscope

  a. Check the focusing and zoom system by pressing the foot-pedal.

  b. Check the X-Y movements.

  c. Check the coaxial and diffuse illumination.

Checking the microsurgical equipment

  a. Infusion cannula, length of infusion sleeves (Fig 5.1).

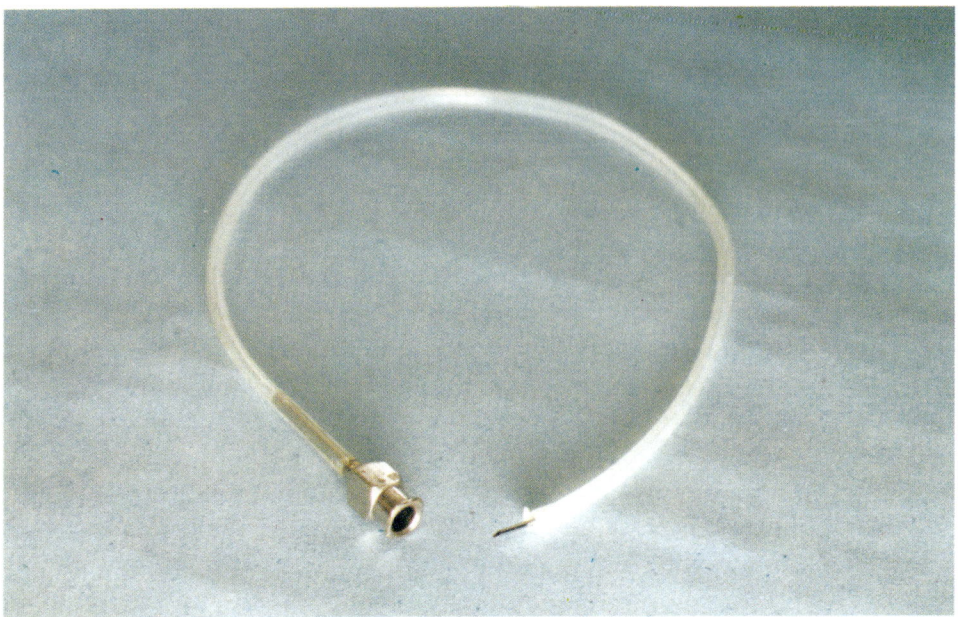

Fig. 5.1 *Infusion cannula*

b. Membrane spatula and picks foreign body forceps (Fig 5.2).

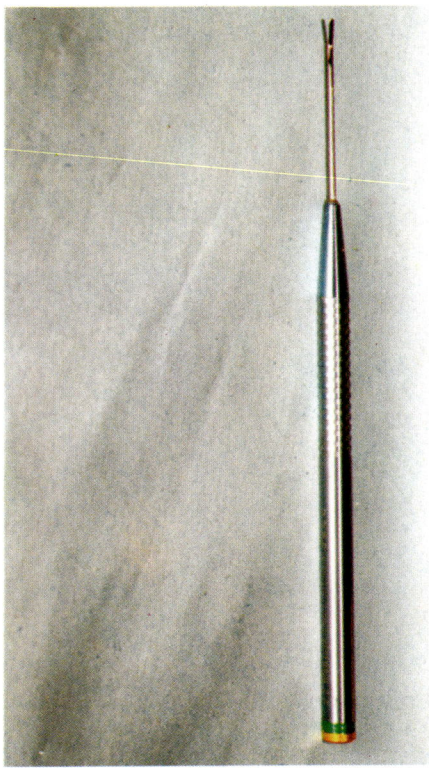

Fig. 5.2 *Membrane spatula*

c. Vitrectomy scissors — horizontal, angled, and vertical (Fig 5.3).

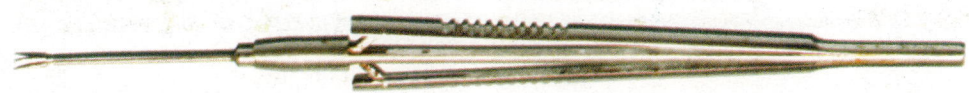

Fig. 5.3 *Vitrectomy scissors*

d. Back-flush needle (Fig. 5.4).

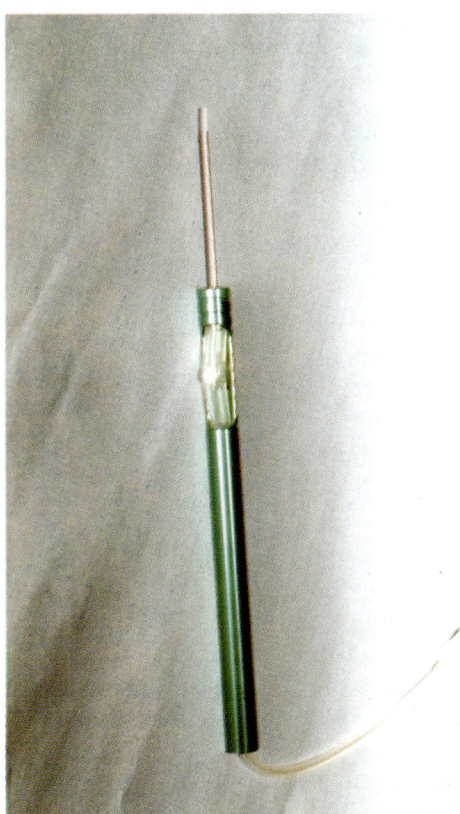

Fig. 5.4 *Back-flush needle*

e. Scleral plugs and scleral forceps.
f. Micro vitreoretinal knife/20 gauge needle.

g. Scleral depressor (Fig. 5.5).

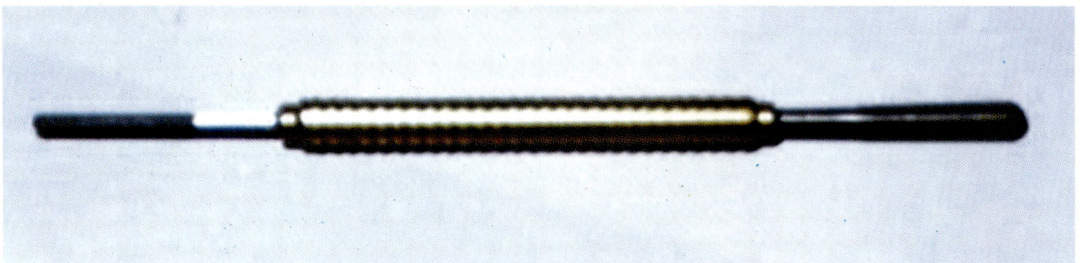

Fig. 5.5 *Scleral depressor*

The OT assistant or scrubbing nurse should check endolaser, diathermy and fluid/air exchange, prior to surgery.

Preparation

Adequate mydriasis is achieved and maintained by topical preparation of atropine and antiinflammatory drop over 24 to 48 hour period and repeated instillation of atropine, and 10 % phenylephrine; one hour prior to surgery. The later should, however, be used with caution because of its potential keratotoxicity which may result in corneal oedema and consequently impede surgery.

Good preoperative mydriasis may be facilitated in the absence of contra-indication, by the addition of adrenaline to the irrigation fluid. It is also dependent on the maintenances of an adequate intraocular pressure throughout the procedure.

As soon as the patient is wheeled into the operation theatre, he/she is started with an IV drip, which should continue throughout the operation if necessary.

The usual aseptic measures must be respected in vitrectomy; it is customary, in particular, to disinfect the eyelid margins and the conjunctival fornices with betadine.

The eye is draped and with a single large surgiwear so that unnecessary spillage of water over the patient's head and on operation table is avoided. The adhesive surgical drape, which is placed on the globe with eyelids open and incised horizontally. Thus the lid margins are covered while the lid retractor is positioned.

Irrigation Fluid

The irrigating fluids, which are currently in use, are ringer lactate and other balanced solution. A certain number of substances may be added to the irrigating fluid.

a. Unless a general contraindication exists, adrenaline adenine (½ or 1 phial of 1/1000 adrenaline to 500 ml of irrigating fluid) is used.

b. In the diabetic, phakic patient, it is better to add glucose (1500 mg of glucose to 500 ml of irrigating fluid), which seems to decrease the risk of development of lens opacities during surgery. Preoperative irrigation is maintained passively and the intraocular pressure is determined by the height of the infusion bag with respect to the eye undergoing surgery. A height of 20 to 25 cm corresponding to an IOP between 15 and 20 mm Hg is sufficed. It is important to avoid high IOP which may cause epithelial oedema and significantly increase, the risk of incarceration in sclerotomies.

CARE OF INSTRUMENTS

Cleaning

Special attention must be given to clean the surgical instrument thoroughly prior to its sterilization. Instruments should be cleaned as soon as possible after their use. Gloves must be worn while handling the instruments to avoid infective material and cuts.

An ultrasonic cleaner is ideal for cleaning instruments. It thoroughly cleans every part of the instrument, including the depths of the cannula; tubes and other unreachable parts, with high frequency sound waves generating bubbles and vacuum zones. This vibrating energy dislodges, dissolves and dispenses blood and organic debris. Chrome-plated instruments should not be cleaned in an ultrasonic cleaner. If ultrasonic cleaner is not available, the instruments are to be first soaked in mild detergent (e.g. Savlon) for half hour and then washed thoroughly under running water using a soft brush.

Storage

The instruments are dried completely before reassembling or storing. Instruments will corrode if they are stored with trapped moisture.

Each instrument has to be checked with the microscope or + 20D lens blank or loop for its working condition. To avoid electrolysis, it is not advisable to mix instruments made of stainless steel with those made of aluminium,[2] brass or copper.

Instrument Sets

Instruments must be placed in a tray with perforated bottom to allow steam penetration around the instruments during autoclaving and to prevent air trapping in the tray. Each delicate instrument must be physically separated from adjacent ones to prevent damage, interlocking or crushing. Piling them on top of each other should be avoided. All attachable parts should be disassembled. Sharp or pointed instruments should be carefully spaced in a tray to prevent contact with other instruments that could damage their surface. The size of the instrument pack should not exceed 15" x 15" and should not weigh over 3 kg.

Disinfections and Sterilisation

The effective use of disinfectants and sterilisation procedures in the operation theatre is critical for the prevention of postoperative infections. The choice of agents and procedures to be used in operation theatre depends on a variety of factors, such as degree of microbial killing required, the nature of the item or surface to be treated and the cost and ease of using the available agents. Because it is unnecessary to sterilize all items in the operation theatre, policies must be formulated regarding indications for cleaning, disinfections or sterilisation on the basis of the intended use. Spaulding[2] described three categories of items such as critical, semi-critical and non critical when determining the methods of disinfection or sterilisation.

The role of acetone[3] in the sterilization of ophthalmic instruments is questionable and is not advisable. Several factors may affect the efficacy of a disinfectant, such as prior cleaning of the object, the organic load on the disinfectant, the physical configuration of the object (e.g., cervices, hinges, lumens), and the temperature and pH of the disinfection process.

Moist heat such as autoclaving at 121° C for 15 minutes at 15 psi of pressure is the most efficient method of sterilisation for all heat-stable critical items. The process can be hastened (3 minutes) by increasing the pressure to 30 lb, when a temperature of 134° C would be achieved. Regular usage of biological indicators have become ensure proper functioning of incorrect wrapping, careless loading, time and temperature failure and tendency to shortcuts or irresponsibility. Every pack that goes through autoclaving must be labeled with colour indicator, which mentions date of autoclaving. Regular servicing of the autoclave is mandatory.

Gas sterilisation using ethylene oxide has simplified the sterilisation of heat labile materials. The operative walls, floor, metal furniture and plastic surfaces should be wiped down with a good phenolic detergent prior to surgery.

REFERENCES

1. Laufmon H: The operative room. In *Hospital Infections*, Eds. Bennelt JV and Brachman PS. Little Brown and Co, Boston, 315-324, 1986.
2. Rutala WA: Guidelines for infection control practice. In APIC guidelines for selection and use of disinfectants. *As J Inf. Control* 18:99-117, 1990.
3. Agrawal V, Sharma S: The efficacy of acetone in the sterilisation of ophthalmic instruments Ins. *J Ophthalmol* 41: 20-22, 1993.

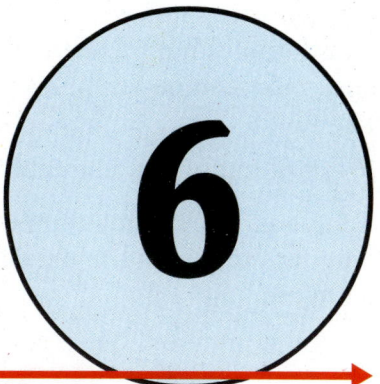

Pars Plana Vitrectomy: Basic Technique

Introduction

The success of surgery for retinal detachment is dependent on attaining closure of retinal break(s), relieving traction on the retina and minimizing the recurrence of traction.[1]

Advances in the surgical instrumentation and vitreoretinal techniques have allowed intra-operative reapproximation of retina to a more normal position. The basic technique of pars-plana is an important step to know for successful outcome of surgery.

The practical use of intravitreal injected liquid materials (viscoelastic liquids, liquid perfluorocarbon and silicone oil) as adjunctive agents to vitreoretinal surgery play an important pre-requisite in facilitating retinal detachment.[1] Preparation of the surgical field, making proper entry site, air–fluid exchange and closer of the site required adequate knowledge for smooth running of the entire procedure.

PATIENT PREPARATION

Mydriasis

Adequate mydriasis is achieved and maintained by the instillation of a topical preparation of atropine and anti-inflammatory drops over a 24 to 48 hour period and repeated instillation, during the hour preceeding surgery. The local eye drops of 1% atropine and 10.0% phenylephrine is instilled: the latter should be used, however, with caution because of its potential keratotoxicity, which may result in corneal oedema and consequently impede surgery.

Good preoperative mydriasis may be facilitated, in the absence of contraindication, by the addition of adrenaline to the irrigation fluid; it is also dependent on the maintenance of an adequate intraocular pressure throughout the procedure.

Preparation of the Surgical Field

The usual aseptic measures must be respected in vitrectomy; it is customary, in particular, to disinfect the eyelid margins and the conjunctival fornices with a weakly diluted solution of betadine.

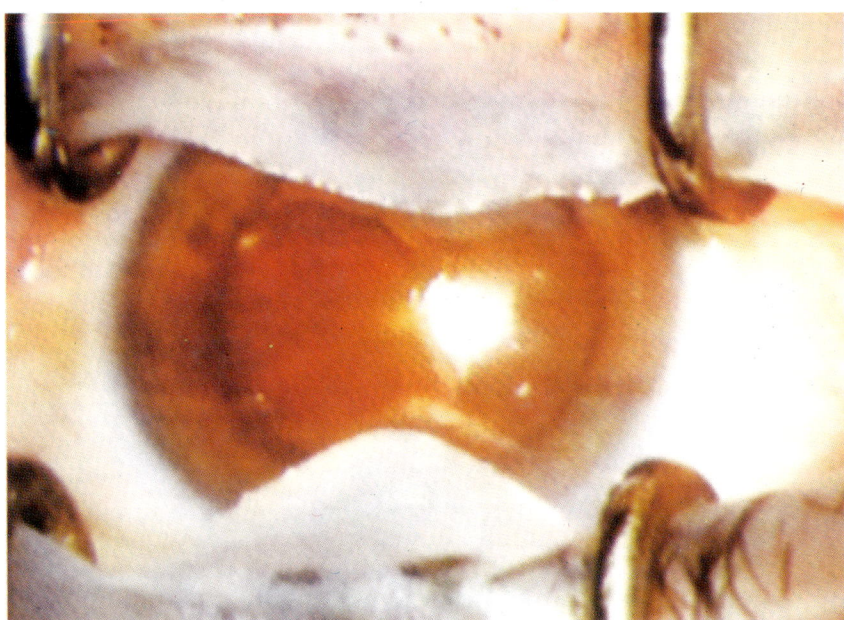

Fig. 6.1 *Positioning of the lid retractors while ensuring that lashes are covered by the surgical drape*

The adhesive surgical drape which is placed on the globe with the eyelids open and incised longitudinally, thus the lashes are covered while the lid retractors are positioned (Fig. 6.1).

Irrigation Fluids

The irrigation fluids in current use are Ringer's lactate and other balanced salt solutions. A certain number of substances may be added to the irrigation fluid. Unless a general contraindication exists, one can routinely use adrenaline, which allows the maintenance of good preoperative mydriasis (1/2 or 1 phial of 1/1000 adrenaline to 500 ml of irrigation fluid).

In the diabetic, phakic patient, one should always add glucose (1500 mg of glucose to 500 ml of irrigation fluid), which seems to decrease the risk of development of lens opacities during surgery. Preoperative irrigation is maintained passively and the intraocular pressure is determined by the height of the infusion bag with respect to the eye undergoing surgery, a height of

20 to 25 cm corresponding to an intraocular pressure between 15 and 20 mm Hg. It is important to avoid any increase in intraocular pressure, which may cause epithelial oedema and significantly increase the risk of incarceration in the sclerotomies.

Conjunctival Incisions

One should carry out a limbal incision with two lateral extensions. The advantages of such an incision are that it is easy to suture, it does not cause visible scarring and it does not hinder an eventual further surgical procedure. The incisions are made at the limbus for 60° temporally and 30° nasally; radial incisions allow exposure of the sclera over the parsplana.

Making the Entry Sites

In all but unusual cases, the vitrectomy is carried out by means of three entry sites, allowing the use of a separate infusion cannula, a light pipe and various 20-gauge accessory instruments. The infusion is usually situated inferior temporally while the two other sclerotomies are situated superior nasally and superior temporally. The distance between the two superior sclerotomies must be large enough to allow access to all parts of the globe during the intervention. If the sclerotomies are too close, this will rapidly result in discomfort for the surgeon. Ideally, two sclerotomies should be made at an angle of about 150° with each other; at the upper borders of the medial and lateral recti (Fig. 6.2). The infusion terminal is normally positioned at the lower border of the medial rectus. They are usually situated 3 mm from the limbus in the phakic patients and 4 mm from the limbus in the aphakic patient so as to avoid accidental trauma to the lens by the infusion terminal or by an instrument (Fig. 6.3).

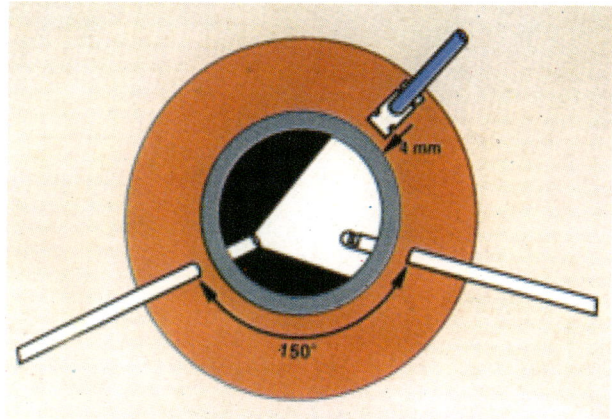 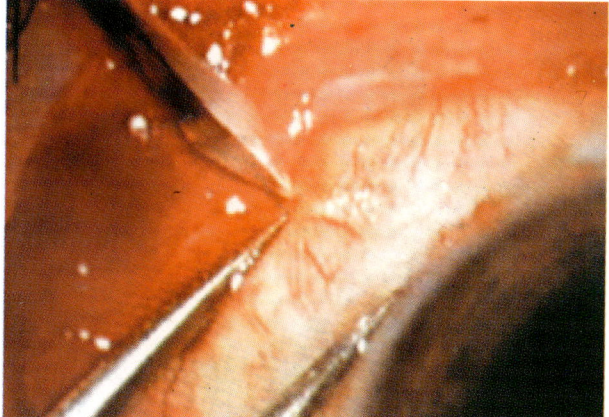

Fig. 6.2 *Diagrammatic representation of the position of sclerotomies*

Fig. 6.3 *The sclerotomy is positioned 4 mm from the limbus using caliper*

The sclerotomies are made parallel to the ora serrata with a calibrated knife, which must perforate sclera, parsplana and vitreous base; directed towards the posterior pole, it should be visible in the pupillary area before being withdrawn (Fig. 6.4).

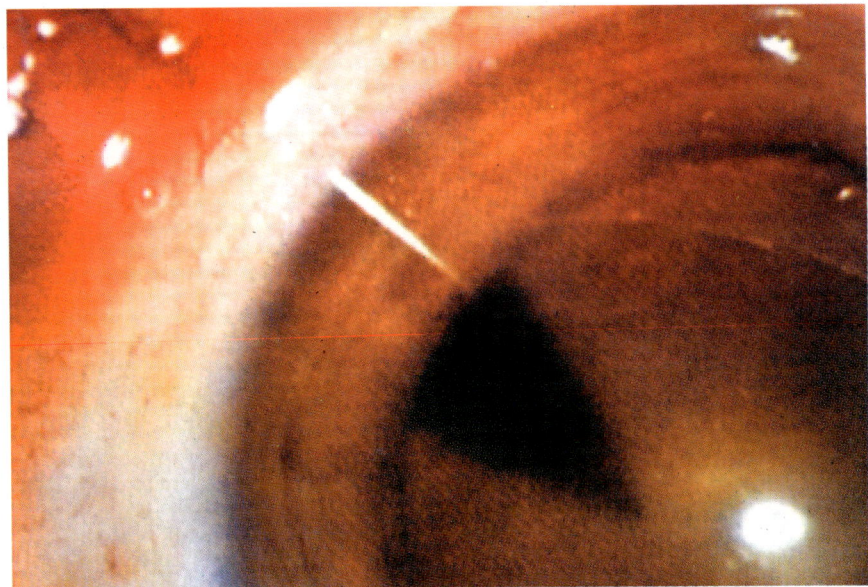

Fig. 6.4 *Micro vitreoretinal knife visible in the pupillary area.*

It is preferable to make the inferiotemporal sclerotomy first and to attach the infusion terminal straight away. First, a U-shaped scleral suture is placed and this will be responsible for anchoring the terminal during the intervention; the terminal is introduced into the eye with its bevel facing upwards and the U-shaped suture is tied, preferably, by a temporary knot. We use a triple-square knot followed by a half-key, which is easily undone at the end of the intervention and allows the sclerotomy to be kept watertight when the terminal is being removed (Fig. 6.5).

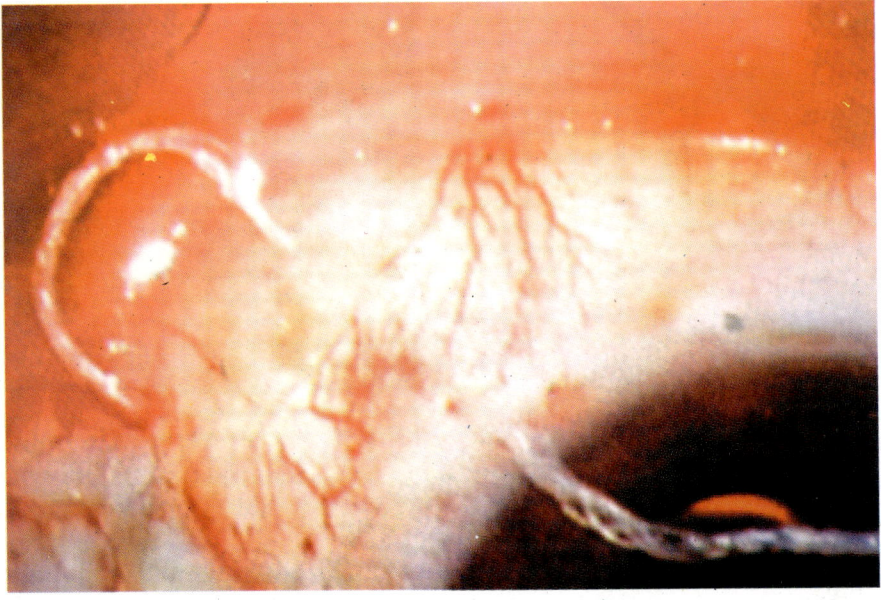

Fig. 6.5 *Placing of a 6/0 vicryl U-shaped superficial scleral suture.*

It is very important to keep the infusion closed while the terminal is being introduced and to open it only when it has been ensured that the terminal has successively cleared the parsplana, in order to avoid producing a choroidal effusion.

The position of the cannula may be checked with a three-mirror lens, a prismatic vitrectomy lens or an indirect ophthalmoscope but it is simpler to visualize it directly with the naked eye, illuminating the pupillary area with an optic filament (Fig. 6.6). If the terminal has not cleared the parsplana, it is imperative to reposition it correctly; in certain cases it is not possible to visualize the terminal at the beginning of the intervention: in this case, the early stages of the vitrectomy must be carried out without endoillumination, infusing via one of the superior sclerotomies by means of a hand piece, which must be visible in the pupil.

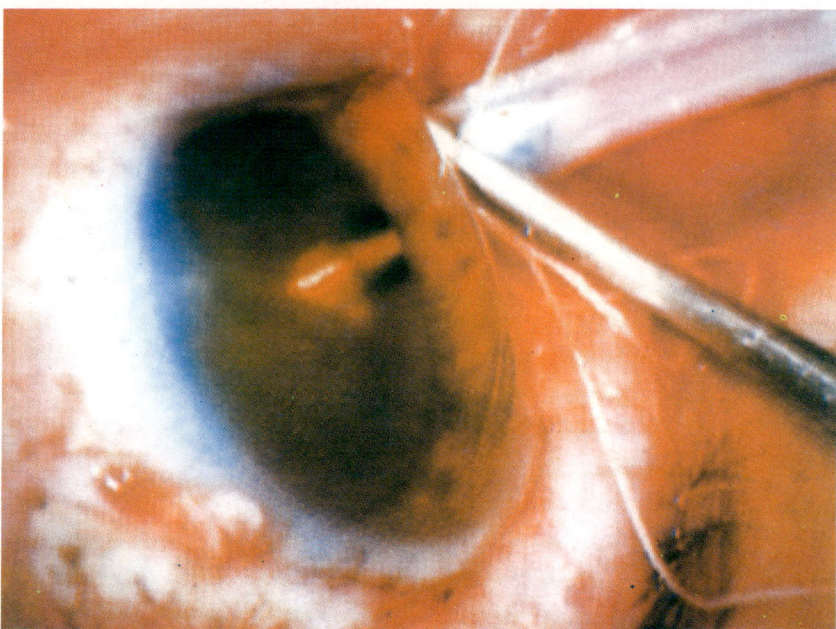

Fig. 6.6 *Checking the terminal for correctly position.*

THE INFUSION CANNULA

One has to remember that the infusion cannula has to be first inserted and last to out (Figs 6.7 and 6.8). The infusion should be started as soon as the tip is visualized and continued till just before the conjunctiva is sutured (Fig. 6.9). The superior sclerotomies are usually made with a calibrated knife after the infusion cannula has been introduced; it is preferable to make them with the infusion turned off, so as to avoid incarceration of the vitreous, or even of the retina (a complication most frequently encountered in an eye with a retinal detachment), in the sclerotomies.

The advantages of inserting infusion cannula first in are:

• No hypotony induced

• No miosis

- No bleeding

- No striate keratopathy

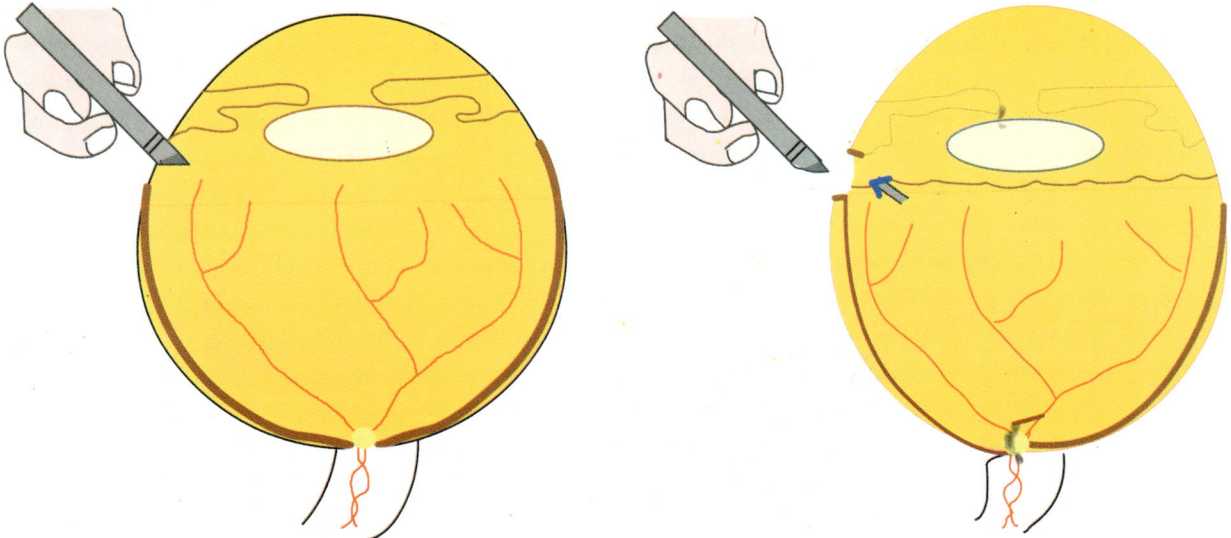

Fig. 6.7 *First in*   **Fig. 6.8** *Last out*

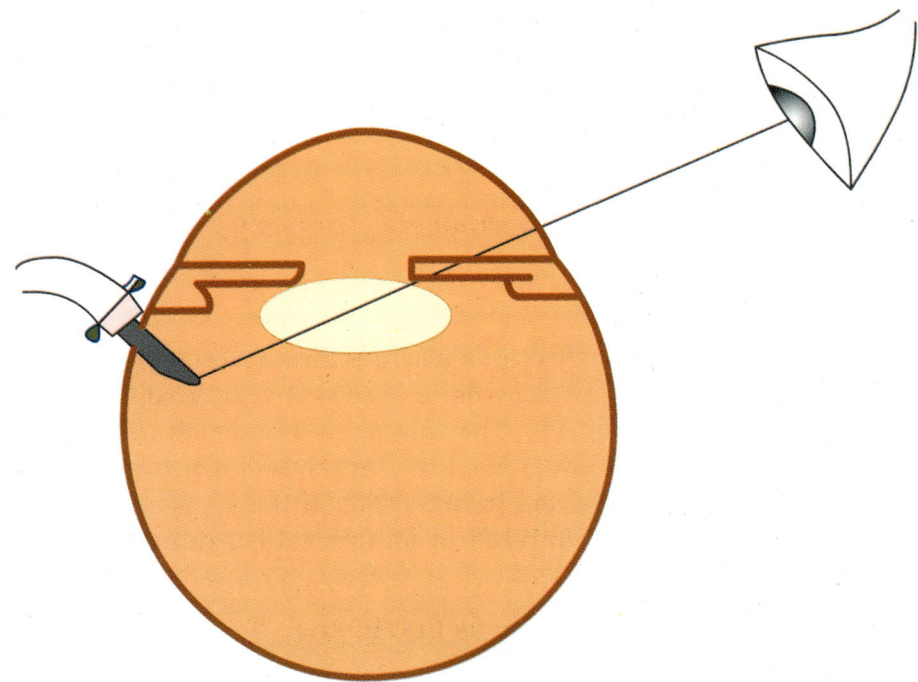

Fig. 6.9 *Always see the tip*

The advantages of inserting infusion cannula last out are:

• No subretinal or choroidal infusion.

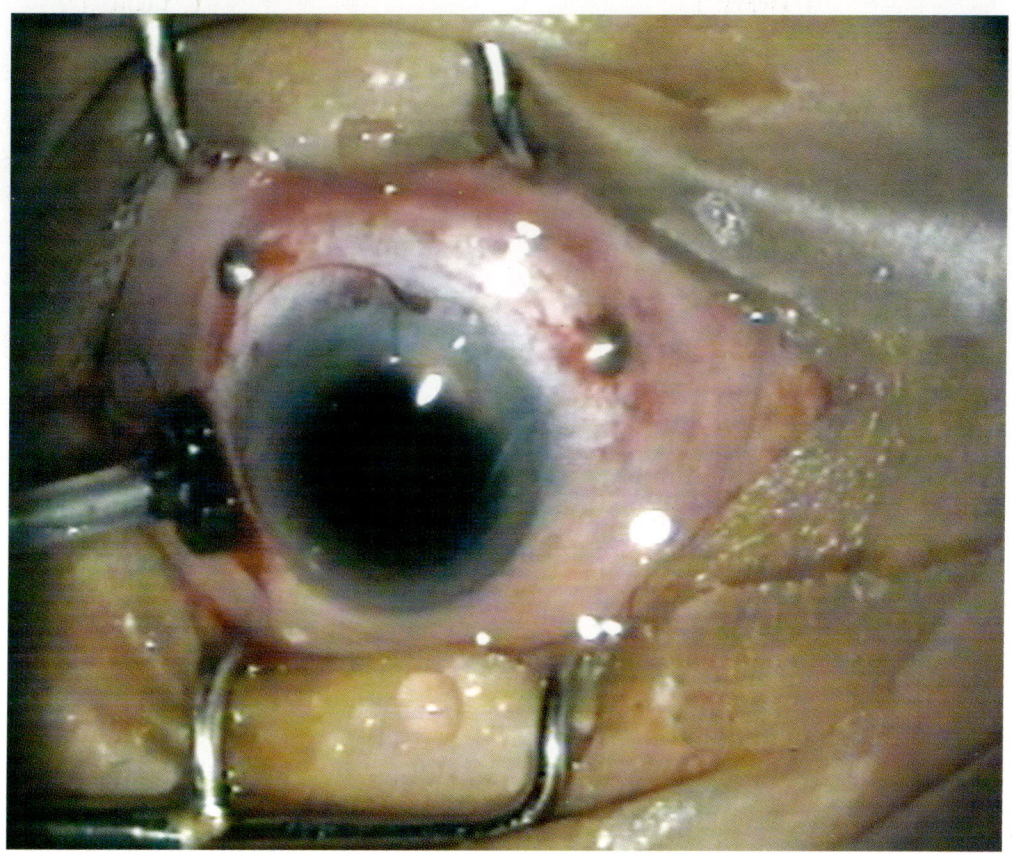

Fig. 6.10 *Sclerotomies temporary closed with scleral plugs*

When during the intervention, the sclerotomies are not being used; they may be temporarily closed with scleral plugs (Fig. 6.10).

INSTRUMENT HANDLING

All instruments are to be held in the fingertips if not along metacarpal joints because of better tactile sensations. The instrument has to be triangular between the three fingertips with the thumb apposing the fingertips which occupy approximately 30-35 percent of handle length (Figs 6.11 and 6.12). While cutting tissue, the probe should be moved towards the tissue (Figs 6.13 and 6.14). This is easier with the new delta suction systems as by accurately controlling the suction to low level the probe orifice can be turned towards the retina. The surgeon should avoid pulling the probe (burned-hand reflex) once the tissue is caught in the probe (Figs 6.15 and 6.16). The ideal cutter should be pneumatically diaphgram-driven, hourglass-shaped, self-sharpening and lightweight to avoid fatigue.

HAND PIECE

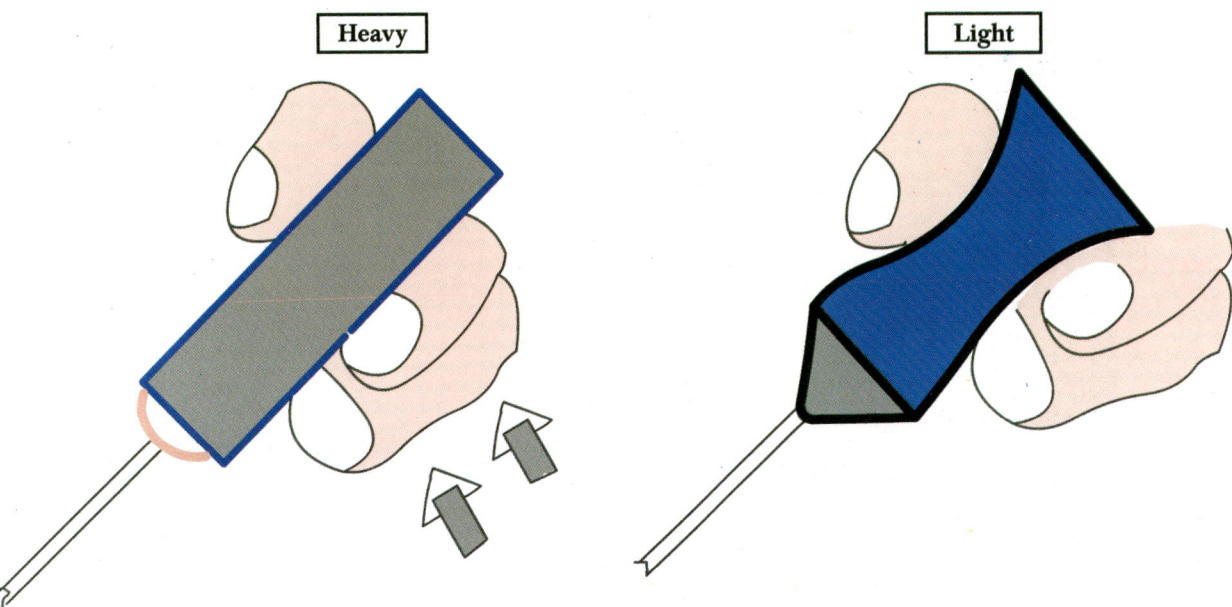

Heavy

Light

Fig. 6.11 *Excessive pressure leads to insensitivity (straight probe)*

Fig. 6.12 *Contoured probe*

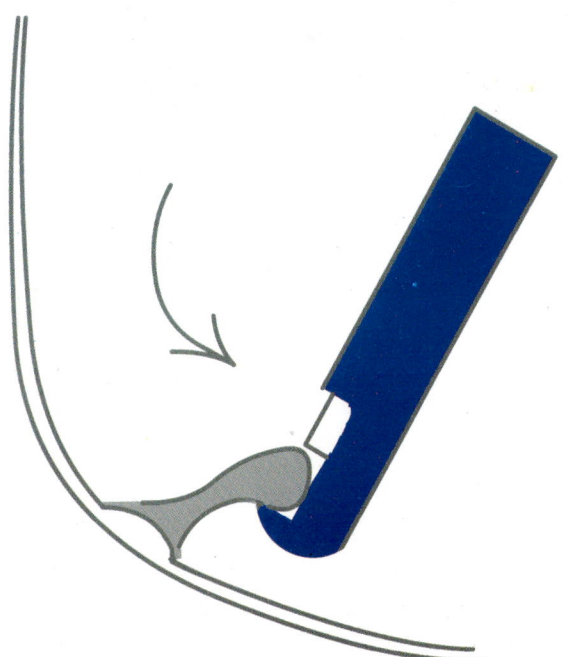

Fig. 6.13 *Wide angle port close to tip*

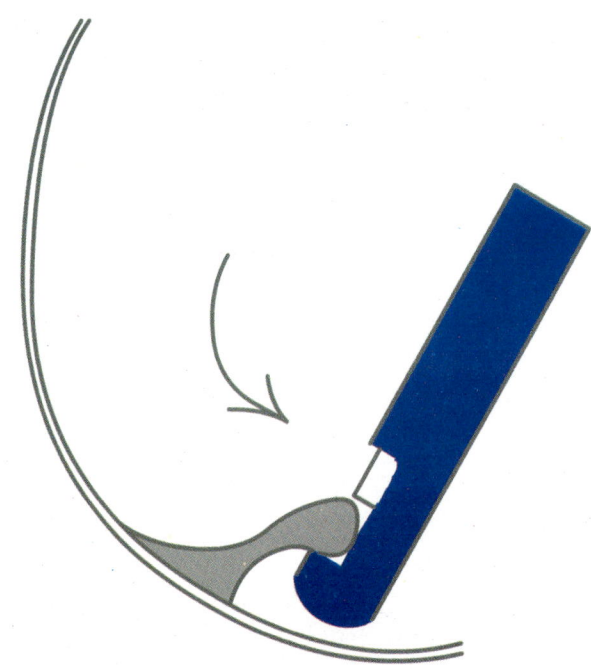

Fig. 6.14 *Port farther from retina requires excessive suction force*

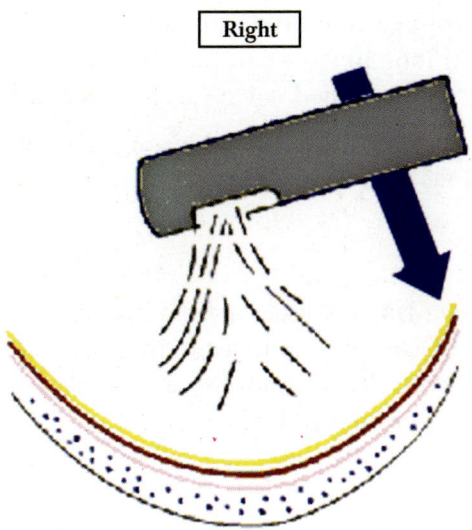

Fig. 6.15 *Cutting while advancing (proper technique)*

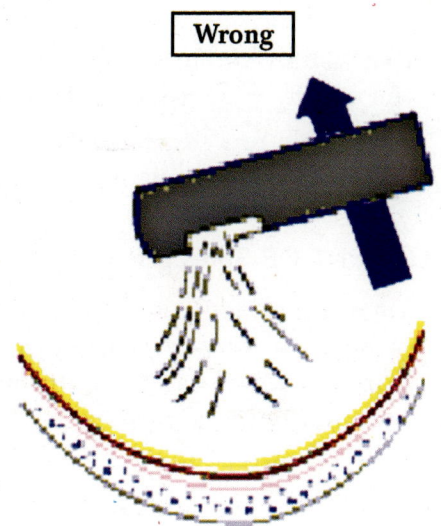

Fig. 6.16 *Cutting while pulling away (improper technique)*

PARS PLANA LENSECTOMY

Cataract may be present preoperatively or may develop during surgery. The lens may be removed by extracapsular technique or by phacoemulsification if intraocular lens (IOL) is desired. Pars plana lensectomy is often a technique of choice when cataract develops intraoperative. Removal of luxated lens by pars plana technique is an excellent procedure in young patients in whom an anterior approach often will create problem with the vitreous.

STEPS FOR REMOVAL OF LENS

- After putting the infusion cannula in inferior temporal quadrant and having made two sclerotomies in upper two quadrants, removal of lens is done in many situations where decompartmentalization is required.

- The lens is initially penetrated peripherally with micro vitreoretinal (MVR) blade. The lens nucleus is perforated and rotated gently to begin breaking up the lens material.

- Removal of lens is performed either by vitrectomy instrument or fragmantome. One can keep the micro vitreoretinal (MVR) blade inside the lens from the other port, to facilitate bimanual cutting and aspiration of lens matter by vitreous cutter or fragmatome. It must be remembered that while removing the lens matter not to be removed the anterior capsule first as it will cause collapse of anterior chamber.

- The most peripheral portion of the lens that is visible through the pupil is done first by moving sweeping motion superiorly and inferiorly until the area just anterior to the posterior capsule is removed. The posterior capsule, which is thin, fragile is removed first and then the anterior capsule is removed. If capsular support for intraocular lens (IOL) is desired, the anterior capsule is allowed to remain. Indentation with cotton-tipped swab allows visibility of the periphery lens and capsule, which can be removed by end-gripping forceps. The peripheral lens matter can also be removed with the cutter by depressing the limbal zone using a soft-tipped cotton applicator.

- The whole procedure can be performed under coaxial illumination of an operating microscope and there is no need of irrigating contact lens.

MANAGEMENT OF SMALL PUPIL

A clear cornea and adequate pupillary opening are essential for successful vitreoretinal surgery. A wide view is particularly desirable for repair of complex detachments such as giant retinal tear, retinopathy of prematurely and proliferative vitreoretinopathy with anterior contraction. Manipulation of intraocular lens is facilitated by wide dilatation.

Non-surgical Treatment of Small Pupils

- Viscoelastic injection sometimes enlarges the pupil.
- Some surgeon injects 0.3 ml of 1:1000 preservative free epinephrines in each 540 ml of bottle of infusion solution to maintain dilatation of pupil.
- Bolos of 0.1 ml of 1:10,000 preservative free epinephrines also may be injected into the vitreous cavity during the procedure to enhance dilation. This technique is more effective in aphakic eyes.

The pupil may dilate poorly, particularly if multiple previous procedures have been performed due to trauma. The iris sometimes is bound down to capsular remnants, an IOL, vitreous, or membranes. Sometimes intraoperative hypotony may produce pupillary constriction.

Surgical Treatment of Small Pupil

In eyes that do not respond adequately to pharmacological dilation, the most reliable technique for achieving wide pupillary dilation is use of flexible nylon iris retractors. The iris retractor consists of flexible hook made of nylon suture material and silastic, which slide, to hold the hook in position (Fig.6.17).

The four self-sealing 0.5 mm stab paracentesis incisions are made in the peripheral, cornea at the 10 O'clock, 2 O'clock, 4 O'clock, and 8 O'clock meridians. The hook is inserted through the paracentesis incision and engages the iris at the pupil margin. Pulling the hook forcibly enlarges the pupil. The position is fixed by adjusting the flexible silastic slide down towards the eye. In most cases the retractors are placed in all four quadrants to obtain a clear 360° view.[4] Once all the retractors are in place it gives wide 360° view. Special lenses, placed in lens ring, may provide a wide field but this requires an image inverter or the microscope. The binocular indirect ophthalmoscope-microscope (BIOM) is a non-contact system that is installed on the microscope and does not require an assistant to manipulate the lens. The working distance from the cornea to the lens is approximately 0.6 inch. About 100° of the fundus is visible so that scleral depression is necessary to work in the periphery. There is some other methods can be used to dilate the pupil surgically.

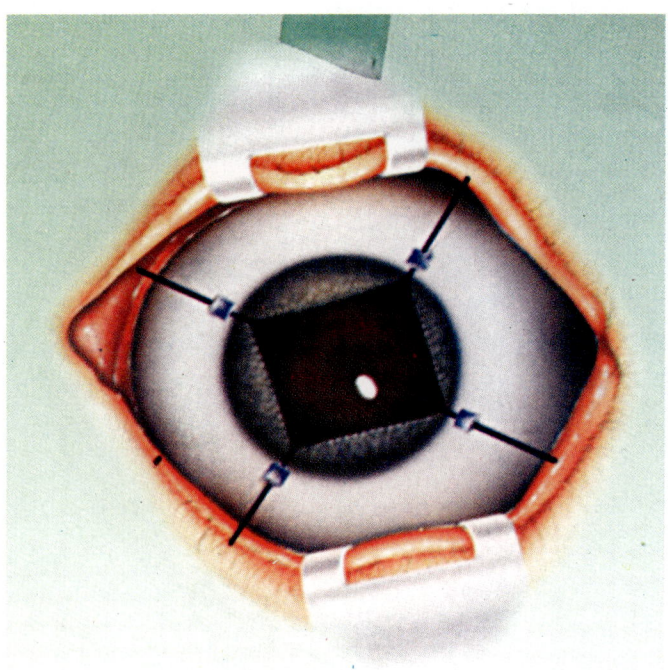

Fig. 6.17 *Iris retractors*

a. *Sphincterotomy or pupilloplasty.*

b. *Mid-peripheral iridectomy.* This begins with a mid stromal; full thickness iridectomy. Viscoelastic is placed above and below the iris and scissors are used to enlarge the iridectomy to the pupillary aperture.

c. *Radial iridectomy for miotic pupil.* The anterior chamber is filled with viscoelastic fluid. With the help of straight venous scissors, incise the iris from the peripheral iridectomy to the pupil margin to expose the entire pupillary area. If pupillary area is not adequately exposed, two small sphincterotomies are done at the 4 O'clock and 8 O'clock meridians.

d. *Multiple sphincterotomies.* These can be done in patients on chronic miotic therapy to dilate the pupil.

STEPS OF VITRECTOMY IN SIMPLE VITREOUS HAEMORRHAGE

I. After performing the three port sclerotomies, the infusion line being in the inferior temporal and the two superior sclerotomies in superior temporal for vitrectomy probe and superior nasal quadrant for endoilluminator. If the lens is cataractus, it may be removed by fragmatome. Initially the light and cutting probe are placed in the anterior third of the vitreous cavity. If lens is clear, these should be placed well behind the lens. Both instruments should be in view at all times. The light source must be manipulated to provide the best view of the vitreous while avoiding reflected glare from the metallic instruments. The working instrument usually is positioned near the edge of the illuminated area to reduce glare (Figs 6.18 and 6.19). (see Vitreous Hemorrhage Flow Chart).

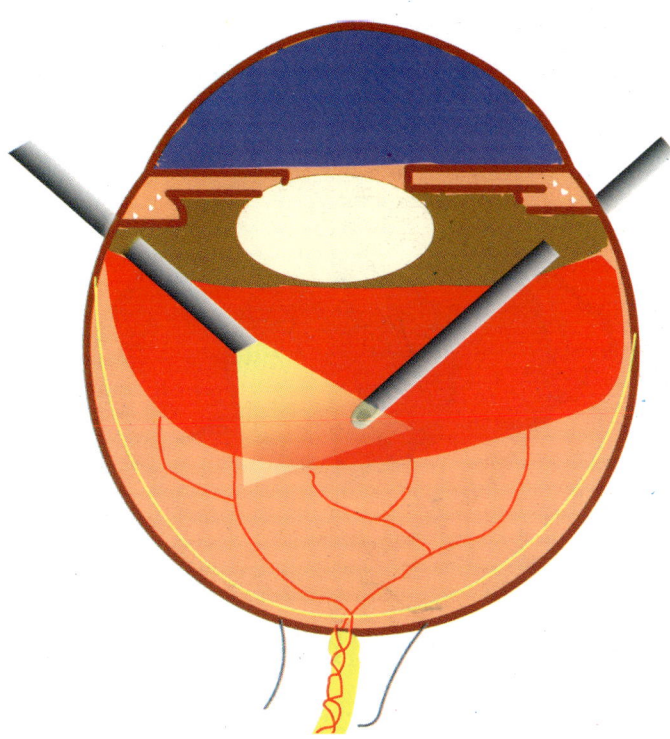

Fig. 6.18 *Light and cutting probe are placed in the anterior two-thirds of the vitreous cavity.*

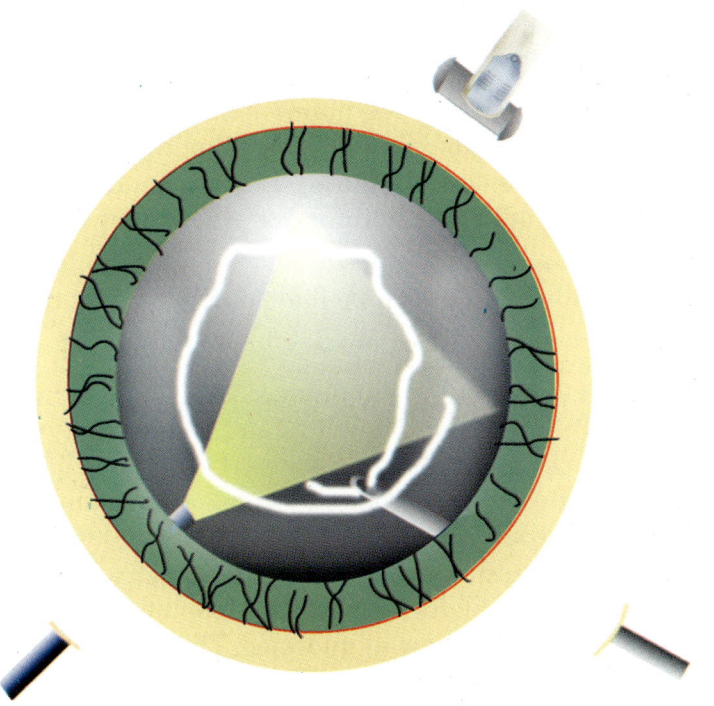

Fig. 6.19 *Both light pipe and cutter are viewed at all times*

II. The vitreous removal is first carried out in the region of the central anterior hyaloids face and then the cutter is moved peripherally to clear the area of anterior vitreous gel. At this stage a low suction rate is necessary. Once the opaque vitreous is removed, the retina can be identified and also it allows improving orientation to the intraocular position of the instruments. The mid-vitreous (central vitreous core) is then removed using high cutting rate and low suction rate (Figs 6.20 and 6.21).

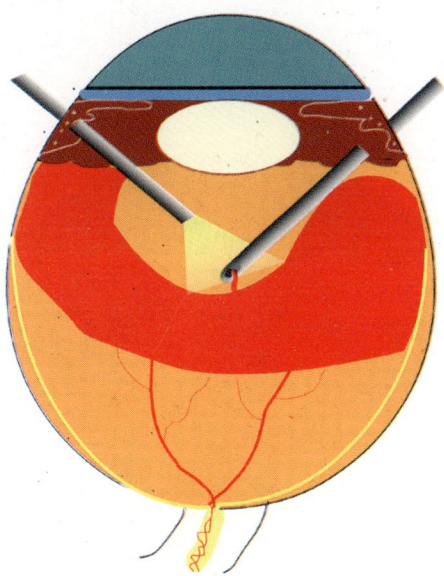

Fig. 6.20 *Central vitreous is removed for proper orientation of intraocular position of instrument*

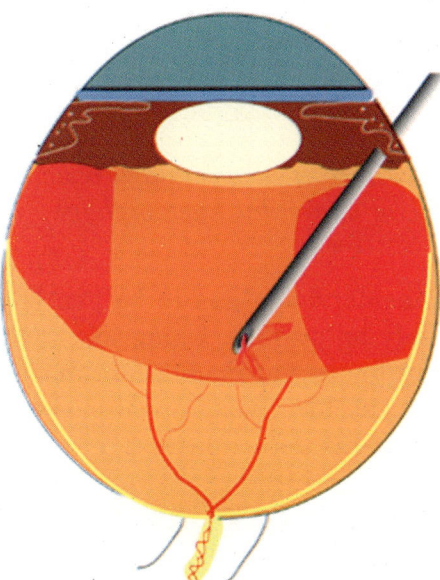

Fig. 6.21 *Vitrectomy carried towards the periphery*

Once the posterior area is identified, the vitrectomy is carried out towards the periphery by using the 30° prism lens, which allows a better view of the periphery and are important points to be remembered that while working towards the periphery the cutting prove always should be visible at the edge of the pupillary opening. In case there is sudden appearance of a new rounded opacity at the edge of the field of view, it should alert the surgeon to the possibility of peripheral retinal detachment or choroidal haemorrhage. Once the situation is appreciated, the cutting and suction should be discontinued (Fig 6.22).

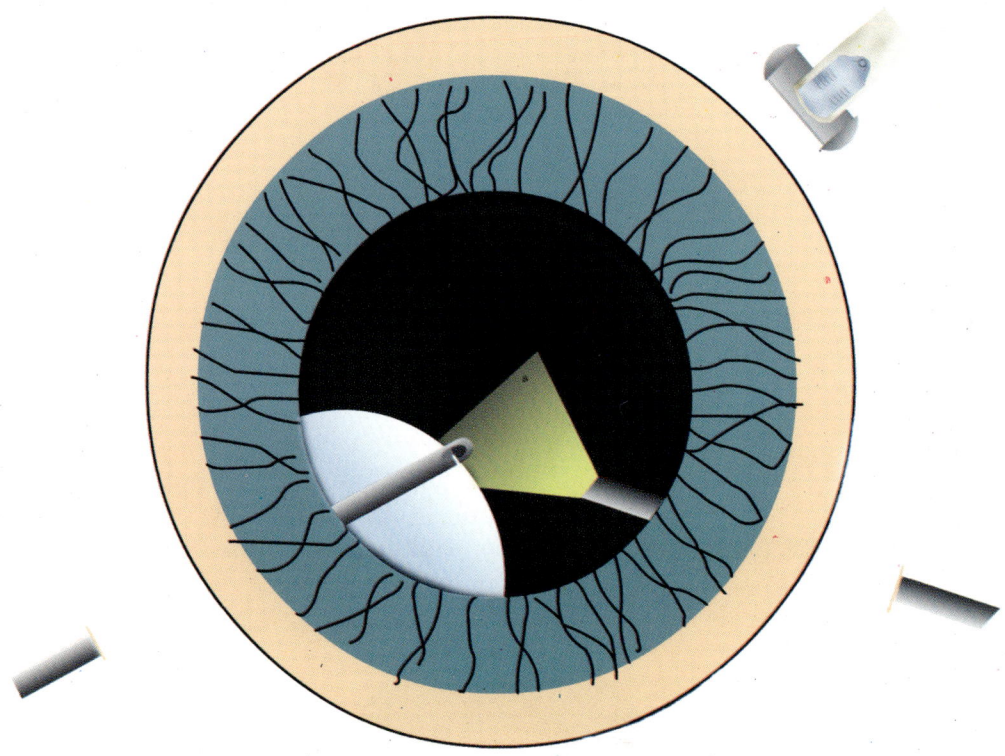

Fig. 6.22 *Sudden appearance of new rounded opacity alerts peripheral RD or choroidal haemorrhage*

III. The posterior vitreous haemorrhage has to be gently cleared as in many areas sub hyaloids haemorrhage may be present. Using low suction and entering the posterior vitreous in nasal quadrant to prevent inadvertent macular damage are keys to successful posterior vitreous removal. Ideally, an opening is created in the posterior gel in the region of the posterior vitreous detachment (PVD) and then gradually the gel is removed.

IV. If sub-PVD blood is present, then vacuum cleaning of the blood is carried out using a fluid needle. Once the retina surface is clearly visible, the area of surface neovascularisation is then treated with endolaser in eyes with proliferative retinopathy. The sclerotomy openings are then closed with 6.0 vicryl sutures.

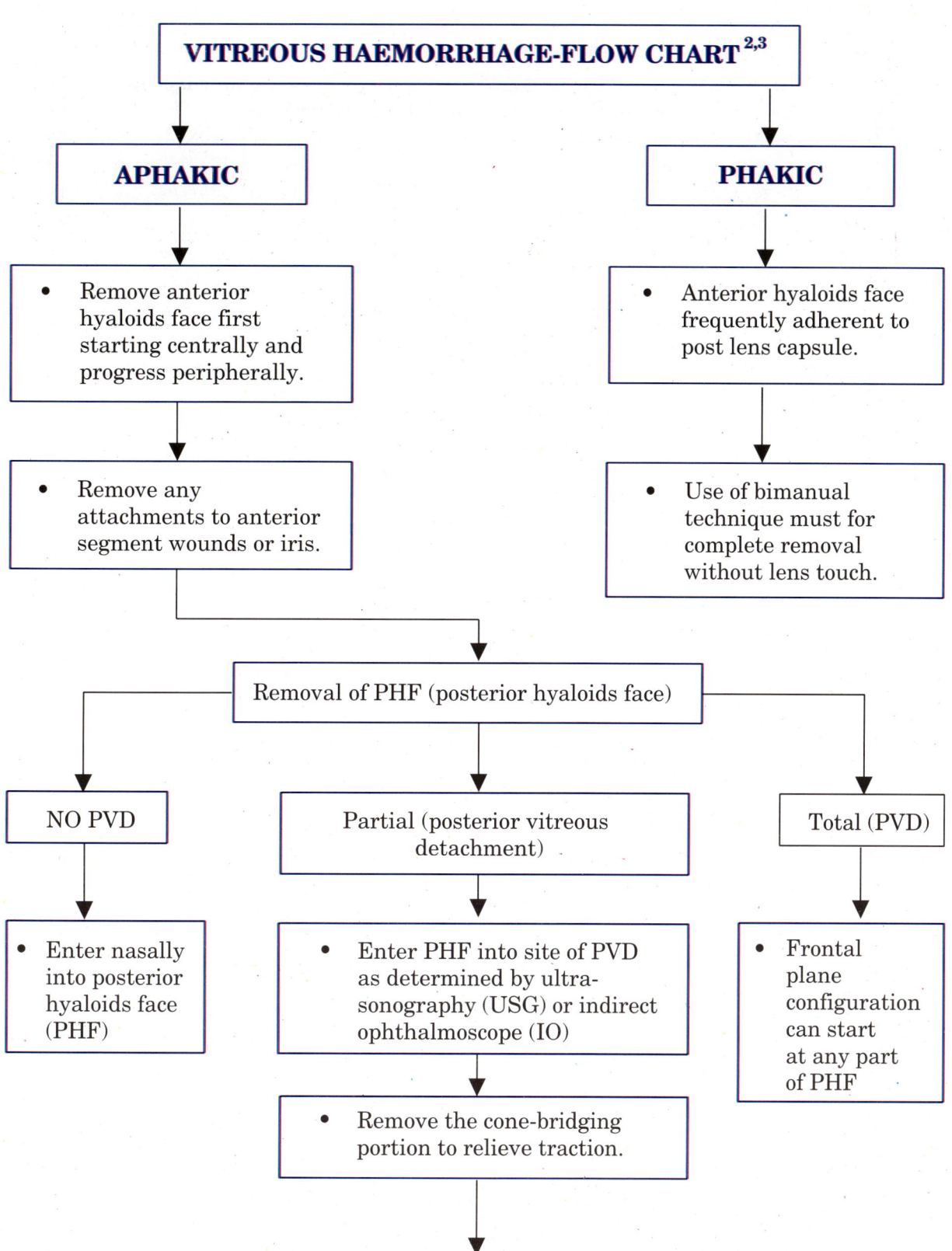

VITREOUS HAEMORRHAGE-FLOW CHART[2,3]

APHAKIC

- Remove anterior hyaloids face first starting centrally and progress peripherally.

- Remove any attachments to anterior segment wounds or iris.

PHAKIC

- Anterior hyaloids face frequently adherent to post lens capsule.

- Use of bimanual technique must for complete removal without lens touch.

Removal of PHF (posterior hyaloids face)

NO PVD

Partial (posterior vitreous detachment)

Total (PVD)

- Enter nasally into posterior hyaloids face (PHF)

- Enter PHF into site of PVD as determined by ultrasonography (USG) or indirect ophthalmoscope (IO)

- Remove the cone-bridging portion to relieve traction.

- Frontal plane configuration can start at any part of PHF

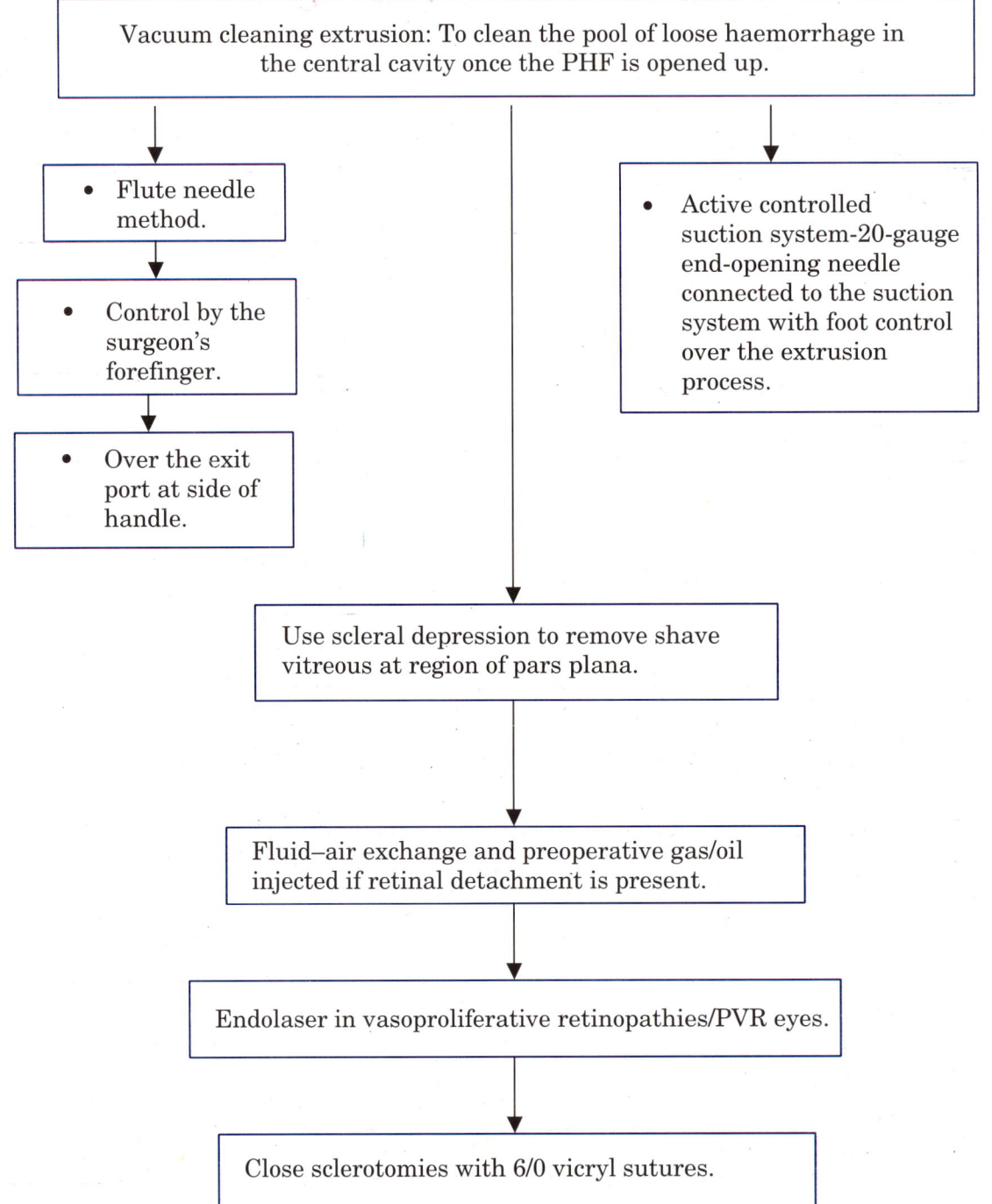

Vacuum cleaning extrusion: To clean the pool of loose haemorrhage in the central cavity once the PHF is opened up.

- Flute needle method.

- Control by the surgeon's forefinger.

- Over the exit port at side of handle.

- Active controlled suction system-20-gauge end-opening needle connected to the suction system with foot control over the extrusion process.

Use scleral depression to remove shave vitreous at region of pars plana.

Fluid–air exchange and preoperative gas/oil injected if retinal detachment is present.

Endolaser in vasoproliferative retinopathies/PVR eyes.

Close sclerotomies with 6/0 vicryl sutures.

Courtesy: Michael R et al.

Vacuum Technique

In vitrectomy, intraocular pressure depends upon the height of the infusion bottle. The ringer lactate runs from an open sclerotomy as long as that opening is below the level of the infusion. When a blunt needle is placed inside the eye (Fig. 6.23), it allows outflow to be directed creating a stream to remove fluid, blood and particles from the eye. Sometime blood accumulates over the retina, which can be removed by vacuum technique, where the needle is attached to the handle with a plastic insert containing a vent hole. Removing the finger from the hole initiates drainage and it may be slowed by partially covering the hole. (Fig. 6.24) Backflush may be created by squeezing down the plastic tube. Longstanding blood, which is not coagulated, can be removed easily by vacuum technique. The flute-needle should be placed above the edge of the blood but one should avoid to place in the centre of the pool because underlying retina may be engaged. The drainage is always efficient at the edge of a blood-pool. When back flush is difficult the connecting tip may be connected to the automatic vacuum for easy removal. Once the clot is free from the retina surface, it may be aspirated and cut with the vitrectomy probe. Recently, a laser probe coupled with aspiration may be used to coagulate the underlying source of bleeding and also suck the blood simultaneously.

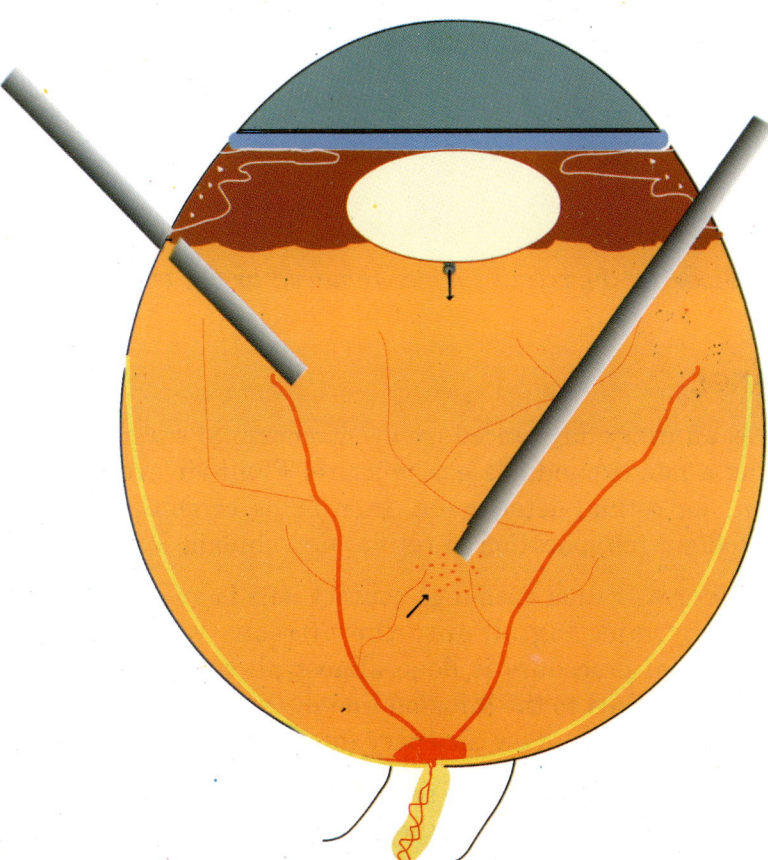

Fig. 6.23 *Flute needle is below the level of infusion thereby allows to remove blood and particles from the eye*

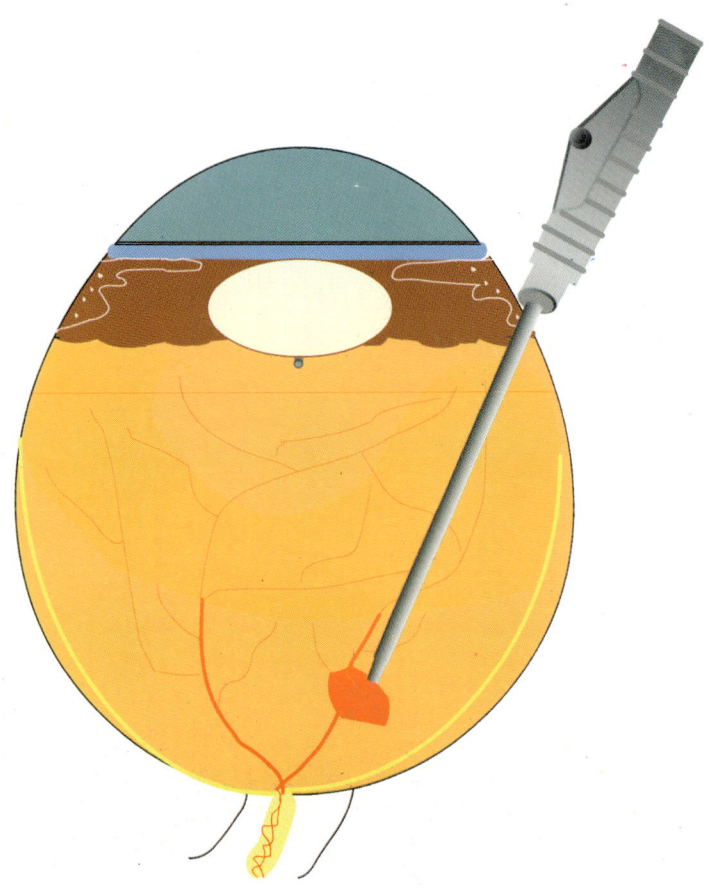

Fig. 6.24 *Blood on the retina surface removed by the technique vacuuming*

FLUID–AIR EXCHANGE

Fluid-air exchange is an every day procedure in vitreoretinal surgery. It often precedes internal tamponade using a non-expandable gas mixture. Fluid-air exchange often takes place at the end of vitrectomy for retinal detachment, then being combined with internal drainage of subretinal fluid, or follows reapplication of retinal detachment by liquid perflurocarbon.

In vitrectomy procedure-air fluid exchange contact lens is an important step (Fig. 6.25). Re-attaching the retina by injecting air into the vitreous while simultaneously draining subretinalfluid is a critical procedure is done almost all cases in vitreoretinal surgery (Fig. 6.26). The air tubing is attached to the infusion line in the inferiotemporal quadrant. The infusion bottle is kept low in order to allow air entry into the vitreous cavity.

A flute needle (backflush) is inserted in through one of the superior sclerotomy along with the endo-illumination source through the other sclerotomy.

The air is switched on and the vitreous fluid removed by placing the flute needle at air fluid interface (Fig. 6.27). When the eye is phakic or has a biconcave IOL, a high minus contact lens must be used to produce a clear view of the posterior segment during the air fluid exchange.

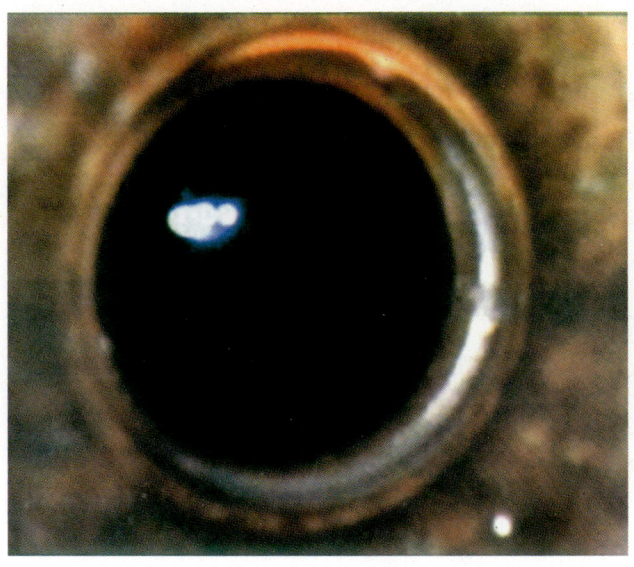

Fig. 6.25 *Contact lens for vitrectomy procedure*

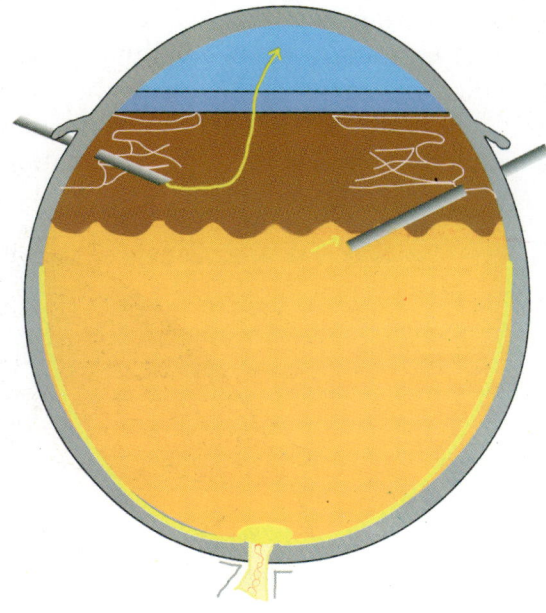

Fig. 6.26 *Air injected into the vitreous while simultaneous drainage of fluid*

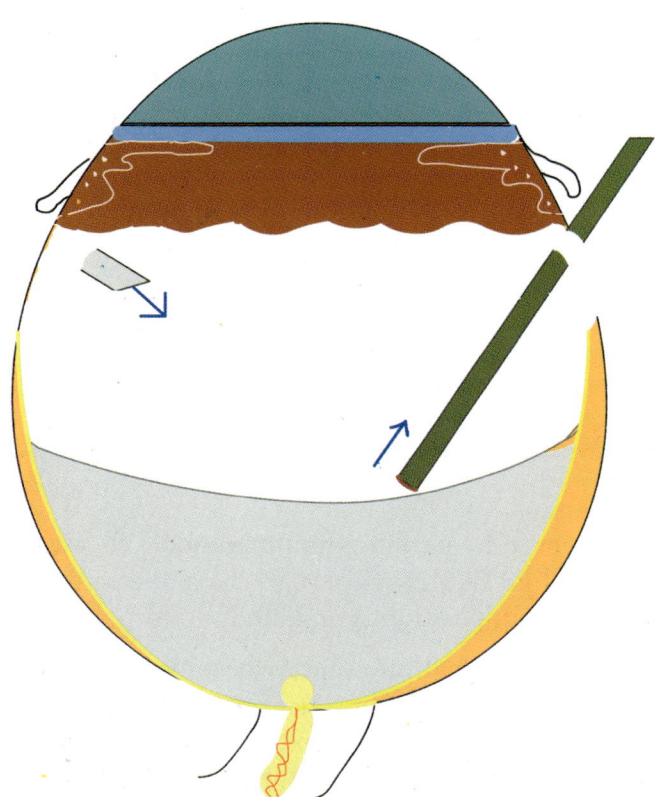

Fig. 6.27 *Fluid is removed by placing the flute needle at air–fluid interface*

In aphakic eyes the retina may be viewed by standard contact lens or no contact lens during the air fluid exchange. At the air-fluid interface the fluid needle is gradually moved down to the deep vitreous cavity and towards the optic disc (Fig. 6.28). The air injection pressure must be sufficient to ensure the easy drainage of intravitreous fluid. Visualization during the procedure is enabled by fibro-optic endo-illumination.

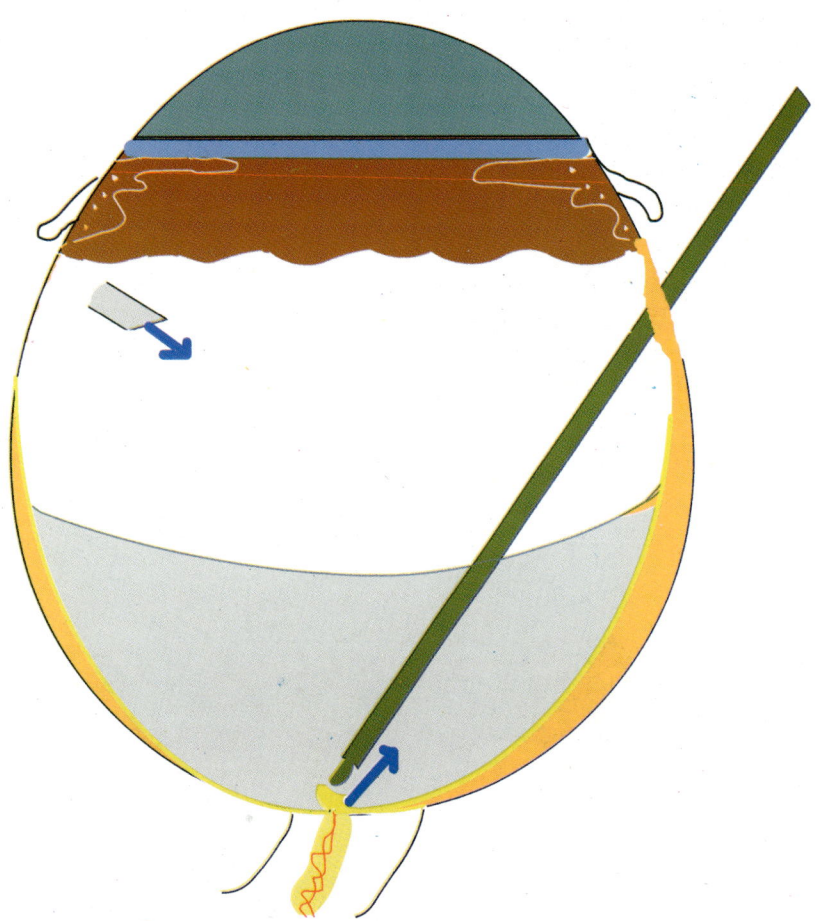

Fig. 6.28 *Flute needle moved down towards the optic disc*

Subretinal fluid is also removed by passing the flute needle through the retinotomy opening into the subretinal space and fluid flows out through the side opening in the back-flush needle handle and the retina falls back in position (Fig 6.29).

If there is a pre-existing retinal break, it s posterior edge is marked with a diathermy spot because it may be difficult to find and treat once the retina is reattached behind the gas-bubble. During the initial part, the flute needle is held next to the break or is placed through the break to drain the subretinal fluid during the initial part of the exchange. A tapered-tip silicone cannula is best for placing through small breaks, to reduce the risk of damage by inadvertently striking the retina or nerve (Fig 6.30).

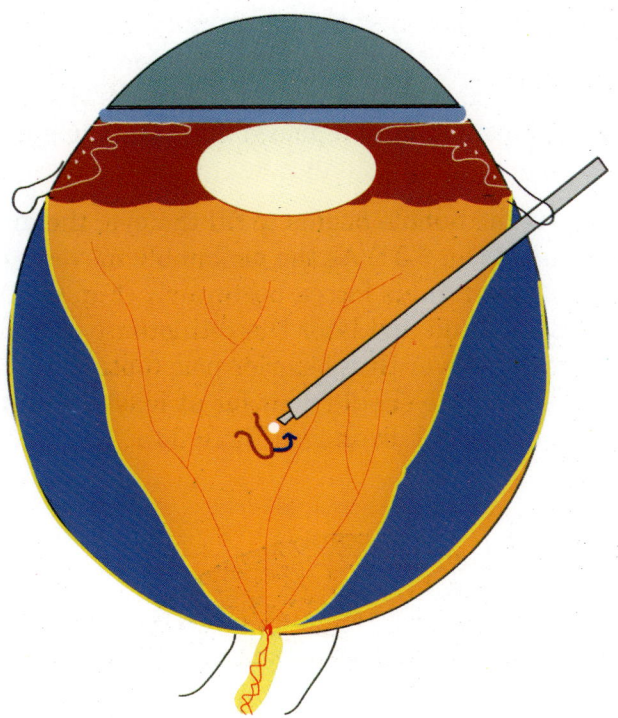

Fig.6.29 *Pre-existing retinal break: posterior edge is marked with diathermy spot*

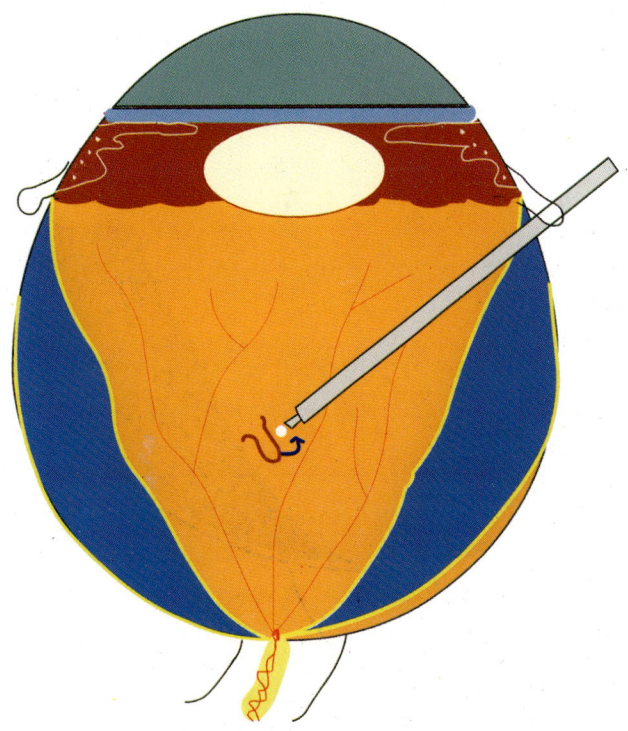

Fig. 6.30 *The flute needle tip is held through the break to drain the sub-retinal fluid*

The retina brought back in apposition with the retina pigment epithelium (RPE) by internally draining the subretinal fluid (SRF) through a retinotomy and replacing the intravitreal fluid air or gases (SF_6 or C_3F_8). In cases with severe proliferative vitreoretinopathy (PVR) and in eyes with giant retina tears, the air is then replaced with silicone oil, which provide long-term tamponade.[5]

During air-fluid exchange as the bubble begins to fill the eye, the anterior retina is flattened against the pigment epithelium. (Fig. 6.31) As the air bubble moves posteriorly, the breaks are closed and any residual subretinal fluid is forced posteriorly (Fig. 6.32). A posterior retinotomy is created to drain the subretinal fluid and later the retinotomy is treated with endolaser. The remaining fluid which accumulates over the posterior pole (optic disc) is drained by placing the silicone tube over the optic nerve. One should wait for at least 15 minutes to allow accumulation of fluid over the optic disc for total drainage (Fig. 6.33).

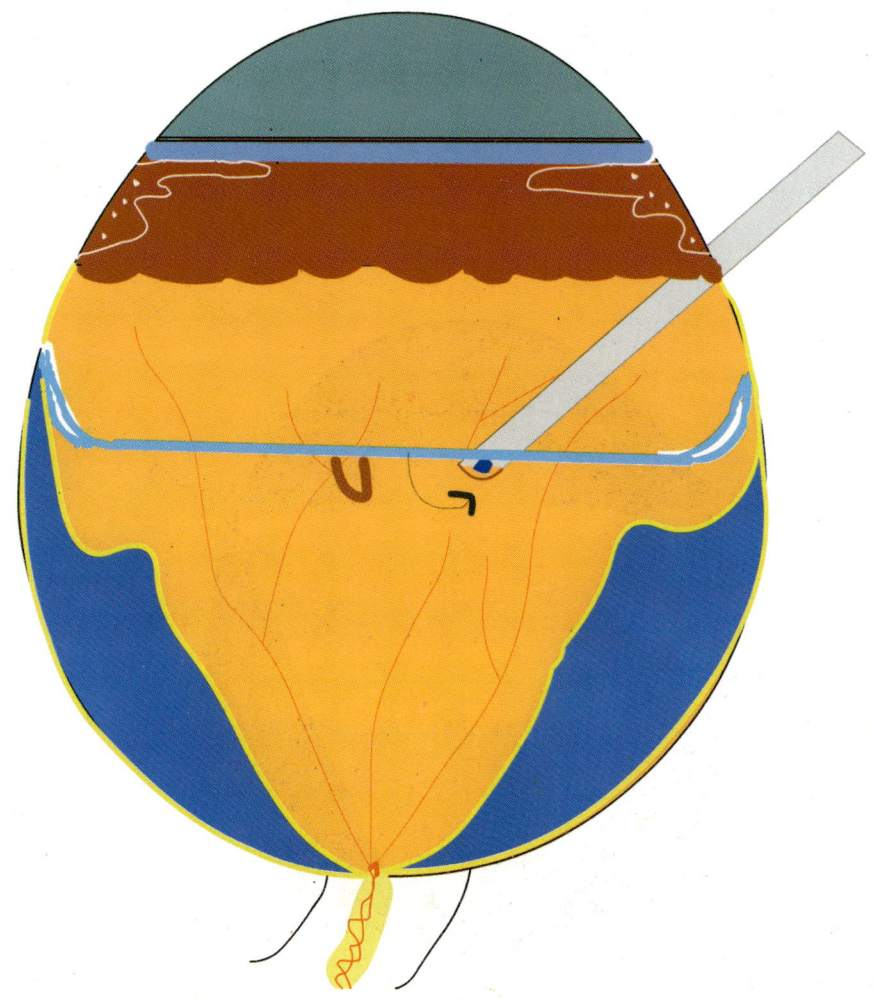

Fig. 6.31 *Anterior retina is flattened against the pigment epithelium*
as the bubbles begin to fill

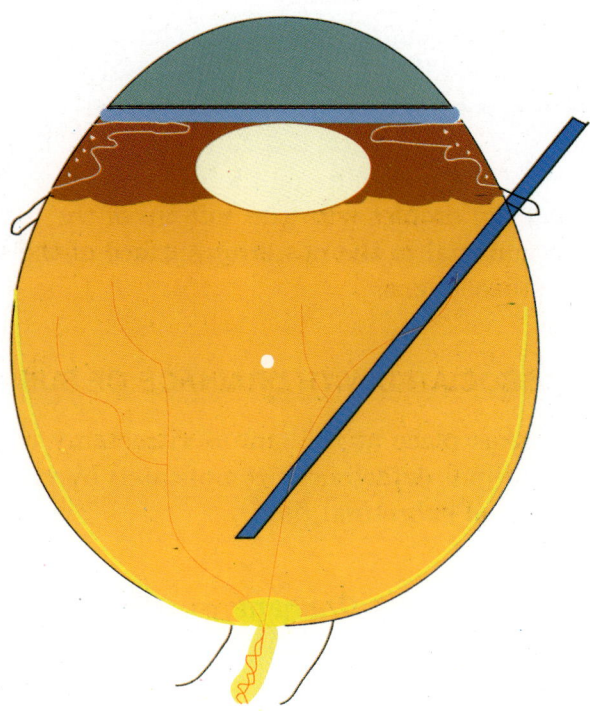

Fig. 6.32 *The break is closed, as the bubble moves posteriorly residual subretinal fluid is forced posteriorly*

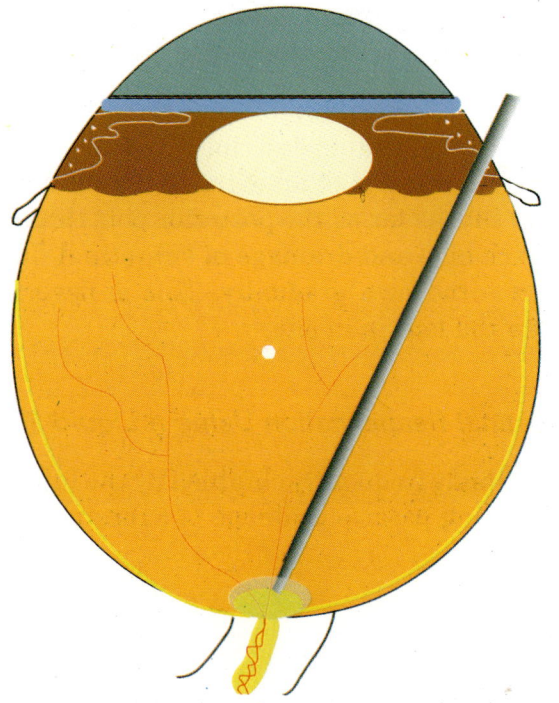

Fig. 6.33 *Remaining fluid drained over the optic nerve head; retina totally settled*

Several problems may arise during the air-fluid exchange. In initial stage the air may form small bubbles (fish eggs) that usually coalesce as the exchange continues. In aphakic eyes there may be irregularities of the posterior cornea, which reduce the visibility, and injecting viscoelastic on the posterior surface of the cornea can restore it. In posterior chamber IOL with open capsule-condensation of the air occurs on the posterior capsule during the exchange and this goes away by stroking the droplet with the soft tip of the cannula. If unsuccessful, then application of viscoelastic material to the posterior surface of the lens is usually helpful. It is difficult to do in case of a silicone lens.

FLUID–AIR EXCHANGE ASSOCIATED WITH DRAINAGE OF SUBRETINAL FLUID

Fluid air exchange often takes place at the end of vitrectomy via the pars plana for retinal detachment, in particular retinal detachment complicated by vitreoretinal proliferation. It is then combined with drainage of subretinal fluid.

Fluid–air Exchange Combined With Drainage of Subretinal Fluid Through a Posterior Dehiscence

This may involve a dehiscence already present (tear of the posterior pole, macular hole) or a drainage retinotomy created deliberately, generally sub-papillary. An endodiathermy probe is useful in creating, without bleeding, a small retinotomy through which complete drainage of subretinal fluid is possible via a tapered end extrusion cannula. Internal drainage must be started sufficiently rapidly to avoid the accumulation at the posterior pole of a large amount of subretinal fluid, which could hamper continuation of the exchange. Retinopexy around the retinotomy is usually performed by endo laser photocoagulation after exchange is complete.

The cannulated subretinal fluid aspirator described by Flynn can be used for simultaneous drainage of subretinal fluid. This consists of an extrusion cannula with a long retractable silicone tip, inserted under the retina as far as the posterior pole through a peripheral dehiscence; it is used for both fluid air exchange and drainage of subretinal fluid. Once the retina is reapplied, the silicone tip is then withdrawn gradually. This is nevertheless a relatively delicate technique, in particular when the lens is in site.

Fluid–air Exchange After Retinal Reapplication Using a Liquid Perfluorocarbon

Retinal reapplication is increasingly frequently obtained by the injection at the end of vitrectomy of a liquid perflurocarbon enabling passive drainage of subretinal fluid via a peripheral dehiscence.

AIR–PFCL EXCHANGE

PFCL–air exchange takes place most often after vitrectomy for retinal detachment, initially reapplied by injection of a liquid perflurocarbon.

LASER PHOTOCOAGULATION

Application of laser photocoagulation is often an essential step in vitrectomy procedure. Laser commonly is delivered through a 20-gauge probe inserted through the standard sclerotomy incision. The intensity and duration of the beam are adjusted to produce a burn of moderate white color. Burns are most predictable and effective when the probe is perpendicular to the retina approximately 2 to 4 mm above its surface. Burns may be placed posteriorly and in the periphery for pan retinal ablation leaves approximately a half burn width between the edges of each burn. Individual retinal breaks may be treated by two or three rows of burns touching each other produce a confluent scar (Fig. 6.34).

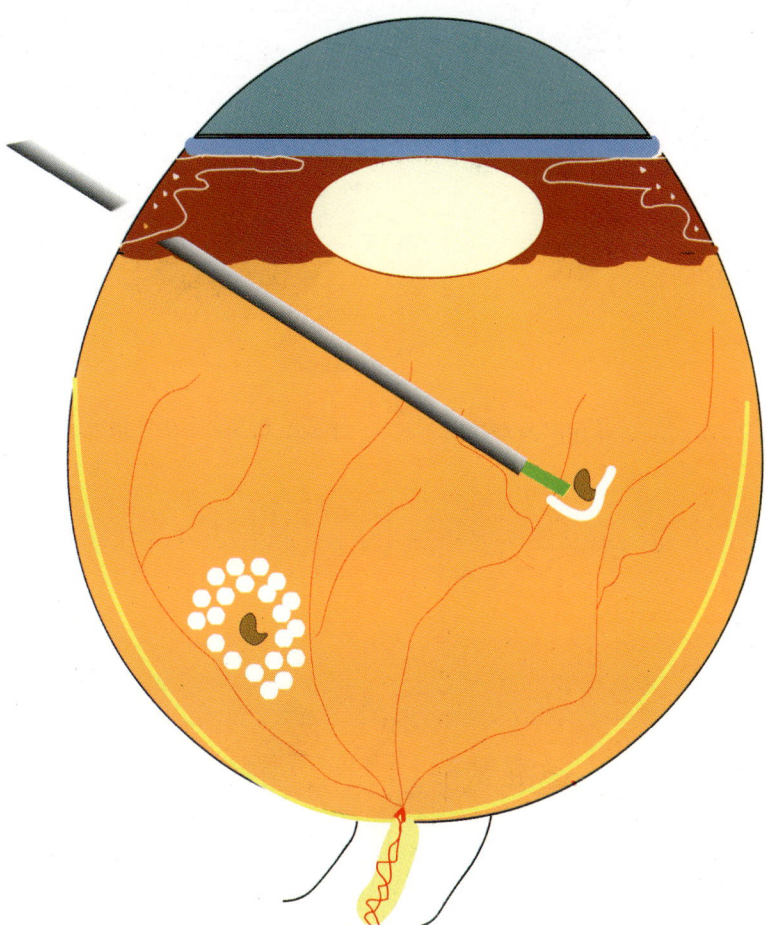

Fig. 6.34 *Application of laser photocoagulation treated by two or three rows of burn around the break*

Treatment on buckle for extensive multiple retinal breaks should be confluent. Peripheral photocoagulation also may be applied by scleral depression or by indirect ophthalmoscope. This allows treatment as far periphery as the ora. Treatment is most effective when the beam is perpendicular to the surface of the retina.

CLOSURE

After the intraocular procedure is completed the individual incisions are closed. The infusion is turned off to avoid extruding vitreous, and one scleral plug is removed (Fig. 6.35). Vitreous is removed from the wound by carefully retracting it a short distance from the sclera and cutting it flush with the scleral surface (Fig. 6.35).

The initial suture bite is taken at one end of the wound using 6.0 vicryl (Fig. 6.36)

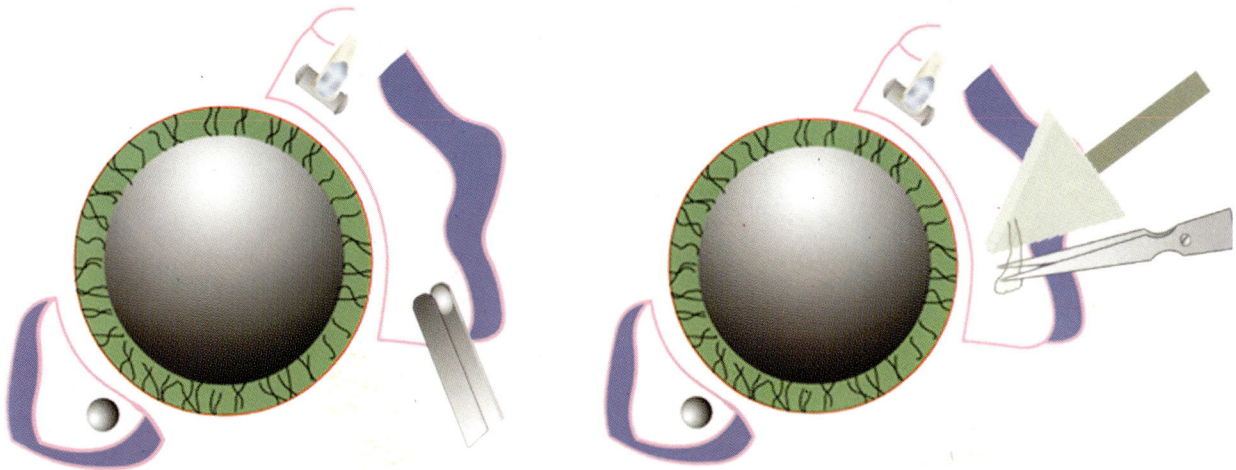

Fig. 6.35 *Infusion turn off and one scleral plug is out*

Fig. 6.36 *Vitreous is removed from scleral wound*

A second bite is taken in the same direction in the opposite end of the wound and the knot is tied to produce a watertight X-closer (Fig. 6.37).

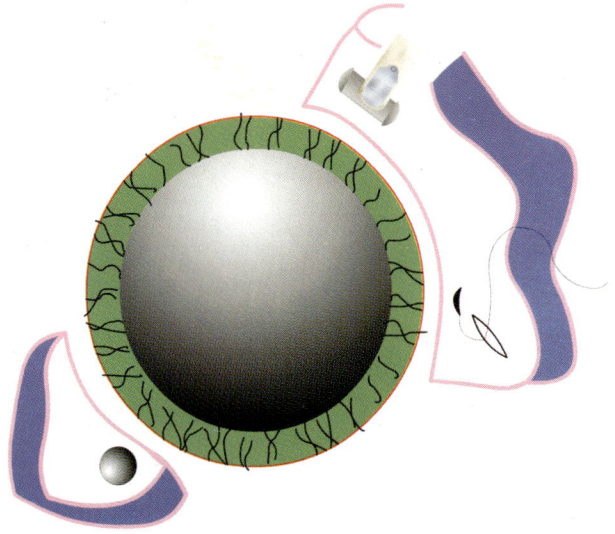

Fig. 6.37 *Initial suture bite at the end of the scleral wound*

The intraocular pressure is brought to normal level by allowing infusion into the eye, and the inferior suture is untied and removed from around the cannula. It is snagged down as the cannula is removed to maintain the intraocular pressure and volume (Fig. 6.38).

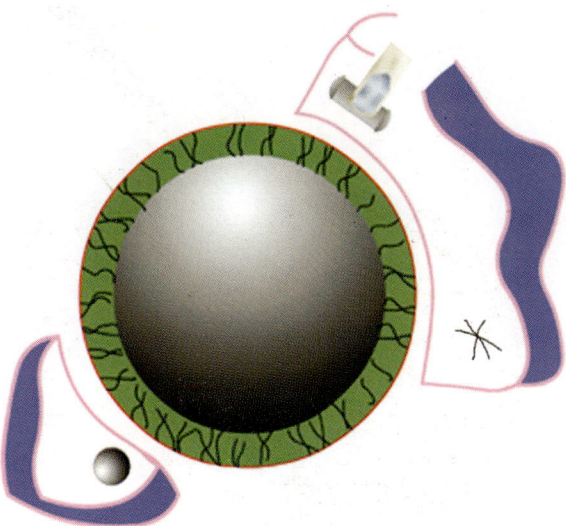

Fig. 6.38 *Second bite is taken in opposite end of the wound knot is tied to produce watertight closure*

If the intraocular pressure is incorrect at the end of the closure, a 27-gauge needle may be inserted carefully through the suture wound. Gas, air or fluid may be injected if the eye is too soft or they may be aspirated if the pressure is too high (Fig. 6.39).

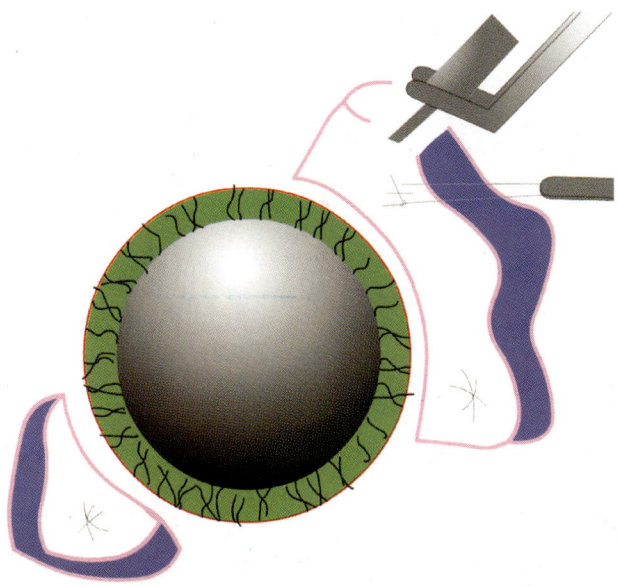

Fig. 6.39 *If the intraocular pressure is low, 27-gauge needle is inserted through the suture wound to inject gas/air/fluid*

Single stitch with 10.0 vicryl at the apex of conjunctiva incisions usually is sufficient for closure (Fig. 6.40).

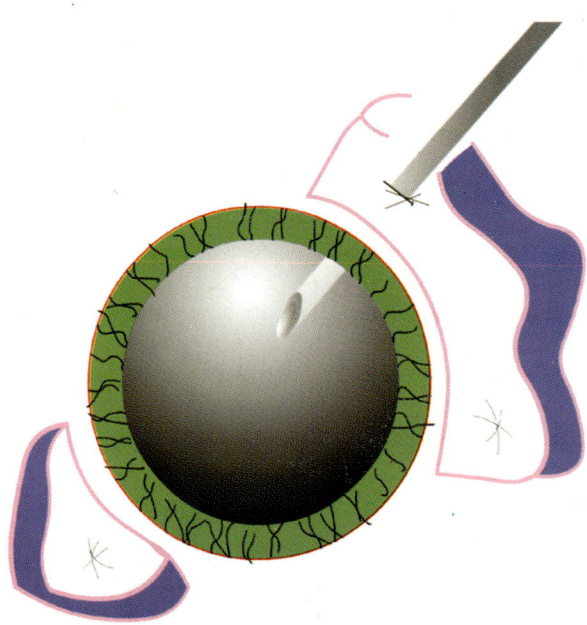

Fig. 6.40 *Closure of conjunctival incision*

REFERENCES

1. Charles S: Principle and technique of vitreous surgery. In Ryan SJ (Ed) *Retina*: Vol. *Surgical Retina*, St Louis, Mosby-Year-Book, 1994.

2. Machemer R, Parel JM, Hickingbotham and D, Nose: Membrane peeler cutter automated vitreous scissors and hooked needle. *Arch Ophthalmol* 99: 152, 1981.

3. MC Cuen Bled, Bessler M, Hickingbotham D, Is bay: Automated fluid gas exchange. *Am J Ophthalmol* 95: 717, 1983.

4. De Juan E JR, Hickingbotham D: Flexible iris retractor. *Am J Ophthalmol* 111: 776, 1991.

5. Glaser BM: Surgery for proliferative vitreoretinopathy. In: Ryan SJ (Ed) *Retina* vol. 3, St Louis, CV Mosby, p 385, 1989.

FURTHER READING

1. Benner JD, Landers MB: Infusion temporary keratoprosthesis for pars plana vitrectomy. *Am J Ophthalmol* 122:579, 1996.

2. Benson W, Blankenship GW, and Machemer: Pars plana lens removal with vitrectomy. *Am J Ophthalmol* 84:150, 1977.

3. Chang S, Lincoff H, Zimmerman NJ et al: Giant retinal tear, Surgical technique and result using perfluorocarbon liquid. *Arch Ophthalmol* 107:761, 1989.

4. Cibispa, Becker B, Okun E, et al: The use of liquid silicone in retinal detachment surgery. *Arch Ophthalmol* 68:590, 1962.

Retained Lens Fragments and Intraocular Lens Dislocation

Introduction

Dropped nucleus into the vitreous is one of the disasters of modern cataract surgery, more so in technique involving phacoemulsification.[1] Maintaining the integrity of the posterior capsule is a must because the incidence of retinal complications is higher when there is posterior capsule disruption.

The disruption of the posterior capsule may occur at any stage of the cataract operation (phacoemulsification), at the beginning, in the mid-stage upon removing the nucleus and in the late stage when aspirating the cortex. Adequate management can provide satisfactory vision.

IDENTIFICATION OF RISK FACTORS

A tear in the posterior capsule is most frequent for surgeon who are beginning in the process of transition of phacoemulsification or who are doing their first cases. It mostly occurs during finishing the phase of aspiration of the residual cortex. The tear is usually located at 12° clock or nearby location. There are some situations where there is high risk of posterior capsule tear, some of which are important.

1. Patients with history of trauma who may have zonular dialysis.

2. Patients with pseudoexfoliation.

3. Hard cataracts with large nuclei.

4. Patients with large axial length.

5. Posterior subcapsular cataracts.

TIME OF REMOVAL OF RETAINED LENS FRAGMENTS AND DISLOCATED LENS

Immediate pars plana vitrectomy offers no visual advantage over delayed vitrectomy in patients with dislocated nucleus.[2] As a matter of fact; some times it is necessary to wait for intraocular pressure to be controlled and for the corneal oedema to resolve. It is now known that the timing of vitrectomy does not have a statistically significant impact on visual outcome. Neither the type of intraocular lens nor the timing of lens implantation significantly altered the final visual acuity in these patients. Most eyes with retained lens fragments do well after vitrectomy[2], with the majority recovering good vision. However, the risk of retinal detachment is increased and visual outcome may be adversely affected if retinal detachment occurs.

EMPHASIZED DURING CATARACT SURGERY

The surgeon must avoid aspirating (without cutting) any presenting vitreous gel. Attempts to retrieve any lens fragments that have started to dislocate posteriorly should be made only with vitrectomy hand-piece. The use of lens loops, forceps, and other instruments that have the potential to engage and pull on vitreous gel should not be used. A complete limbal vitrectomy should be performed before any lens placement and the absence of vitreous to the wound or other anterior structures should be confirmed at the time of wound closure. Last, indirect ophthalmoscopy with scleral depression should be performed at the end of the procedure to identify any retinal tear because these may require at least laser or cryo retinopexy.

LOSS OF LENS FRAGMENTS INTO THE VITREOUS

Whatever may be the regions, once the posterior capsule ruptures during cataract surgery particularly phacoemulsification technique, loss of lens fragments into the vitreous are very common. Posterior dislocation of intraocular lens do occur in day-to-day practice.[4] The vitreous surgeon commonly faces multiple pieces of lens sizes at the vitreous which are trapped inferiorly and are lying on the retina surface (Fig.7.1).

During core-vitrectomy, many of the lens-pieces may be engaged and removed by the help of the cutting probe; the cortical fragments can be removed easily, as they are soft in nature (Fig.7.2).

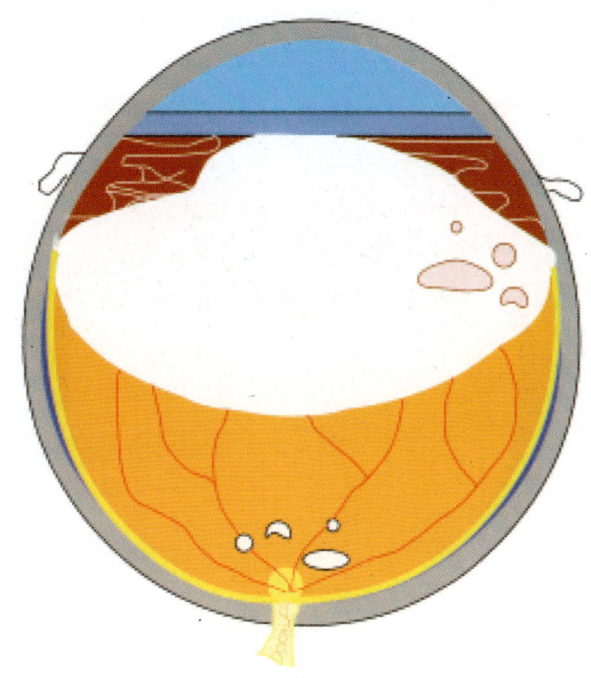

Fig. 7.1 *Multiple pieces of lens fragment of various sizes*

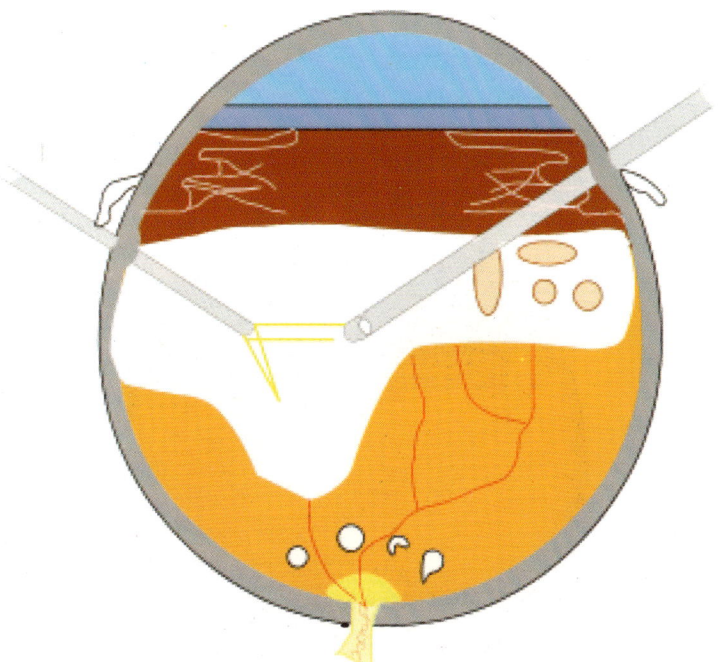

Fig. 7.2 *Core-vitrectomy with removal of cortical fragments*

Hard nuclear fragment may require intravitreal emulsification when lens fragments adhere to the back of the iris or intraocular lens, it should be removed.

By scleral depression with the help of cotton-tipped swab, it is often useful to remove lens material lodged in and around vitreous base (Fig.7.3).

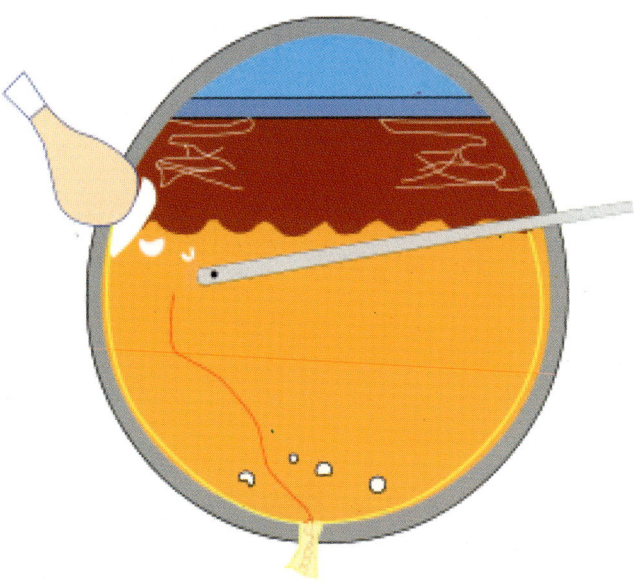

Fig. 7.3 *Depression of vitreous base by cotton-tipped swab to remove lens fragment from periphery*

Sometimes it is necessary to lift the lens fragment into the mid vitreous where they are fragmented with low pressure and simultaneous suction. To protect the underlying retina, perflurocarbon liquid may be injected posterior to the lens fragments, or lens nucleus to allow floating on its surface (Fig.7.4).

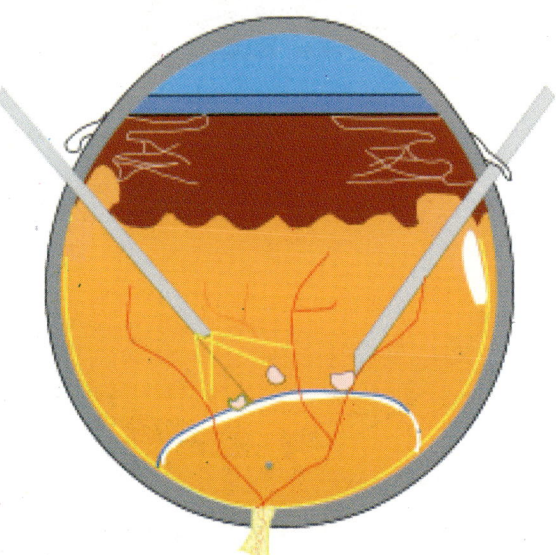

Fig. 7.4 *Fragments are allowed to float over PFCL and are removed by cutter — more helpful when associated with RD*

Use of perfluorocarbon (PFCL) is helpful whenever there is a retinal detachment because perfluorocarbon stabilize the retinal position during removal of lens fragment or dislocated intraocular lens (IOL).[3] During injection of perfluorocarbon, there is a great tendency of lens fragments to go behind the bubble. For that region, small amount of perfluorocarbon should be injected. When large bubble is injected, the anterior surface of perfluorocarbon bubble becomes convex and fragment tends to slide posteriorly thereby visibility becomes poor and difficult.

Residual hard nuclear fragments are seldom stabilized by the help of light source in one hand and the vitrectomy probe should be activated to remove the fragments by aspirating them into the cutting probe (Fig.7.5).

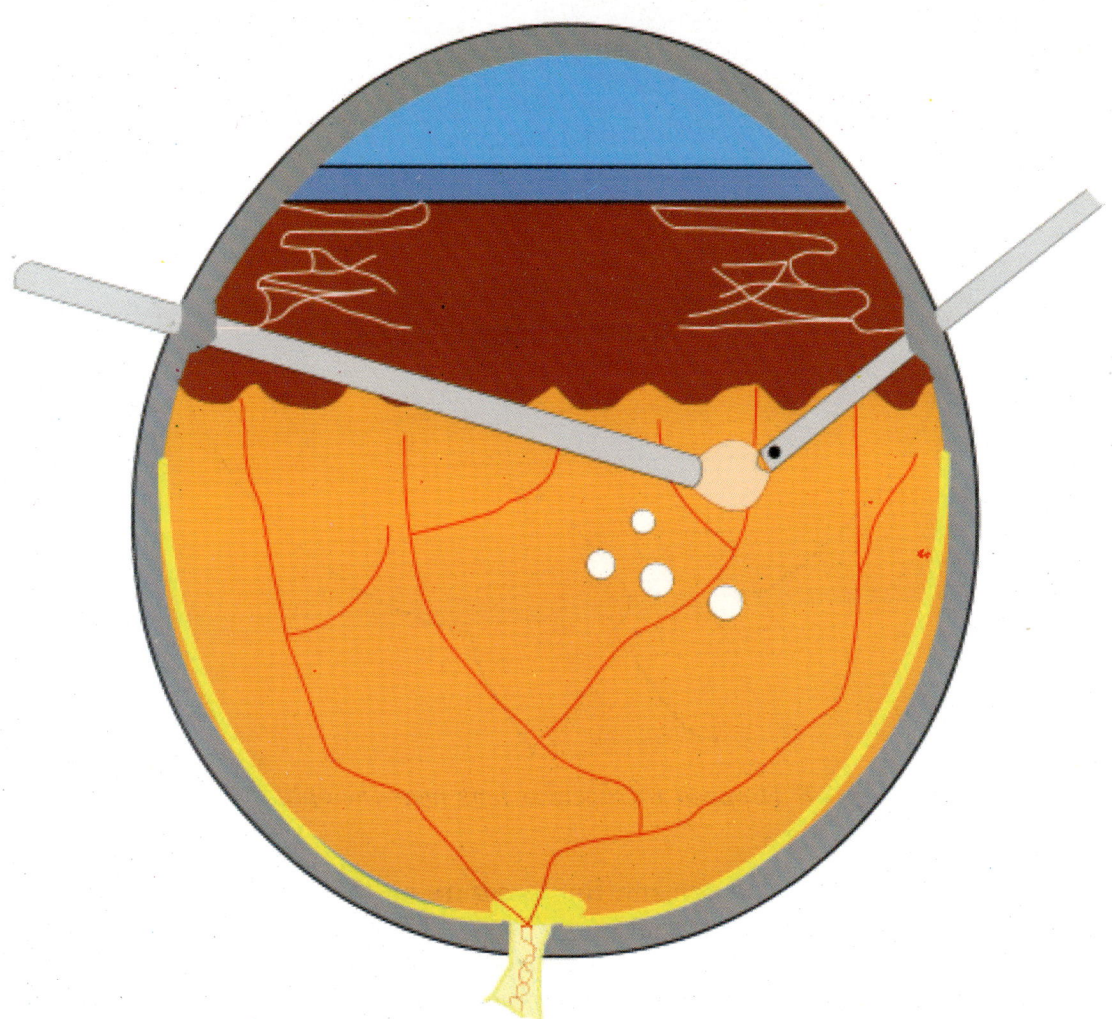

Fig. 7. 5 *Hard nucleus fragments stabilize against light pipe and are removed by vitrectomy probe*

Whenever entire lens is dislocated into the posterior segment, the entire vitreous should be removed to avoid traction on the retina in subsequent maneuvers (Fig 7.6).

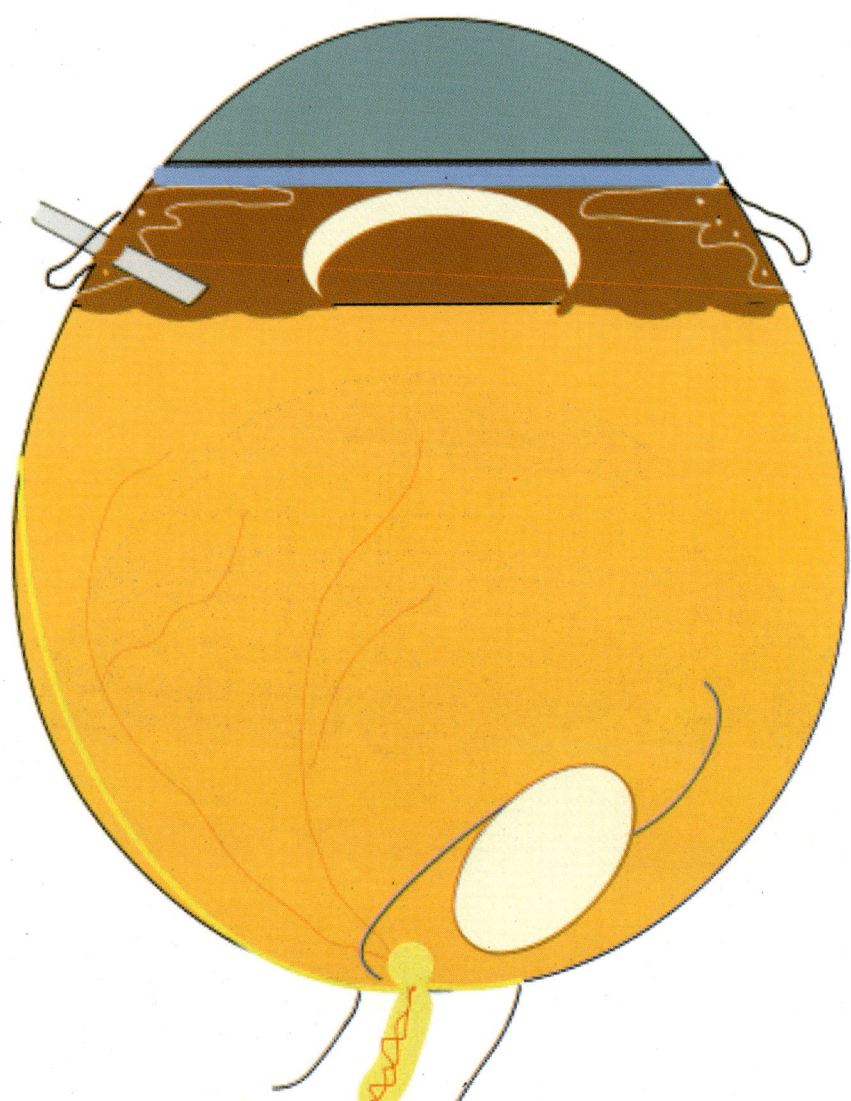

Fig. 7.6 *Dropped intraocular lens near the optic disc.*

As there is always fear of the transmitting pressure on the retina, the lens must not be fragmented on the retinal surface. It is always wise to lift the lens nucleus with the help of 20-gauge cryoprobe through the sclerotomy and lift to the pupillary area. The lens should be fixed near the equator with the help of ice-ball and removed by vitrectomy probe or fragmentation hand-piece. Direct illumination from the microscope provides adequate light. In case small pieces of nuclear fragments fall inside the vitreous cavity, these can be removed with the help of suction and fragmentation probe.

Intraocular lens may be dislocated into the vitreous cavity, either during or after the surgery.

The management of dislocated intraocular lens comprises its removal and replacement by an anterior chamber or posterior chamber lens. Consideration should be given to remove when there is inadequate capsular support. If the lens is an incorrect size or has been damaged or silicone oil infusion anticipated, adequate planning is necessary for reposition of intraocular lens. Initially a complete vitrectomy is performed. The haptic of the lens frequently is caught in the vitreous base and must be carefully dissected free so adequate planning, like complete vitrectomy, lens mobilization and lens fixation are necessary for successful out come.[4] After lens mobilization, it can be fixed in the sulcus without suturing or to suture it into position. The procedure is undergone in three steps initially complete vitrectomy, lens mobilization and lens fixation, all these steps should be planned properly for successful outcome.

The posterior dislocated intraocular lens must be mobilizing carefully to avoid damage to the underlying retina. The light source may be used to elevate the lens initially and grasped with forceps in the central vitreous cavity. The optic or haptic can be grasped with serrated-forceps. Adequate care should be given while grasping the haptic because it may be broken in some cases. It is always available to grasp the optic while removal of intraocular lens. Whenever there is coexisting retinal detachment (RD), perfluorocarbon (PFCL) is always injected to lift the intraocular lens and also stabilize the retina posteriorly.[5] Wide angle viewing system and good pupillary dilation are often useful to observe the position of the lens while it is being elevated. The intraocular lens may be removed through limbal route by retracting iris. Whenever there is sufficient capsular support, the intraocular lens may be deposited easily.

Although multiple suturing techniques have been described, a few important points should be taken into consideration.

   a. Transclera technique is preferable to iris suturing.

   b. Suturing the haptic to the internal sclera is usually preferable rather suturing through position holes.

   c. Knob should bury beneath a scleral flap to reduce transconjunctival erosion and inflammation.

   d. Prolene suture are preferred because permanent suture fixation probably will be necessary.

   e. In most techniques, limbal-based 2 to 3 mm wide scleral flaps are created. When two sutures are planned, area should be selected just above and below 3 and 9 O'clock position to avoid the long posterior ciliary vessels.

REFERENCES

1. Kim JE et al: Retained lens fragments after phacoemulsification. *Ophthalmology* 101: 1827, 1994.
2. Borne MM et al: Outcomes of vitrectomy for retained lens fragments. *Ophthalmology* 103: 971, 1996.
3. Lewis H, Blumem Kranz M.S., Charug S: Treatment of dislocated crystalline lens and retinal detachments with perfluorocarbon liquids. *Retina* 12: 299, 1992.
4. Lewis H, Sanchez G: The use of perfluorocarbon in the repositioning of posterior dislocated intraocular lenses. *Ophthalmology* 100: 1055, 1993.
5. Chan CK: An improved technique for management of dislocated posterior chamber implants. *Ophthalmology* 99: 51, 1992.

Surgical Treatment of Macular Surface Disorder

MACULAR HOLE

Introduction

Modern vitreoretinal surgery is now one of the most effective tools for treating macular diseases. Recent advances in the pathogenesis, classification and surgical intervention have generated a renewed interest in macular hole, macular pucker and subretinal neovascularisation entity. Better indicators of visual outcome as well as refinements in the surgical technique have led to greater success of macular surgery.[1]

It is now recognized that most cases retina hole occurs in the absence of antecedent injury and is referred to as idiopathic. Gass[2] and Junction[3] proposed a theory where by shrinkage of adherent cortical vitreous and subsequent tangential vitreous traction first causes a circumscribed foveolar detachment (stage 1) followed by early retinal dehiscence (stage 2), then enlargement of macular hole with vitreofoveal separation (stage 3) and finally complete posterior vitreous detachment (stage 4).

Proliferation of fibrous astrocytes and Mueller cells[4] occurs with the formation of a macular hole.

Clinical features

Idiopathic macular holes occur most frequently in women in sixth decades of life. Table 8.1 summarizes the biomicroscopic finding of various stages of macular hole. According to Gass[5] (stage 1A and stage 1B) lesion represent focal foveal detachments secondary to vitreous traction (Table 8.1).

Table 8.1 Biomicroscopic classification of idiopathic macular holes		
Stage	**Biomicroscopic findings**	**Anatomic interpretation**
1-A. (Impending Hole)	Central yellow spot Loss of foveolar depression No vitreo foveolar separation	Early serous detachment of foveolar retina
1-B. (Impending or Occult hole)	Yellow ring with bridging interface Loss of foveolar depression No vitreo foveolar separation	Some for small ring. For larger ring, central occult foveolar hole with centrifugal displacement of foveolar retina and xanthophylls, with bridging Contracted prefoveolar vitreous cortex. Cannot detect transition from impending to occult hole.
2.	Eccentric oval, crescent, or horseshoe Retinal defect inside edge of edge of yellow ring	Hole (tear) in contracted prefoveolar vitreous bridging round retinal hole, no loss of foveolar retina.
	Central round retinal defect with rim of elevated retina with prefoveolar opacity	Hole with pseudo-operculum, detachment
	Without prefoveolar opacity	Hole, no posterior vitreous detachment from optic disc and macula
3.	Central round >400 mm diameter retinal defect, no Weiss' ring, rim of elevated retina with prefoveolar opacity	Hole with pseudo-operculum, no posterior vitreous detachment
	Without prefoveolar opacity	Hole, no posterior vitreous detachment from optic disc and macula
4.	Central round retinal defect rim of elevation Weiss' ring with prefoveolar opacity	Hole with pseudo-operculum, and posterior vitreous detachment from optic disc and macula
	Hole prefoveolar opacity	Hole and posterior vitreous detachment from optic disc and macula
Source: Modified From Gass[5]		

A 100–200 mm diameter yellow spot is the earliest changes observed with progression striate are often seen surrounding the yellow ring within several weeks to months, a full thickness dehiscence develops. This dehiscence often starts eccentrically, then opens in a "can opener" fashion to form a crescent retinal defect, which becomes a horseshoe-shaped hole and finally a round hole with an operculum. In some cases, the dehiscence starts centrally, with gradual enlargement of the hole and no operculum develops. A ring of detachment usually surrounds the hole.

As the hole enlarges, vision usually decreases and within several months it progress to a fully developed hole that measures approximately 500 mm in diameter when present, the operculum is suspended over the hole by the vitreous cortex with time, the flowing changes may be observed: round yellow deposits, on the central retinal pigment epithelium, epiretinal membranes causing contracture of the internal limiting membrane; depigmentation of the pigment epithelium under the cuff of elevation, and a pigmentary demarcation ring defining the outer margin of the retinal detachment. Posterior vitreous separation from the macula and disc develops in a small percentage of cases. Eyes with idiopathic macular hole occurs loss vision secondary to tissue loss, cystic changes retinal cuff elevation with photoreceptor degeneration. Clinical observations have led to the impression that macular hole and cuff enlarge secondary to persistent tangential traction from the vitreous, tangential traction from the epiretinal membranes, and the development of large cystic spaces within the surrounding cuff.

Diagnosis

A full thickness macular hole is the most accurately diagnosed clinically using a fundus contact lens and slit lamp biomicroscopy. Supplement tests that may assist in or allow for more accurate diagnosis include Amsler Grid testing, testing for Watzke–Allen sign, and fluorescein angiography.

The Watzke Allen test and to a greater degree the laser aiming beam test is that they are simple to perform, can be done in the clinic and easily accessible.[6]

Watzke Allen sign testing in all patients with clinically defined macular holes can show a break or thinning of the slit beam optical coherence tomography has been found to be effective in distinguishing full thickness macular holes from partial thickness holes, macular holes, and cysts.[7]

The cross-sectional view provided is an alternative to clinch pathologic corelation and allow lesions to be traced longitudinally over time. The micro scale resolution is useful for quantitatively assessing hole diameter and the amount of retinal thickening and oedema surrounding a hole allowing sensitive monitoring of hole progression or recovery after treatment.

MACULAR HOLE SURGERY

Full thickness idiopathic macular hole is an important cause of central visual loss. It is now established that macular hole formation begins with the degeneration of the inner retina at the muller cell, cone-vitreous cortex interface. The macular hole enlarges due to the contraction of the internal limiting membrane (ILM), then by muller (glial) cell migrate on to the internal limiting membrane. Women suffers approximately 67% more with macular hole or impending holes in compare to male.[1] Most of the macular hole patient presents with poor visual acuity. Removal of internal limiting membrane is a useful surgical approach to close an idiopathic macular hole. Removal of internal limiting membrane is some time difficult but when it stains with indocyanine green removal of internal limiting membrane is easier and it facilitate to close the macular hole. Now, it is known that surgical intervention for stage 2 (Johnson and Gass classification) macular holes leads to significantly better vision at 6 months after surgery in comparison to natural history.[2] The aim of the surgery to eliminate of the anterior–posterior and tangential traction that initially creates and later maintains the hole.

When to Perform Surgery in Macular Hole

Whether timely surgery on a stage 1st hole will prevent development of a full thickness hole has not yet been determined. If a macular hole is beginning to develop, surgery may be pre-mature at this point.

Early signals of age related macular degeneration mimic some of cases with macular hole. Therefore careful ophthalmoscopy is necessary to establish a definite diagnosis. Goldman lens with binocular slit-lamp, the eye surgeon can usually differentiate the conditions. If doubts about the diagnosis remain, a fluorescein angiogram can distinguish among various condition that present with these same symptoms: cystoids macular oedema, subretinal neovascularisation, Central Serous Retinopathy (CSR) that some time occurs late, retinal pigment epithelium (RPE) detachment, and macular hole formation.

If macular hole has formed only a small amount of fluorescein is visible in the center of fovea.

The slit beam sign is also a helpful diagnostic tool. A slit beam is projected through the goldmann lens precisely on the fovea and the patient is asked to draw what he or she sees. To a person developing a macular hole, the edges of the beam will not seem parallel, and they may appear to bend. If the patient has a complete macular hole, he/she may see and draw an interruption in the line.

To perform macular surgery if the hole increase from stage 1st to stage 2nd or greater. Early intervention can provide measurable visual improvement in more than 2/3 of the eyes.

Surgical Technique

Standard three-port pars plana vitrectomy procedure is usually done. Complete posterior cortical vitrectomy is followed by careful identification, engagement, elevation and removal of the posterior cortical vitreous layers. Surgical removal of cone-vitreous is done followed by detachment of the hyaloid membrane. It should be removed by active suction near or above the optic disc with the help of a flexible silicone cannula (Fig. 8.1).

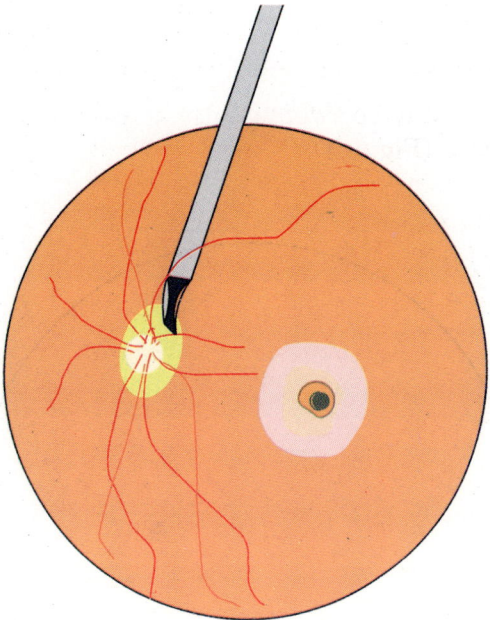

Fig. 8.1 *Active suction above the optic disc hyaloids face is visible*

Engagement of vitreous is difficult to see because the vitreous is clear when the vitreous is engaged the silicone tip s bands giving the "fish strike sign" like a fishing rod being bent. As the hyaloids is elevated, the circle of previous attachments over the disc becomes visible. The hyaloid face itself has variable visibility from one eye to another. The hyaloids should be stripped free from the macula surface and as far beyond the vascular arcades towards the equator as possible. Hyaloid removal within the arcade is most critical (Fig. 8.2).

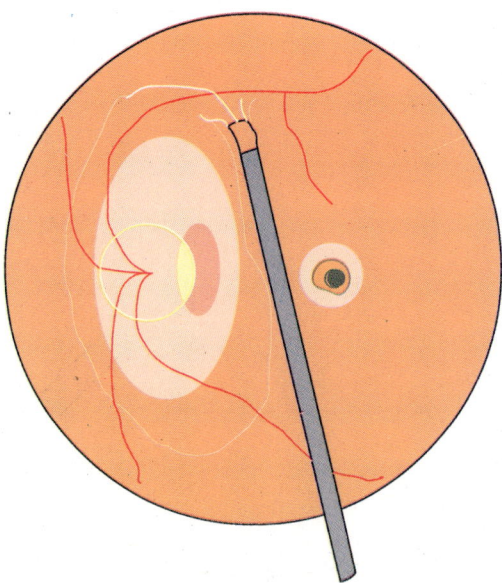

Fig. 8.2 *Removal of hyaloid within the arcade*

After removal of the posterior hyaloid, one can explore edge of the hole with a band microvitreoretinal blade, searching for gossamer invisible membrane (Fig. 8.3).

A diamond dusted probe also may be swept gently across the retinal surface to engage invisible tissue on the retinal surface (Fig. 8.4).

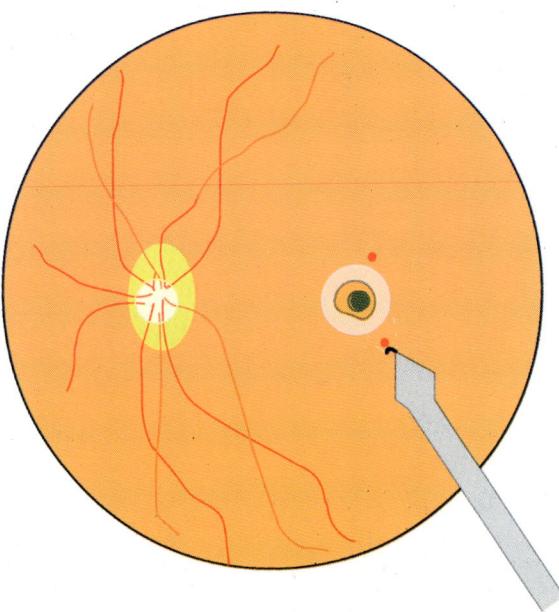

Fig. 8.3 *Explore the edge of the hole with micro vitreoretinal blade*

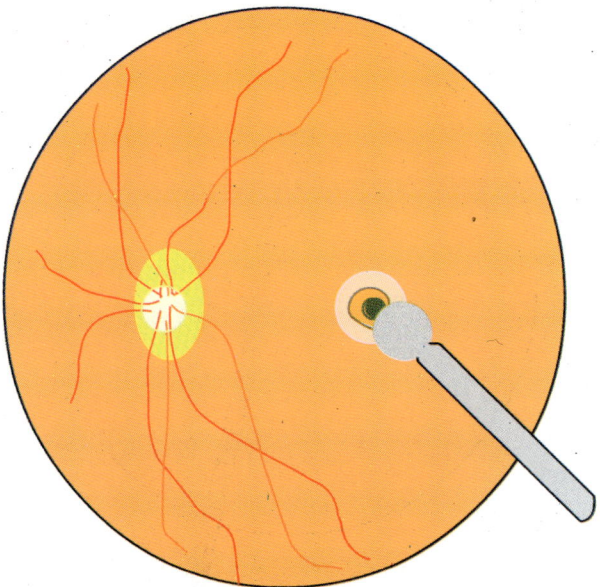

Fig. 8.4 *Diamond-dusted probe engages invisible tissue on the retinal surface*

Removal of the internal limiting membrane is incised with a straight or a bent tip of the micro-vitreoretinal blade approximately one mm from the fovea center. The edge of the internal limiting membrane is elevated and removed and blocked when possible using blade or grasping the internal limiting membrane with fine forceps .The edge of the hole also may be suctioned gently to look for residual vitreous, but care should be taken not to aspirate the edge of the hole (Fig. 8.5).

An air fluid exchange followed by long-acting gas completes the procedure (Fig. 8.6).

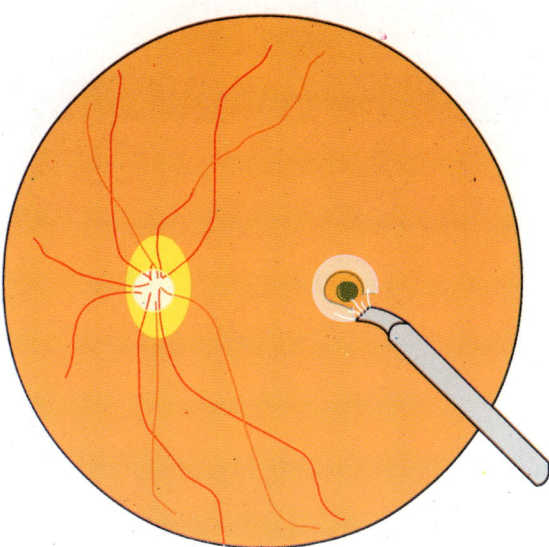

Fig. 8.5 *Edge of the hole suction to look for residual vitreous .*

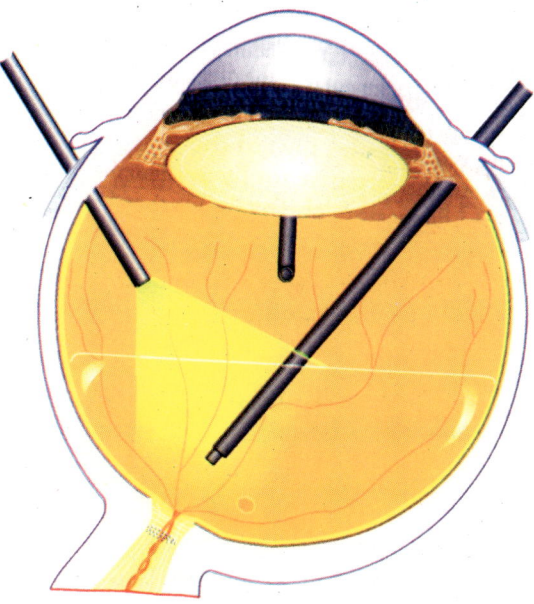

Fig. 8.6 *Long-acting gas completes the procedure*

Removal of ILM

Internal limiting membrane (ILM) can be visible by staining sterile 0.5% 1CG (approximately 0.1 ml of 5 mg per ml of distilled water) has to be squirted over the macular area. The vitrectomy ports were temporarily plugged with scleral plug for about 2–3 minutes. The vitreous cavity once the media clarity improves; one should proceed to remove the ILM.

An optical starting point for internal limiting membrane (ILM) peel is chosen around approximately 4-degree clock within the arcade vessels but away from the fovea. The site is usually chosen to lie outside the maculopapillae bundle (Fig. 8.7).

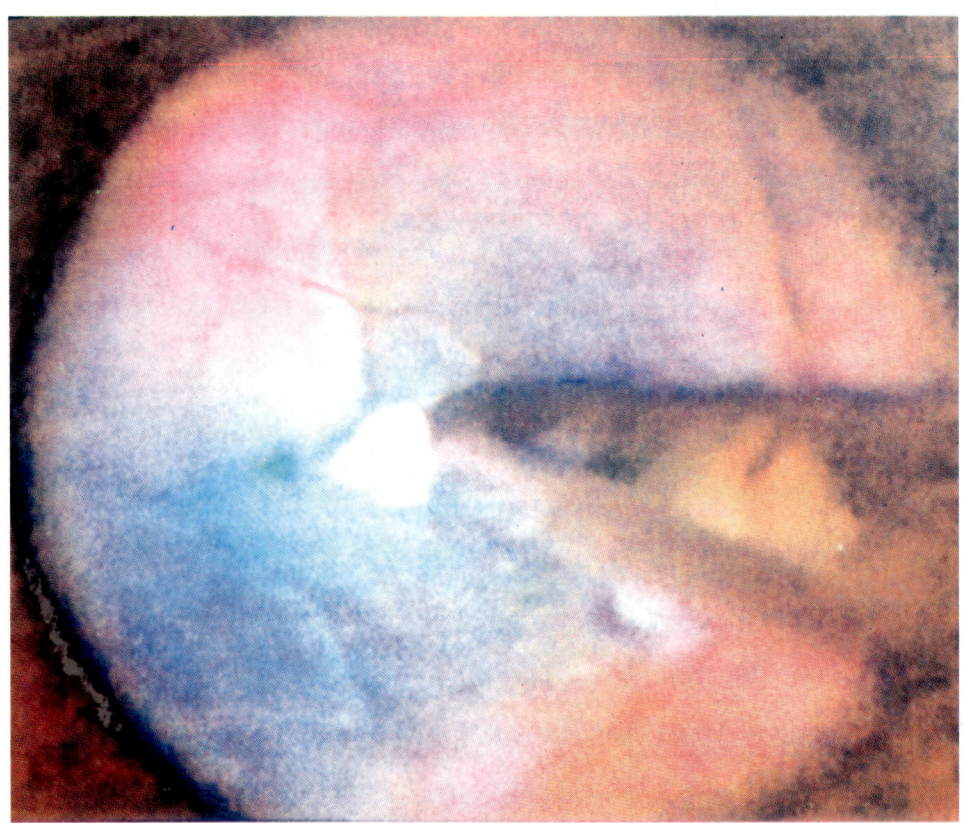

Fig. 8.7 *Intraoperative view showing ICG stain raised ILM flap held by end-opening forceps*

Lifting of internal limiting membrane (ILM) is easier with diamond dusted membrane scraper. Once the edge is elevated, it can be grasped with end opening forceps (DORC) and the tearing of edge is done in a circular motion like the capsulorhexis is done in cataract surgery. The internal limiting membrane when stained with ICG the staining of the internal limiting membrane (ILM) is easy and can be done as a single piece but at times, tearing become incomplete, the ILM is simply re-grasped at the new edge and the rhexis is resumed. It the fovea is noted to be undertaken little traction during this procedure, the peeling fovea traction is resolved and the tearing may be continued in a similar fashion.

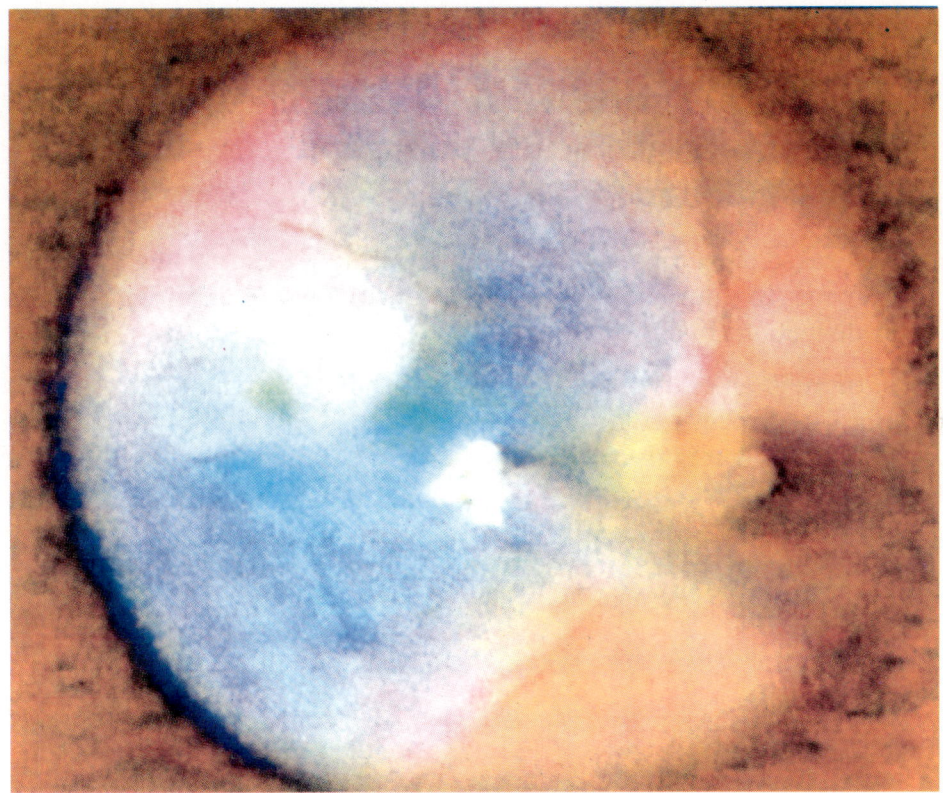

Fig. 8.8 *Internal limiting membrane peel over the fovea*

The most important thing one should be kept under constant observation of the hole while working close to fovea (Fig. 8.8).

The peeling of the internal limiting membrane should be around 2-disc diameter. The small circle of ILM (operculum) if still remaining over the foveola, is not periphery of the retina is examined preferable by wide angle viewing system with scleral depression.

The vitreous cavity is filled with C_3F_8 gas and the sclerotomies are closer with 6.0-vicryl suture. The patients are advised to follow prone position for one to two weeks at least twelve to sixteen hours per day. Constant observation of intraocular pressure is mandatory; the removal of ILM may remove tangential traction from the macular hole and thus aid its closure with this procedure. Visual and anatomic success improves in all stages of recent and chronic macular holes.

Since the natural history of macular hole is poor, and spontaneous closure of the hole occurs in only 5% of cases.

Surgery is important and the visual outcome improves if internal limiting membrane peeling is performed along with posterior cortical vitrectomy and long-term intraocular gas tamponade. The surgery itself contributes only partly to the success. The postoperative position following surgery is absolutely necessary in prone position for two weeks, which provides the best chance for long-term macular hole closure with improved vision.

The gas bubble floats to the back of the eye and maintains gentle pressure over the macular hole, thus keeps the hole completely closed and also encourages new tissue to grow across the hole, providing a permanent seal. The prognosis of the macular hole surgery depends upon the size of the hole as well as post-operative position of the patients following surgery.

MACULAR PUCKER (MACULAR DISTORTION)

Macular pucker is caused most commonly by the membrane on the surface of the retina without attachment of vitreous. In vitreomacular traction, characterized by direct traction on macula creating macular distortion (Fig. 8.9).

In some cases, there is an easily identified edge of the membrane that can be engaged with membrane pick forceps. Force is gently exerted both anteriorly and in the direction of the surgeon watching the attachment of the membrane to the retina carefully as the membrane cleaves the retina (Fig. 8.10).

When there is no visible edge, the tip of the MVR blade can be used initially to engage the membrane (Fig. 8.11).

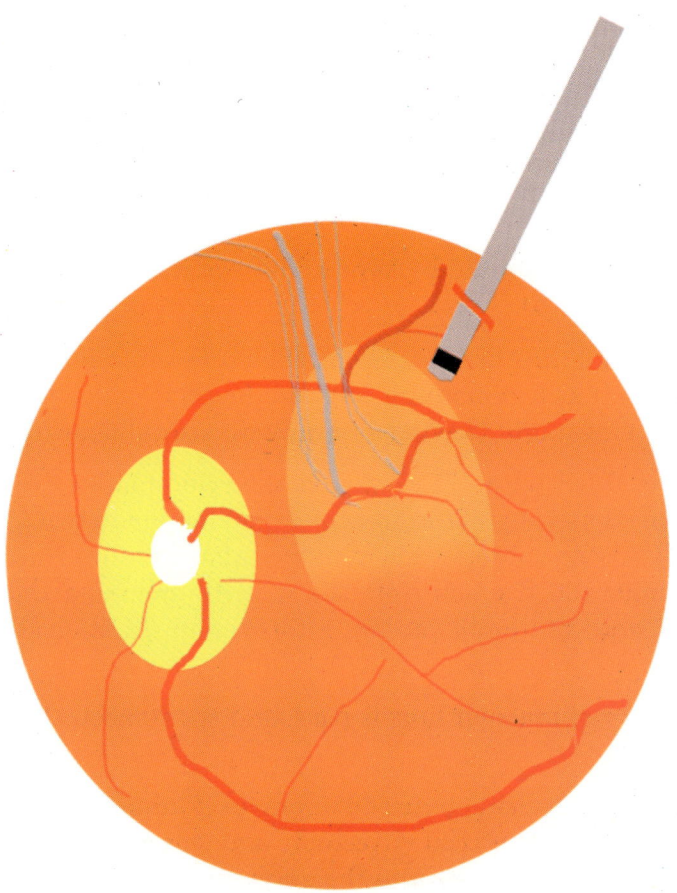

Fig. 8.9 *Macular pucker causing distortion of the macula*

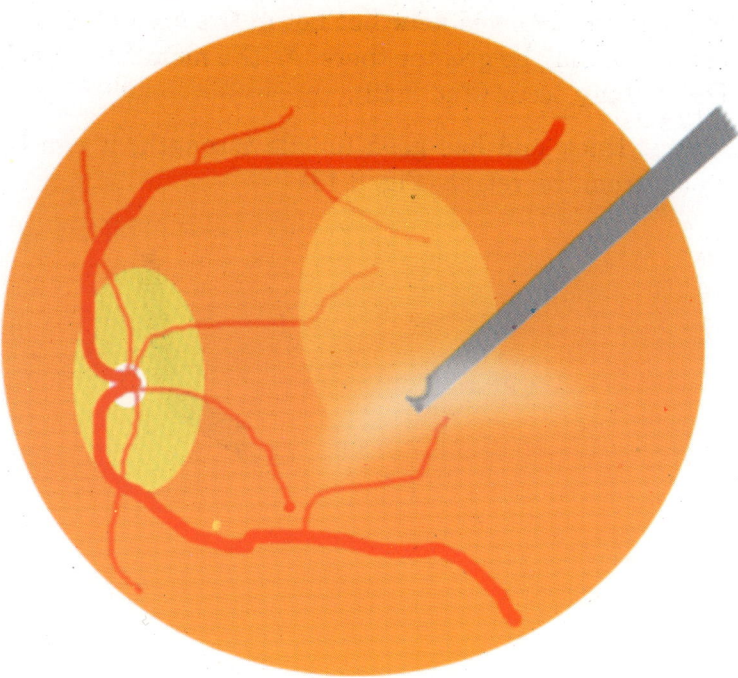

Fig. 8.10 *Membrane identified by membrane picks*

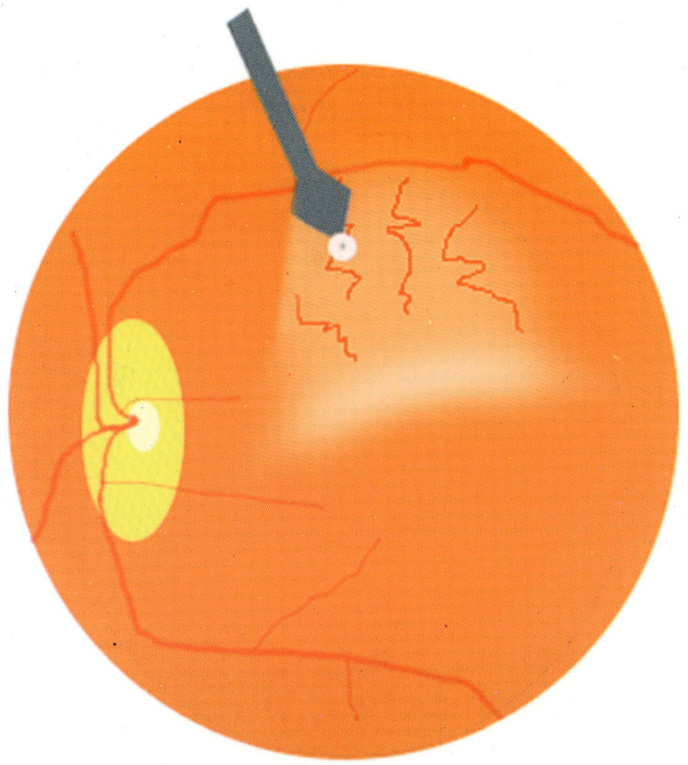

Fig. 8.11 *Microvitreoretinal blade is used to engaged the membrane away from the macula*

A site is selected away from the fovea near but not in the area of maximal distortion of the retina because the adherence may be greater there. As the membrane is elevated small, punctuate retinal hemorrhages may occur (Fig. 8.12).

When the membrane is thick and has good tensile strength, it can be grasped with fine forceps and slowly peeled from the retina (Fig. 8.13).

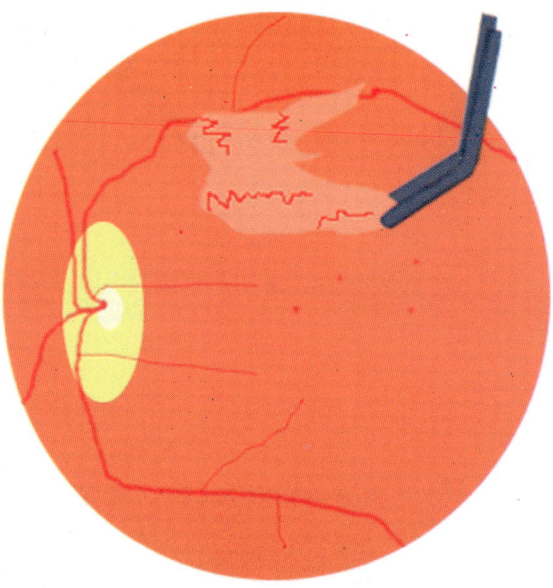

Fig. 8.12 *Membrane is grasped with fine forceps peeling results punctuate retinal haemorrhage*

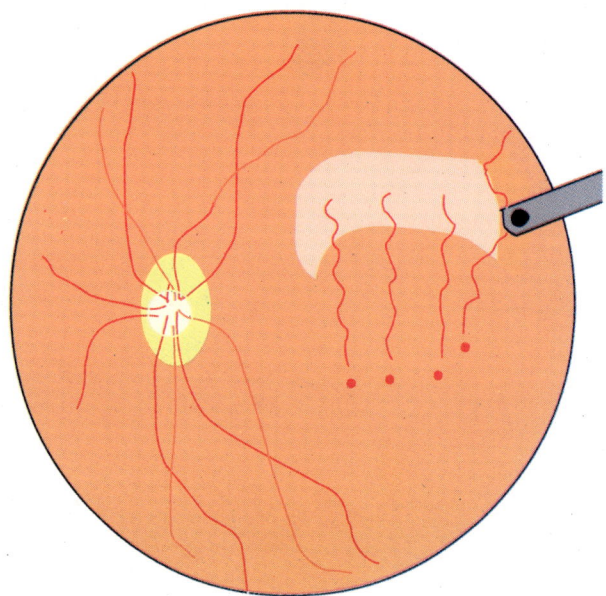

Fig. 8.13 *Membrane removed by cutting probe*

The membrane should be peeled from the retina as far as possible, but usually at least to the vascular arcade. It then removed directly with the cutting probe.

REFERENCES

1. Johnson R, Gass J Idiopathic: Macular holes: Observations, stages of formation, and complications for surgical intervention. *Ophthalmology* ; 95; 917-24, 1988.

2. Kim JW, freeman WR, Azen SP, EL Haig W, Klein DJ, Bailey IL: Prospective randomized trail of vitrectomy or observation for stage 2 macular holes. *Am J Ophthalmol*; 121; 606-14, 1966.

3. Brooks Hill, Jr: Macular hole surgery with or without internal limiting membrane peeling. *Ophthalmology*; 107; 1939-49, 2000.

4. Gayer DR, De Bistros S, Denier-west M, Fine SL: Observation for stage 2 macular hole. *Am J Ophthalmol*; 121; 605-14, 1996.

5. Siaarda RN: Macular hole. *Intra Ophthalmol Clin* 35; 105-22, 1995.

SUBRETINAL NEOVASCULARIZATION

Introduction

Modern vitreoretinal surgery is now one of the most effective tools for treating posterior segment diseases. In the last several years, there has been a surge of interest in submacular surgery, which allows removal of submacular choroidal neovascular membranes and haematomas. Removal of scar tissue and blood that interfere with retinal function is the main stay of vitreous surgery. With refinement in techniques and instrumentation, extensive surgical manipulation within the vitreous cavity can now be performed with resulting improvement or stabilization of visual function. Innovative and exciting developments in the relatively new field of macular surgery offers great promise to patients with many diseases that were previously thought to be incurable. During the past few years, increasing attention has been given to applying similar techniques in the submacular area, which allow removal of choroidal neovascular membranes and heamorrhage.[1]

Subfoveal Choroidal Neovascularization

Choroidal neovascularisation (CNV) is the principal cause of loss of central visual function in adults. Age-related macular degeneration (ARMD) and presumed ocular histoplasmosis syndrome (POHS) are frequent causes of choroidal neovascularisation.[2] It disrupts normal macular anatomy, leak serum and or formed overlying photoreceptors[3], When fibrovascular membranes grow beneath the center of the fovea avascular zone, the visual prognosis is generally poor. Laser photocoagulation has been demonstrated to be effective in the management of extrafoveal and juxta-foveal membranes of various etiologies. The macular photocoagulation study and other investigators have demonstrated a marginal benefit of laser treatment and limitations of laser treatment is the concomitant damage to overlying neuron sensory retina.[4] This is particularly harmful when the membrane is under the center of the fovea because central vision is almost always significantly reduced after treatment.[5]

Surgical removal is an alternative means of eradicating subfoveal choroidal neovascularisation (CNV) with potentially less damage to neuron sensory retina and selection determines the success outcome of the best surgical prognosis, as preservation of the RPE is a critical factor in the subsequent recovery of central vision. Surgical removal of subfoveal choroidal neovascular mem-

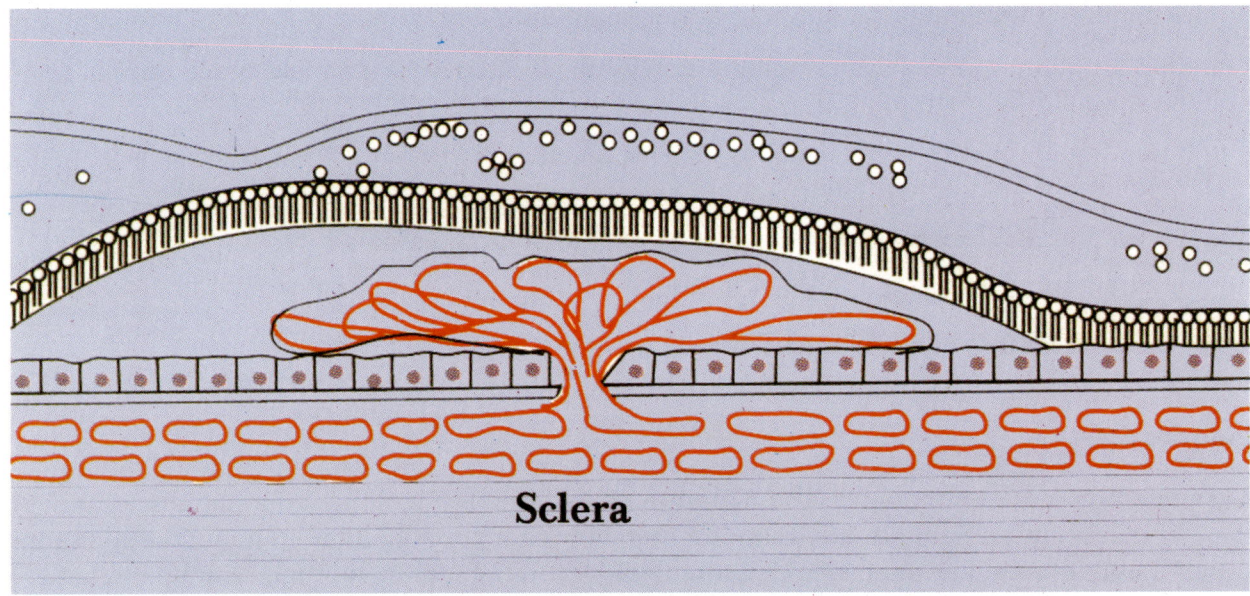

Fig. 8.14 *Subretinal neovascularisation where vessels grow through focal defect in the retinal pigment epithelium*

brane is advised if it appears to lie anterior to the RPE (Fig. 8.14).

Contact lens examination of the macular and 2x colour stereo view and stereoscopic fluorescein angiography helps in determining the location of the membrane.

Instrumentation

Some special instruments are required for removal of subretinal neovascularisation.

    a. Angled subretinal pick
    b. Infusion cannula
    c. Sub-retinal forceps: Horizontal
                             Vertical
    d. Sub-retinal scissors: Horizontal
                             Vertical

Surgical Technique

A standard three-port pars plana vitrectomy is performed. In this technique, the vitreous is removed and the posterior hyaloid stripped as it is done for macular hole surgery. The subretinal space is entered with a fine, 36-gauge sharp pick. The site of entry is planned to give a good range for subretinal manipulation using the dominant hand. For right-handed surgeon this is usually temporally or superior temporally for a right eye. For left eyes the retinotomy may be supero nasal or intranasal to the fovea but not in the papillomacular bundle. If an intranasal retinotomy is desired, the nasal sclerotomy should be placed as close as possible to the horizontal meridian. The retinotomy site must be closed enough to the membrane to manipulate and grasp it with subretinal forceps. The 33-gauge needle is inserted under the retina and balanced salt solution is slowly injected by the assistant to raise a small bleb that separates the retina from the under-lying membrane (Fig. 8.15).

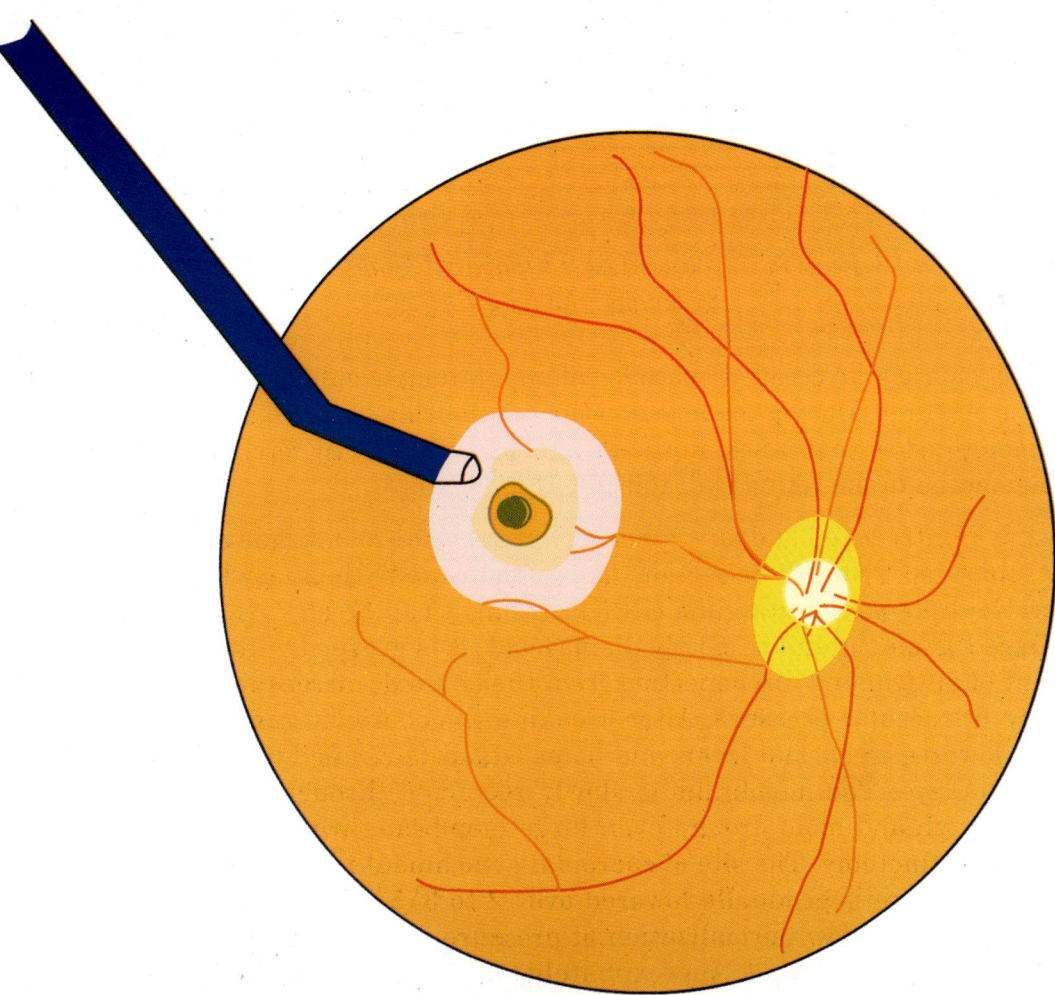

Fig. 8.15 *With 30 gauge needle balanced salt solution is slowly injected to create a space for manipulation*

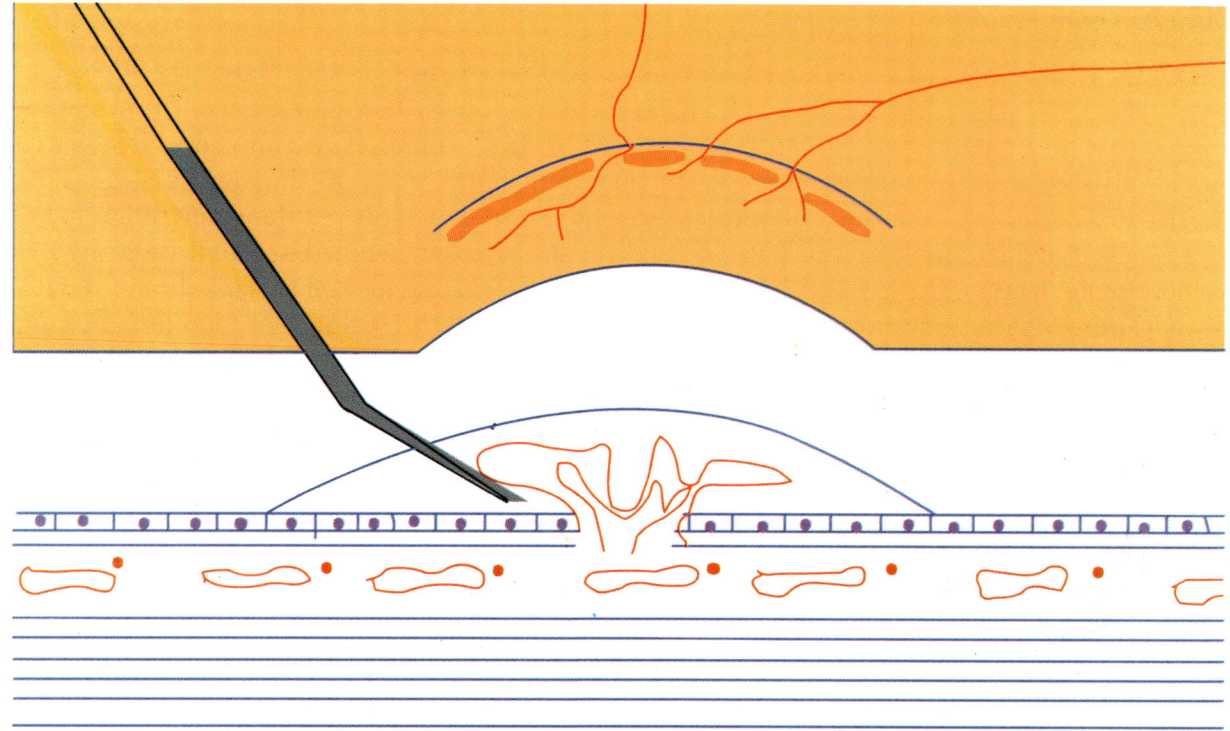

Fig. 8.16 *Peak is introduced and separated from the retina adhesion to remove the vascular tuft*

The bleb is enlarged to create a space for manipulation, avoiding injecting so much that the membrane is obscured. During the injection the relationship between the membrane and retina is closely monitored so that a hole in the retina is not created by forcibly breaking the attachment of membrane to the retina hydraulically (Fig. 8.16).

The pick is reintroduced and any adhesion between the membrane and overlying retina is carefully separated by blunt dissection. The membrane is then slowly teased from the underlying retinal pigment epithelium (RPE) so that it can be elevated to be grasped by the forceps. Once the membrane is mostly disinserted, it is grasped with subretinal forceps. At the moment of anticipated disconnection from the choroid, increasing the infusion pressure elevates the intraocular pressure. After breaking the choroidal connection, the pressure is very slowly lowered to normal levels and homeostasis is verified before removing the membrane from the eye. The membrane is slowly retracted through the retinotomy site. The retina will stretch and mold around even large membrane with only a modest increase in the size of the retinotomy. The site of choroidal attachment is monitored for bleeding, while the infusion pressure is gradually lowered over 2 to 3\5 minutes. If any blood appears at the ingrowth and the slow normalization of pressure is repeated. An air–fluid exchange is performed to flatten the retina. Approximately 80-90% of the eye is refilled with fluid subsequently, leaving a 10-20% bubbles so that the retinotomy may be tamponade overnight with the patients in the facedown position. Laser photocoagulation may be required for the retinotomy.

Complications

Complications[7] which might be encountered in subretinal neovascularisation surgery are may lead to the following.

1. Iatrogenic macular hole

2. Avulsion of fovea during membrane removal

3. Subretinal haemorrhage

4. Retinal detachment

5. Cataract

Postoperative management

Postoperative patients are examined at 24 hrs and at 1 week after surgery for signs of infection, retinal detachment or elevated intraocular pressure. The view usually adequate immediately for the presence or absence of subfoveal RPE. Occasionally, residual subretinal blood will obscure the underlying tissues for a longer period of time. Fluorescein angiography is repeated as soon as the media clarity allows establishing a new base line for monitoring recurrence. Non-uncommonly, the site of the original choroidal on growth stalk may demonstrate recurrence after this site is not subfoveal and therefore slit lamp laser photocoagulation can be employed to ablate recurrence. Since the membrane recur in approximately one-third of cases within 6-months, close follow-up is essential.

REFERENCES

1. Lopez PF, Grossniklaus HE, Lambert HM et al: Pathologic features of surgically excised subretinal neovascular membrane in age related macular degeneration. *Am J Ophthalmol* 112: 647-656, 1991.

2. Ruby AJ, Jampol LM, Goldberg MF et al: Choroidal neovascularisation associated with choroidal hemangiomas. *Arch Ophthalmol* 110: 658-661, 1992.

3. Gass JDM: Pathogenesis of disciform detachment of the neuroepithelium senile disciform macular degeneration. *Am J Ophthalmol* 63: 617-644, 1967.

4. Macular photocoagulation study group laser photocoagulation of sub-foveal neovascular lesions of age-related macular degeneration. *Arch Ophthalmol* 111: 1200-1209, 1993.

5. Macular photocoagulation study group, laser photocoagulation of sub-foveal recurrent neovascularisation in age-related macular degeneration: Results of a randomized clinical trial. *Arch Ophthalmol* 109: 1220-1231, 1991.

6. Green WR: Clinicopathologic studies of treated choroidal neovascularisation membranes: A review and report of two cases. *Retina* 11: 328-356, 1991.

7. Capone A JR: Submacular surgical procedure. *Int Ophthalmol Clin*; 35: 83-93, 1995.

FURTHER READING

1. Ibanez HE et al: Surgical management of sub macular hemorrhage a series of 47 consecutive cases. *Arch Ophthalmol* 113: 62, 1995.

2. Mein CE, Flinn HW Jr: Recognition and removal of the posterior cortical vitreous during vitreoretinal surgery for impending macular hole. *Am J Ophthalmol* 111: 611, 1991.

3. Mel berg NS et al: Vitrectomy for the vitromacular traction syndrome with macular detachment. *Retina* 15: 774, 1995.

4. Thomas MA, Ibene HE: Instruments for sub macular surgery. *Retina* 14: 84, 1994.

5. Wendell Rt et al: Vitreous surgery for macular hole. *Ophthalmology* 100: 1671, 1993.

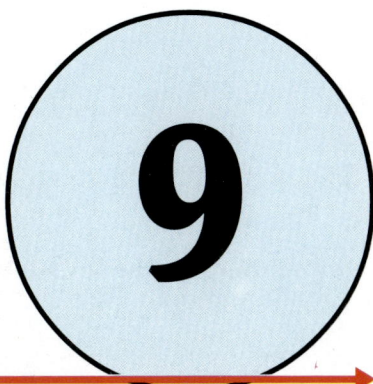

Diabetic Vitrectomy

Introduction

The main serious vision-threatening complications of diabetic retinopathy occurs in patients who have not had laser therapy or in whom laser photocoagulation has been unsuccessful or is inadequate.

ANATOMIC CONSIDERATIONS

In proliferative diabetic retinopathy there are multiple complications. These complications may be simple vitreous haemorrhage, fibrovascular proliferation, epiretinal membrane, tractional, retinal detachment and retinal breaks. These complications may be present singly or may be combined to produce various complex surgical problem.[1]

Out of all surgical presentations, simple vitreous haemorrhage produces the least surgical problem (Fig. 9.1).

It may be present with posterior vitreous detachment and no fibrous visible fibrous proliferation on the retina surface. In some cases vitreous haemorrhage may be present with persistent attachment of the posterior hyaloid to the retina (Fig. 9.2).

This focal adherent produces least surgical problem during operation.[2] Anterior to posterior traction commonly is found within eyes with vitreous haemorrhage or in eyes with clear media and retinal detachment. The anterior attachment of traction always includes the vitreous base but may extend more posteriorly as well. Posterior attachment usually includes both the optic nerve and areas of fibrovascular proliferation on the posterior retinal surface, particularly along the vascular arcades (Fig. 9.3).

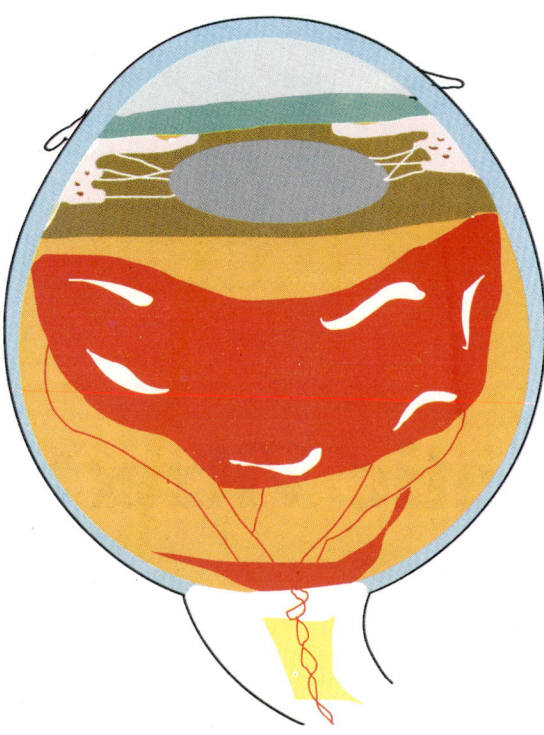

Fig. 9.1 *Vitreous haemorrhage with posterior vitreous detachments.*

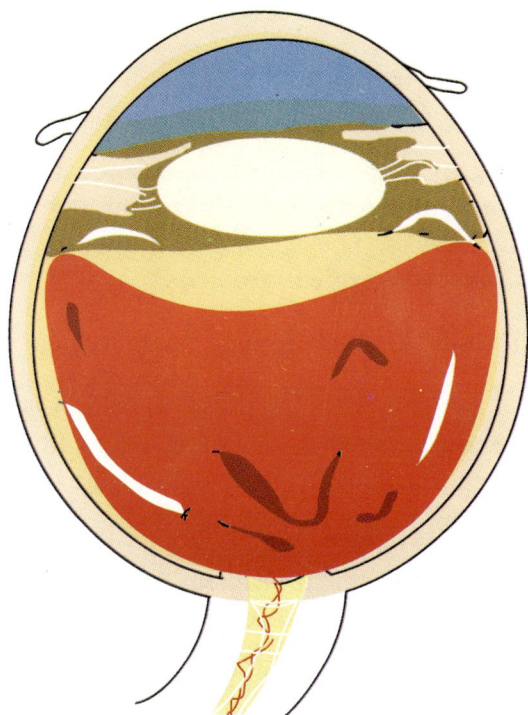

Fig. 9.2 *Vitreous haemorrhage with inactive regressed fibrovascular proliferation*

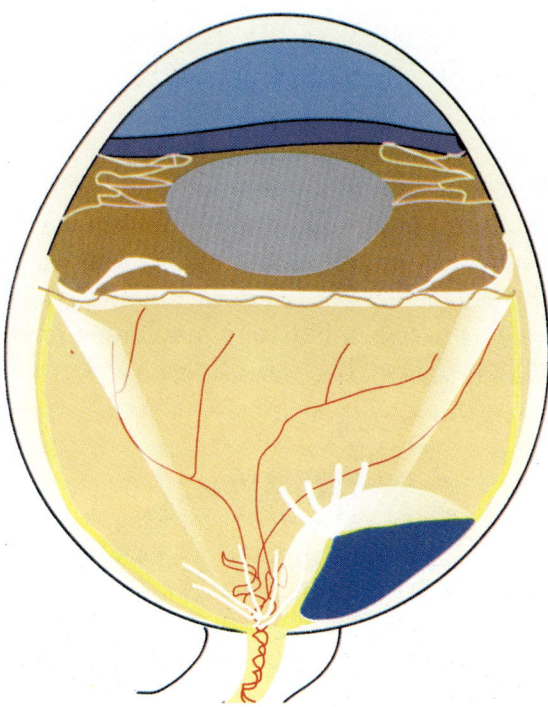

Fig. 9.3 *Anterior posterior traction with retinal traction detachment*

Fibrovascular proliferation typically bridges between multiple attachment points on the posterior retina, especially along the vascular arcades. It often grows from the optic nerve confluently along both vascular arcades to procedure a "wolf-jaw configuration (Fig. 9.4).

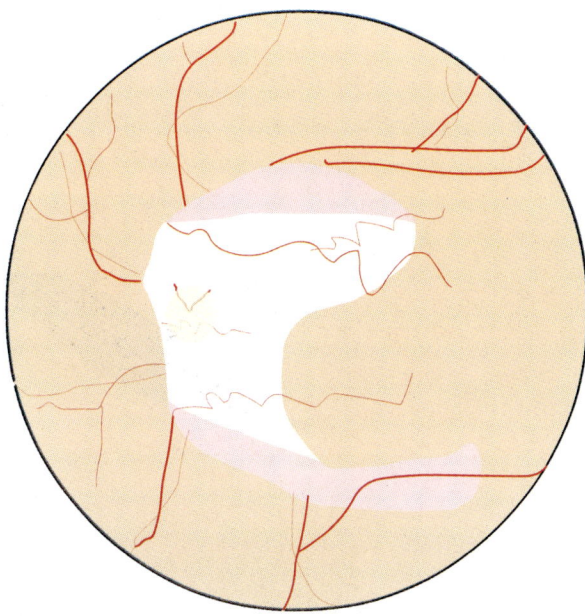

Fig. 9.4 *Fibrovascular proliferation involving optic nerve and vascular arcades*

Massive fibrovascular proliferation may grow over the posterior pole, including all four vascular arcades; anterior displacement of this tissue produces a "tabletop" detachment (Fig. 9.5).

Dissection planes usually are found temporal to the macula between the arcades where adherence of the hyaloid to the retina and fibrovascular proliferation are less common. Contraction of the vitreous, producing shortenings between the vitreous base and the attachment of the vitreous to fibrovascular membranes on the retinal surface, coupled with contraction of the membranes themselves produces traction retinal detachment. These detachments are usually posterior and involve the vascular arcades, but they may be extensive and spread for into the periphery or involve the periphery alone (Fig. 9.6).

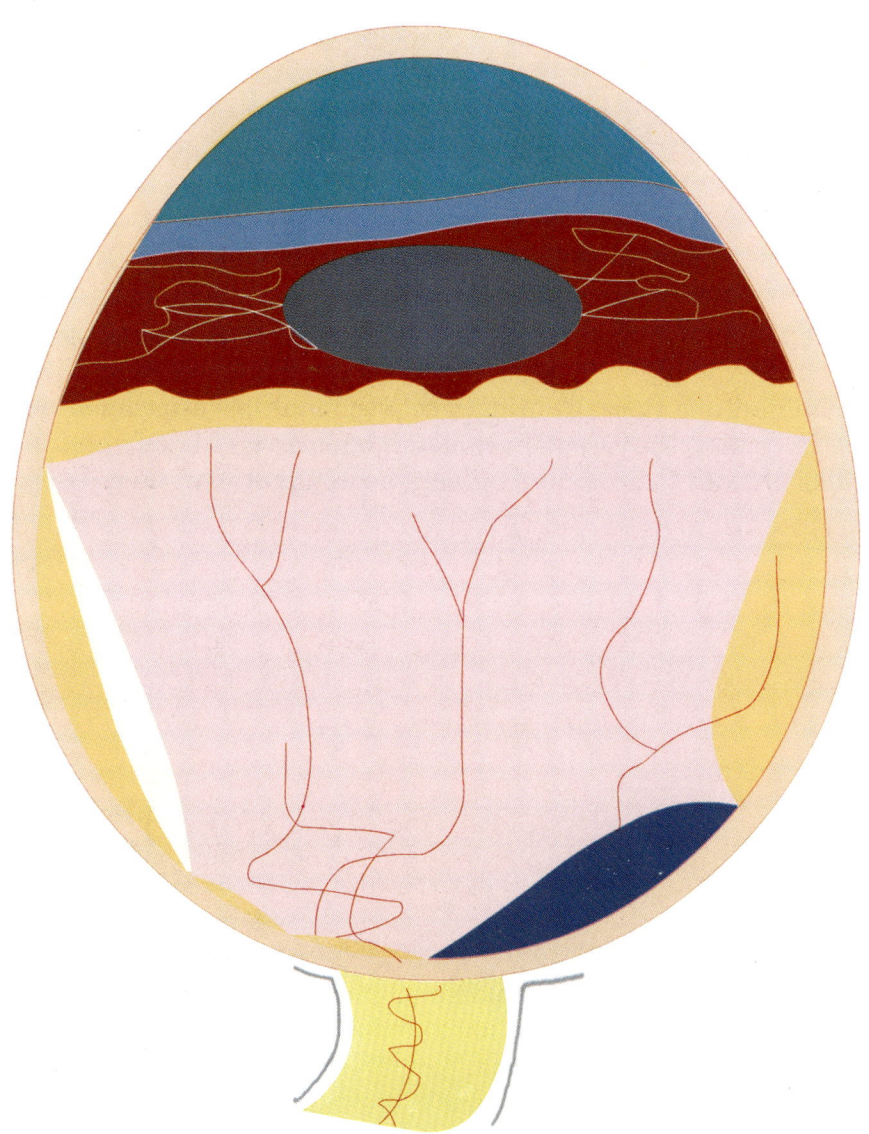

Fig. 9.5 *Extensive fibrovascular proliferation with retinal detachments*

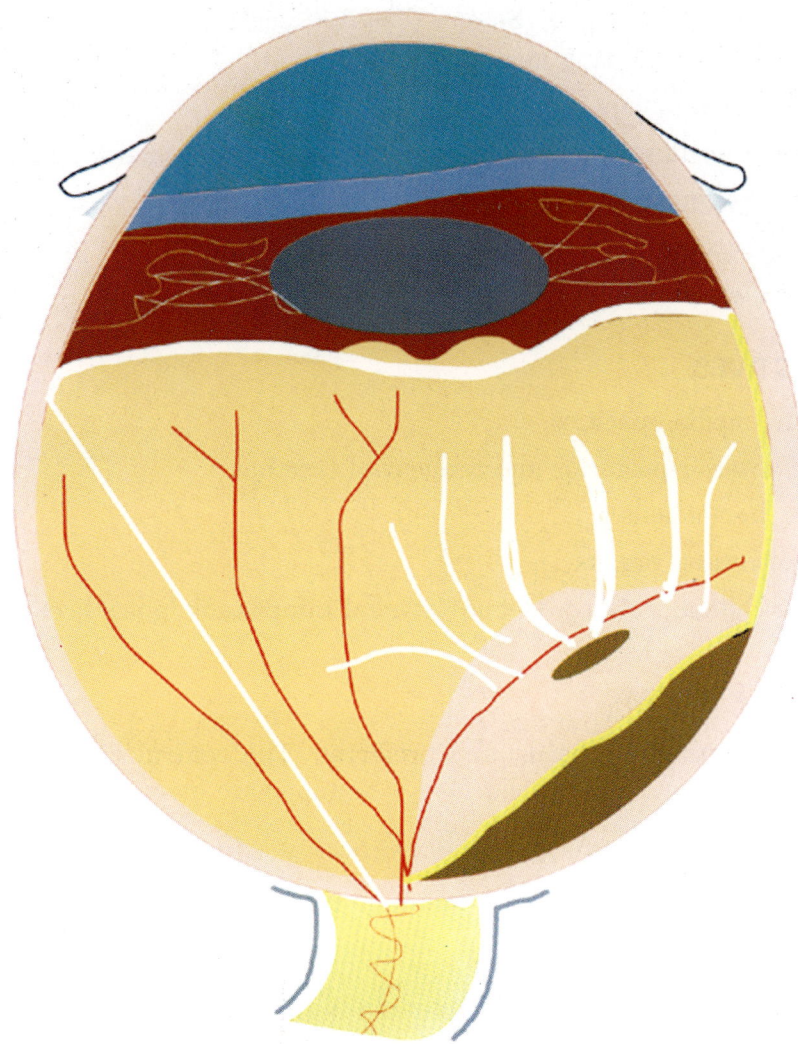

Fig. 9.6 *Tractional rhegmatogenous detachment near the vascular arcade*

Traction-rhegmatogenous detachments result when traction is found in the presence of retinal breaks. These detachments are recognized by their bullous configuration as opposed to the taut elevation of traction detachments alone. Retinal breaks are typically near the vascular arcades in atrophic retina. They are usually round or oval and often may be found in the retina on the peripheral edge of an area of fibrovascular proliferation. With the development of modern vitrectomy techniques, the indication of vitreous surgery for complications of diabetic retinopathy is increasing.

INDICATION OF DIABETIC VITRECTOMY

1. Non-clearing vitreous haemorrhage.
2. Traction retinal detachment.

3. Combined tractional-rhegmatogenous retina detachment.
4. Progressive fibrosis causing macular ectopia.
5. Dense premacular haemorrhage.
6. Persistence of florid retinopathy despite adequate photocoagulation.
7. Anterior hyaloid neovascularisation.
8. Hemolytic glaucoma.
9. Diffuse macular odema.

SURGICAL OBJECTIVES

1. Clearing the media opacities.
2. Release of anterior-posterior and tangential traction.
3. Intraocular hemostasis.
4. Detection of retinal breaks.
5. Fluid gas exchange, retinopexy and internal tamponade (gas/silicone oil).

BASIC DIABETIC VITRECTOMY

Standard three ports vitrectomy is usually preferred. The central vitreous is removed with vitrectomy probe. If the anterior hyaloid face is semiopaque or opaque or taut, it should be removed first (Fig. 9.7).

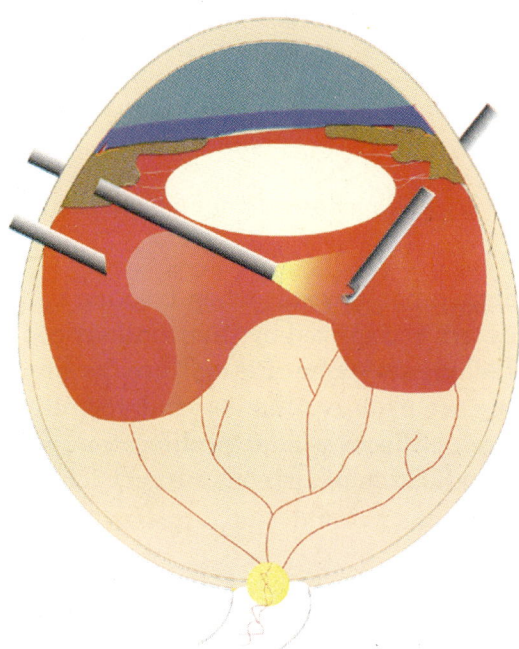

Fig. 9.7 *Central vitreous removed with vitrectomy probe*

If it is clear and the lens is to be left in place, it should be retained unless there is an element of anterior loop traction or compartmentalization requiring removal. If the posterior hyaloid face is opaque, the vitreous probe should be entered away from the macula. Liquid blood may be pooled in the posterior segment, obscuring details of the retina and membrane. Vacuum removal improves visibility for subsequent surgical maneuvers (Figs. 9.8 and 9.9).

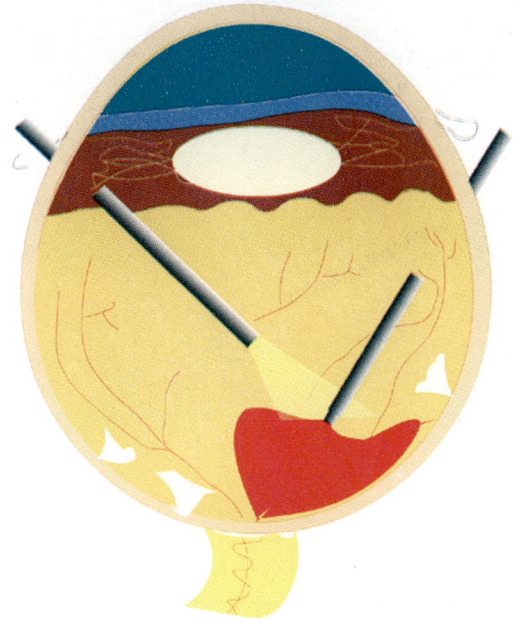

Fig. 9.8 *Liquid blood pooled from the posterior segment*

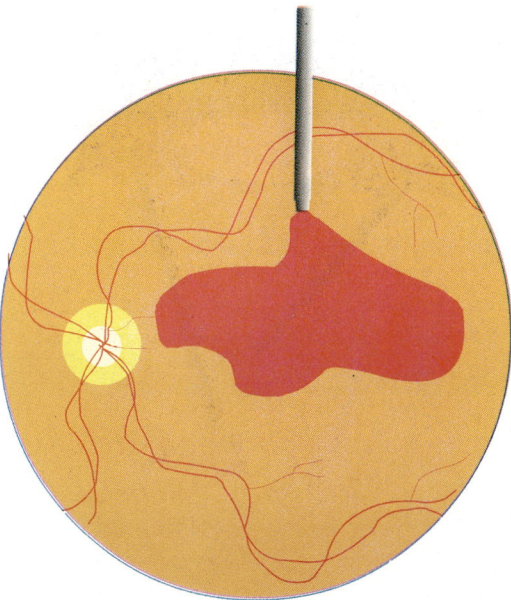

Fig. 9.9 *Vacuum removal improves visibility of the retina and membrane*

Anterior traction should be removed before proceeding delamination or membrane segmentation (Fig. 9.10).

Whenever there is thin membrane, it should be elevated gently with a pick or spatula and separated by vitreous cutter (Fig. 9.11).

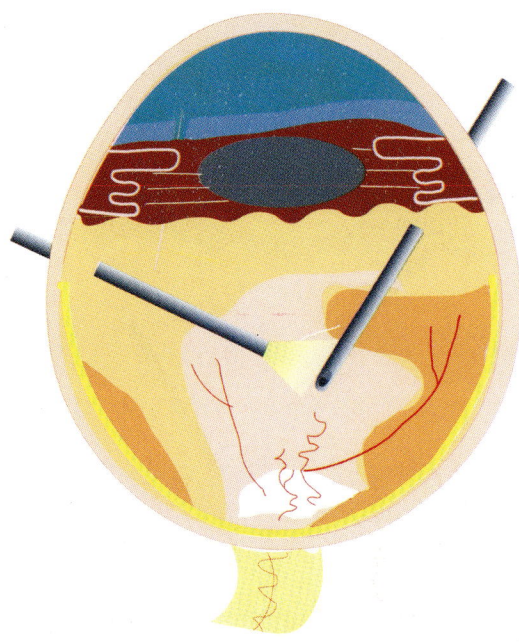

Fig. 9.10 *Anterior traction removed before delamination*

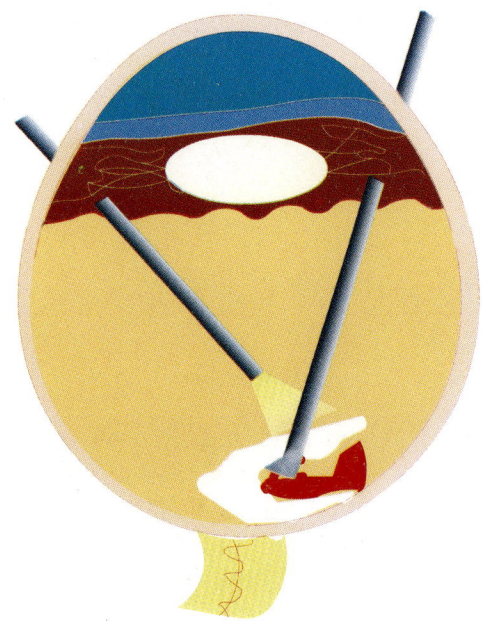

Fig. 9.11 *Elevation of membrane by retina picks*

Small surface bleeders or small breaks occasionally may result from membrane stripping. Diathermy also used to mark the edge of iatrogenic or pre-existing breaks, so they can be identified once the retina is reattached during the fluid gas exchange procedure.

SEGMENTATION ON FIBROVASCULAR PROLIFERATION

Fibrovascular membrane may bridge between the optic nerve and retinal epicenters or between two retinal epicenters. Scissors with blades oriented perpendicular to the retinal surface may be used to segment these membranes (Fig. 9.12).

Diathermy to the membrane before segmentation when significant vascularisation is present may reduce bleeding from the cut ends. A fibrovascular tissue is removed close to the retinal surface with vitreous cutting instrument, leaving island of residual tissues on the retinal surface (Fig. 9.13).

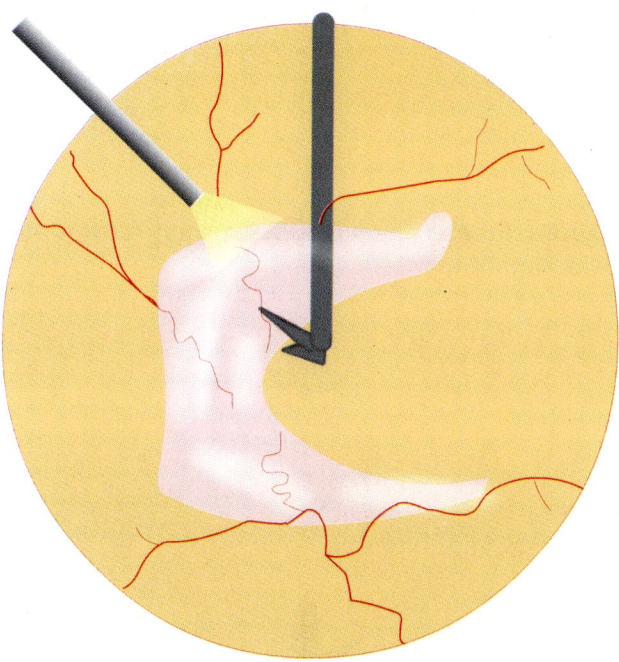

Fig. 9.12 *Vertical scissors are used to segment the membrane*

DELAMINATION OF DIABETIC MEMBRANE

When large area of membrane is present over retinal surface, surgeons prefer to remove as much as possible. This technique has been termed 'delamination'. In a majority of cases, the core vitreous surgery requires no specific attention. If there is posterior hyaloid face (PHF) opaque, it should be truncated before proceeding to delamination. With broad sheets of fibrovascular tissues along the temporal vascular arcades, horizontal scissors are introduced that cut parallel to the plane of the retina, working from the posterior pole towards the equator (Fig. 9.14).

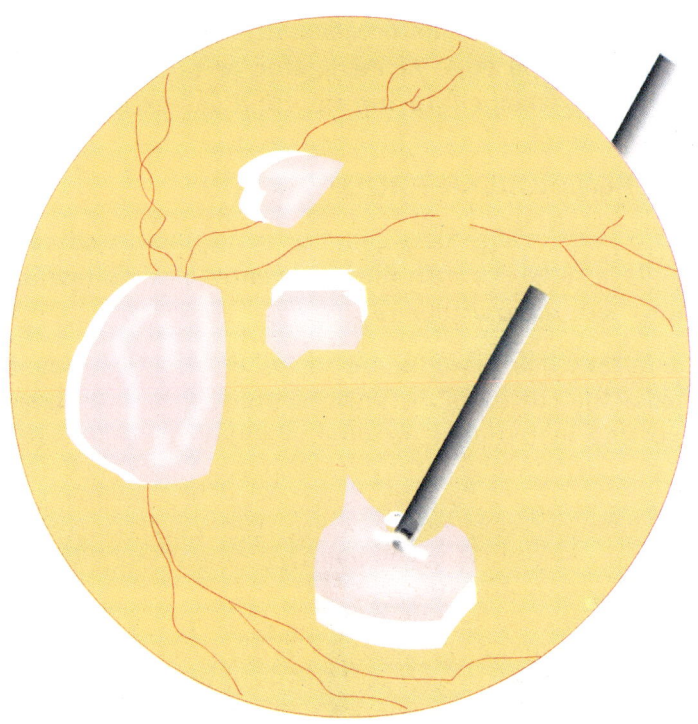

Fig. 9.13 *Islands of residual tissues on retinal surface*

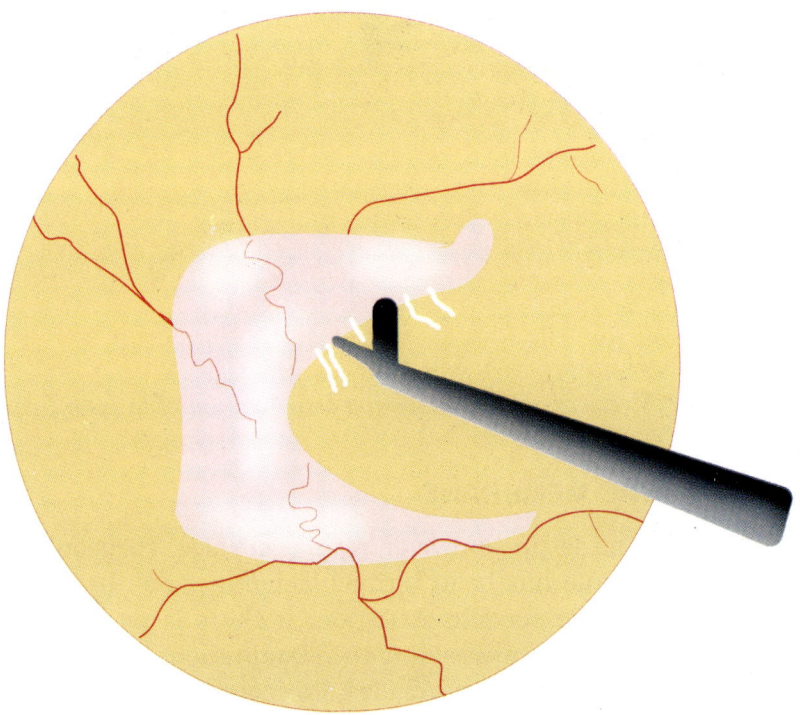

Fig. 9.14 *Broad sheets of fibrovascular tissues approached from posterior pole .*

The fibrovascular tissues are attached more firmly on the peripheral side and easily served when the approach is from the posterior pole. The main object of delamination is to separate the fibrovascular membrane from the retina, cutting the multiple small attachments between the two tissue plana (Fig. 9.15).

When there is partial posterior vitreous detachment (PVD) and the epiretinal membrane is continuous with the PHF, delamination should precede PHF truncation.

When there are bands, blunt dissection technique using spreading of the scissors blade easily defines the cleavage planes (Fig. 9.16).

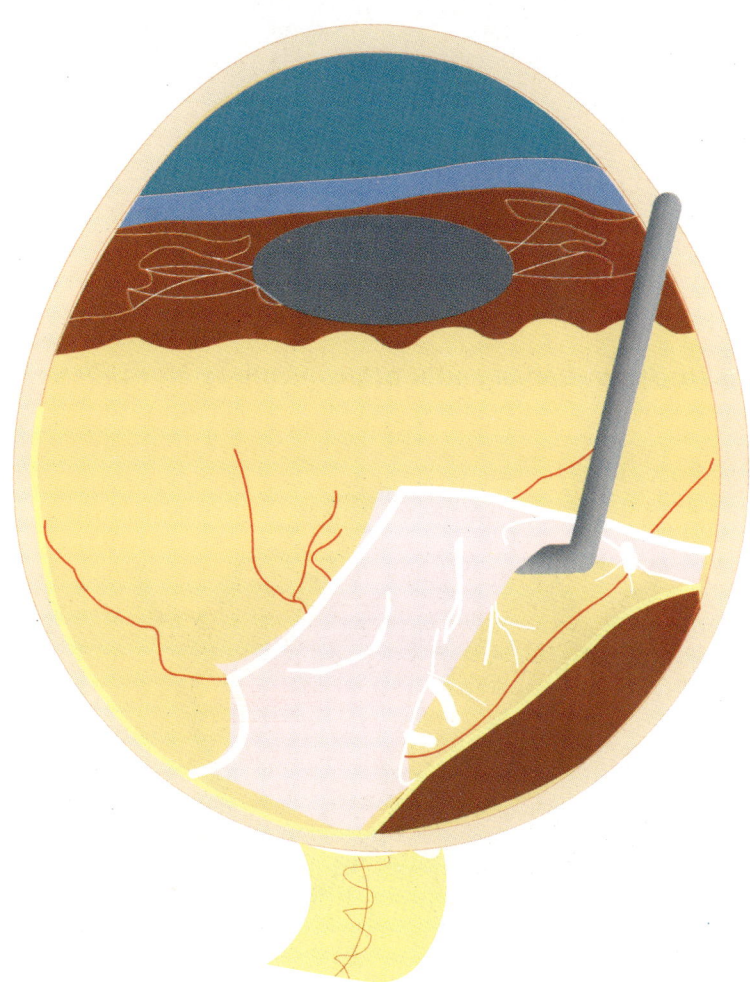

Fig. 9.15 *Multiple small attachments between tissue planes-delaminated*

Once the cleavage planes are achieved, viscoelastic is introduced to define cleavage planes and also to control intraoperative bleeding. At the end of the procedure, the retinal surface is entirely free of membrane (Fig. 9.17).

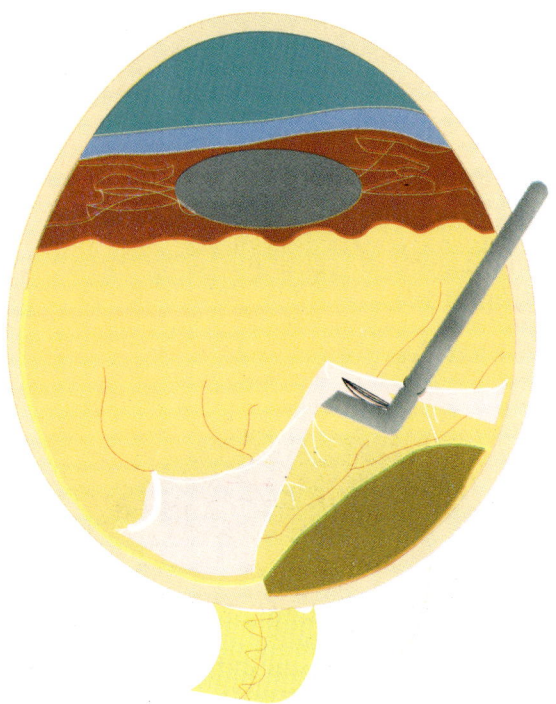

Fig. 9.16 Separation of small attachments by blunt dissection

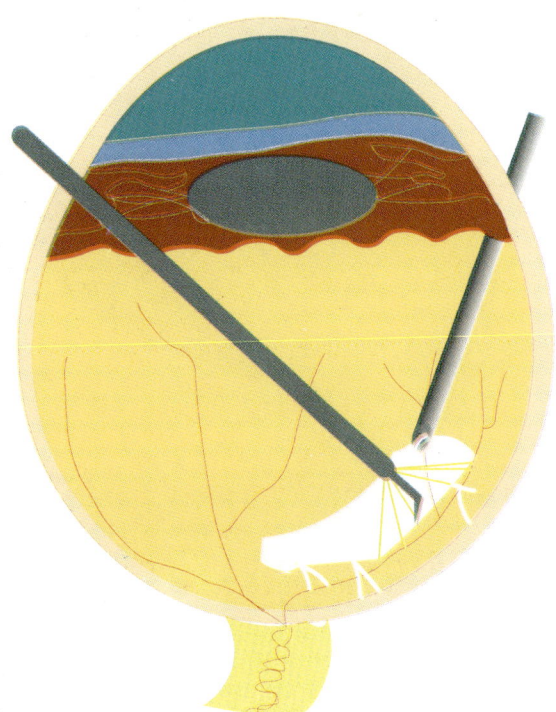

Fig. 9.17 Membranes are removed by cutting probe to free from retinal surface

ENBLOC TECHNIQUES IN DIABETIC MEMBRANE

In enbloc technique, the central vitreous is first removed to ensure good visibility (Fig. 9.18).

In this technique delamination is modified by allowing some area of anterior posterior or vitreous traction to remain when the dissection process has begun.[3] The traction acts as a third hand, elevating the membrane and helping to develop dissection planes. Once the membranes are removed, the retina falls back posteriorly, exposing new area of adhesion to be served (Fig. 9.19).

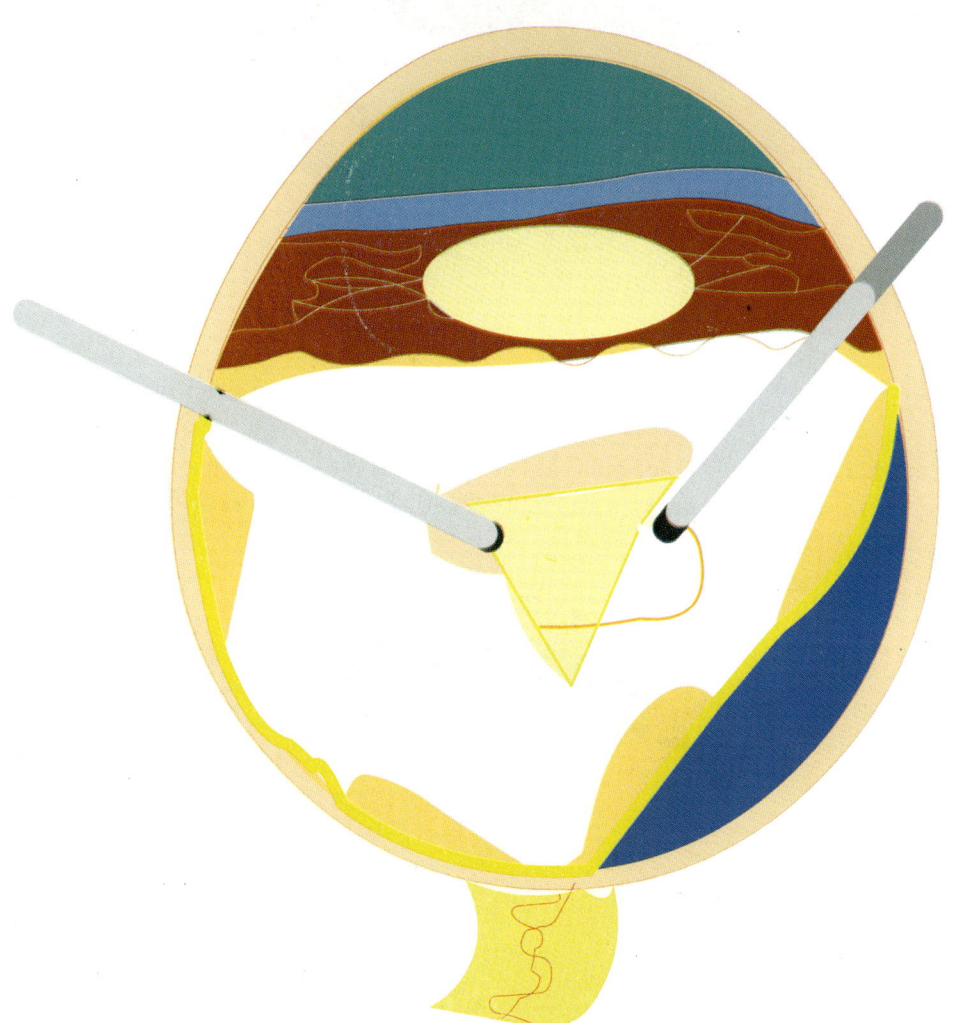

Fig. 9.18 *Removal of central vitreous to improve visibility*

With the help of vitreous cutter now the membrane is removed. In the final stage, all traction is released and membrane is drawn anteriorly where the vitreous cutter removes it. The retina settles posteriorly but dose not become entirely attached until fluid is removed posteriorly through a retinal break.

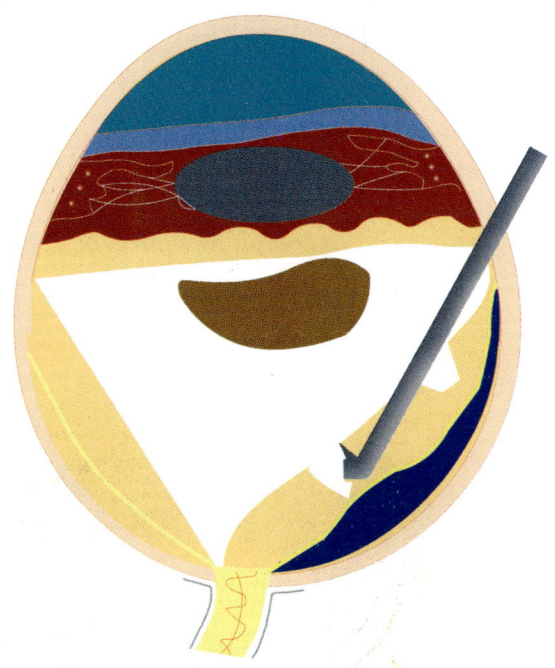

Fig. 9.19 *Retinal falls back posteriorly to expose new area of adhesion*

Further dissection removes traction from retinal surface. At the end all tractions are released and the membrane is drawn anteriorly where the vitreous cutter removes it (Fig. 9.20).

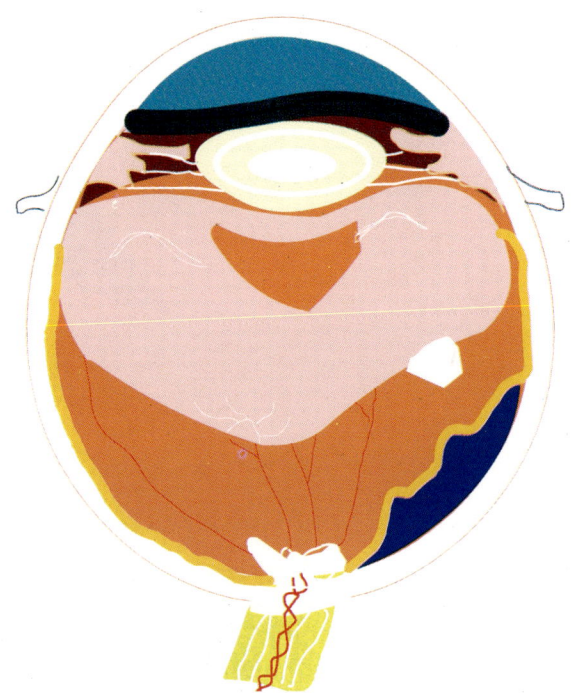

Fig. 9.20 *Traction removed from retinal surface*

The retina settles posteriorly but does not become entirely attached until fluid is removed posteriorly by active transport and by osmotic pressure or is drained through a retinal break (Fig. 9.21).

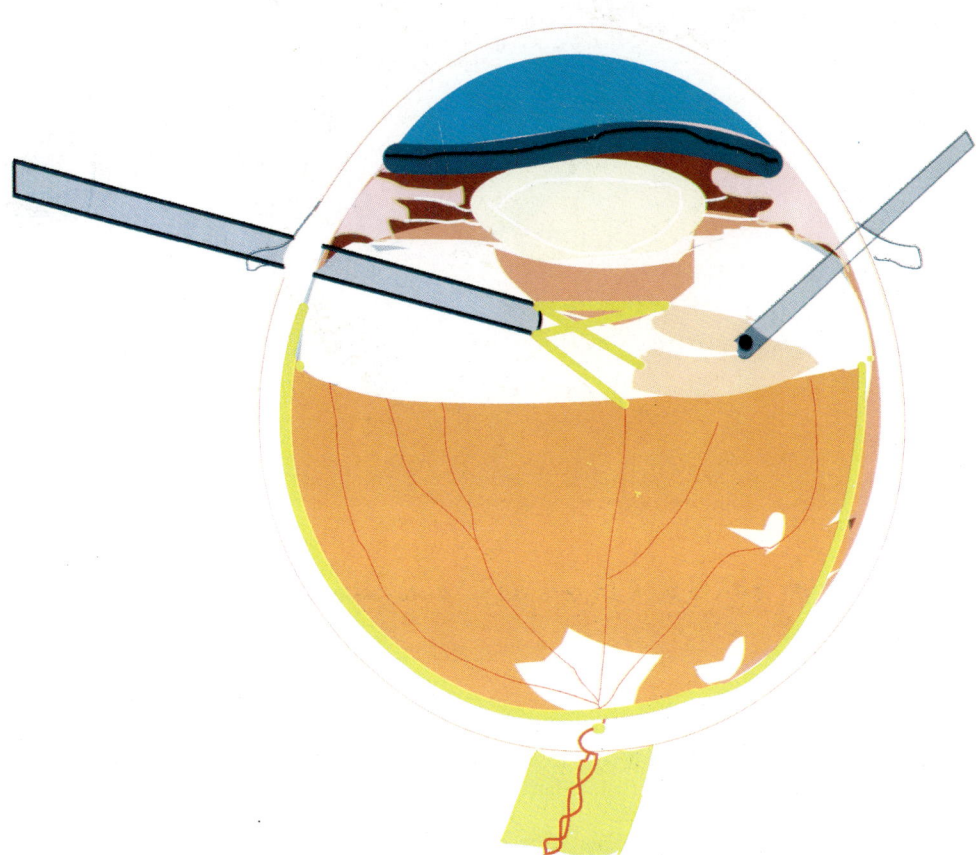

Fig. 9.21 *The retina settled completely*

DIABETIC MEMBRANE DELAMINATION: BIMANUAL DISSECTION TECHNIQUE

Recent development of bimanual technique is quite encouraging in vitreoretinal surgery. Two hands are used simultaneously for delamination of tissues[4]. The basic approach is to retract tissue gently with one instrument while cutting it with either vertical or horizontal scissor in other hand.

The light pipe with pick on the end allows retraction of the tissue while illuminating tissue to be cut and with other hand cutting the tissue on the retina (Fig. 9.22).

In some cases, light pipe fitted with diathermy is used, which helps to coagulate the bleeding vessels. Once the tissue or membrane elevates over the retina, motorized vertical scissors helps in dissecting the tissue without producing any retinal tear or hole. The light pipe with pick lifts the fibrovascular tissue gently and allows proper identification of larger retinal vessels, which may otherwise be inadvertently severed with the scissors technique (Fig. 9.23).

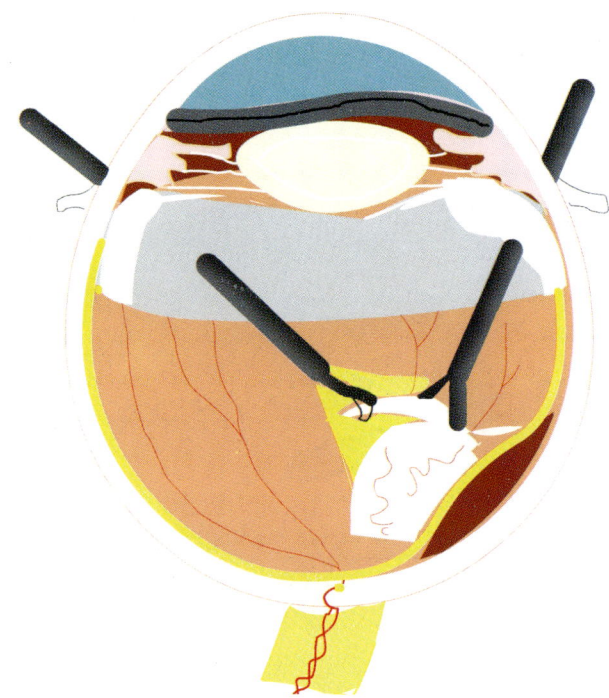

Fig. 9.22 *Light pipe with a pick in one hand and cutting tissues with other hand*

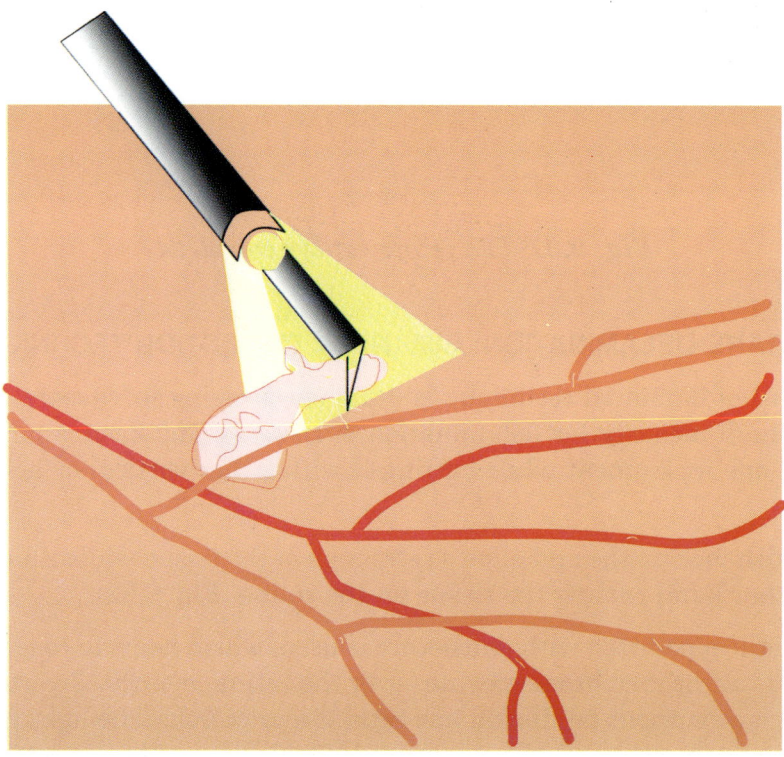

Fig. 9.23 *Lifting the fibrovascular tissue allows identification of large retinal vessels*

ANTERIOR HYALOIDAL PROLIFERATION

Anterior hyaloid proliferation is a complication usually found in postvitrectomy diabetic eyes. It occurs when fibrovascular tissue grows from the peripheral retina along the anterior hyaloid face, pars plana and ciliary body (Fig. 9.24).

The peripheral retina is drawn anteriorly by dense membrane, and the ciliary body and anterior retina may become detached (Fig. 9.25).

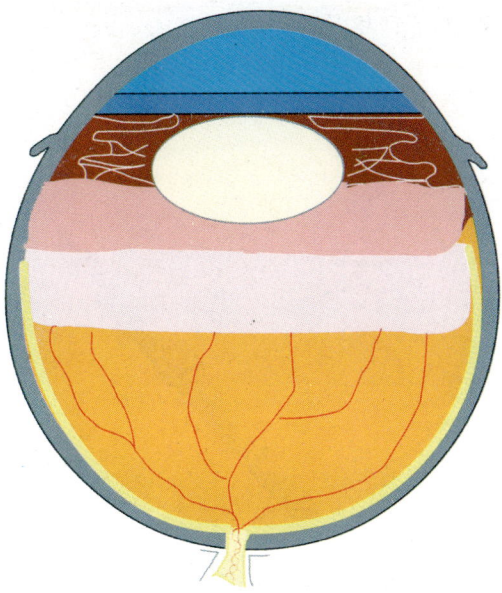

Fig. 9.24 *Fibrovascular tissue grows from peripheral retina.*

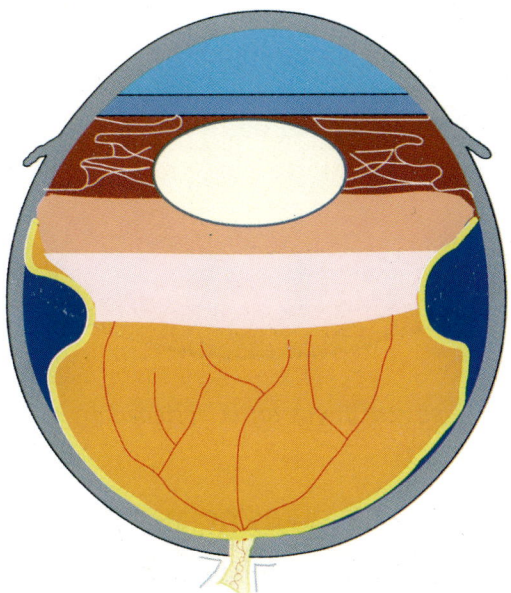

Fig. 9.25 *Ciliary body detached from retina*

After lensectomy to gain access to the area of anterior fibrovascular proliferation, diathermy is applied to the elevated tissue.

The vitreous base is shaved close to the retina with the vitreous cutter. The anterior retina is folded onto itself to create a "taco" configuration. The anterior rotation of the retina is relieved by opening the taco with sharp dissection with a micro vitreoretinal blade. Two-handed dissections with scissors or lighted pick also is useful for relieving traction. After dedulking the remaining tissue, any residual traction is relieved by making radial cuts into the ring of proliferative tissue with end cutting scissors (Fig. 9.26).

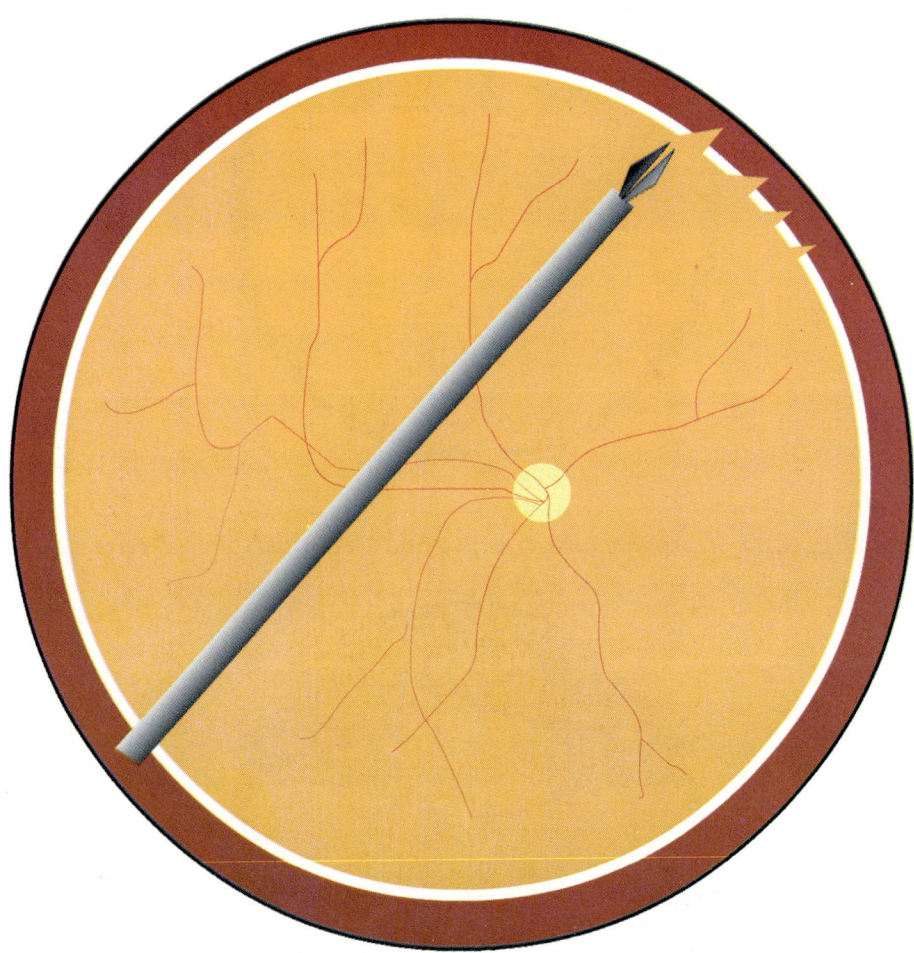

Fig. 9.26 *Residual traction is relieved by radial cuts.*

INTRAOPERATIVE COMPLICATIONS OF DIABETIC MEMBRANE DISSECTION

The important intraoperative complications in diabetic membrane dissection are surface bleeding and retinal tears. Whenever there is active bleeding during dissection, it should be treated by diathermy (Fig. 9.27).

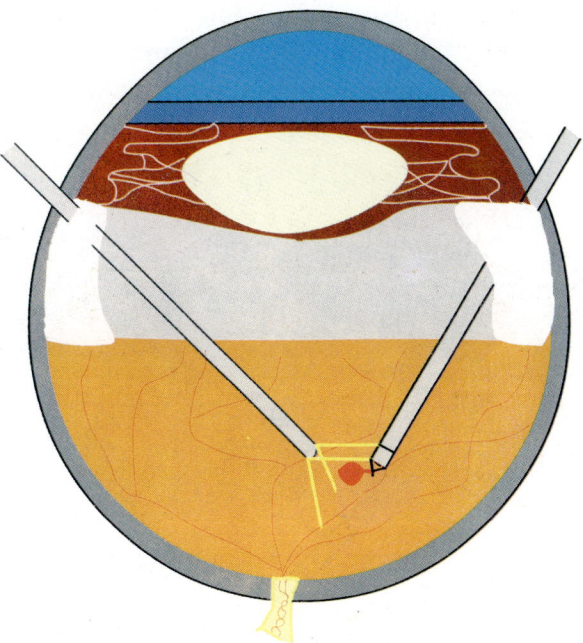

Fig. 9.27 *Active bleeding during dissection treated by diathermy*

After removal of the membrane, sometimes blood clotted and adherent close to the retina surface. Flute-needle with silicone tip can remove the clotted blood without damaging the retinal tissue (Fig. 9.28).

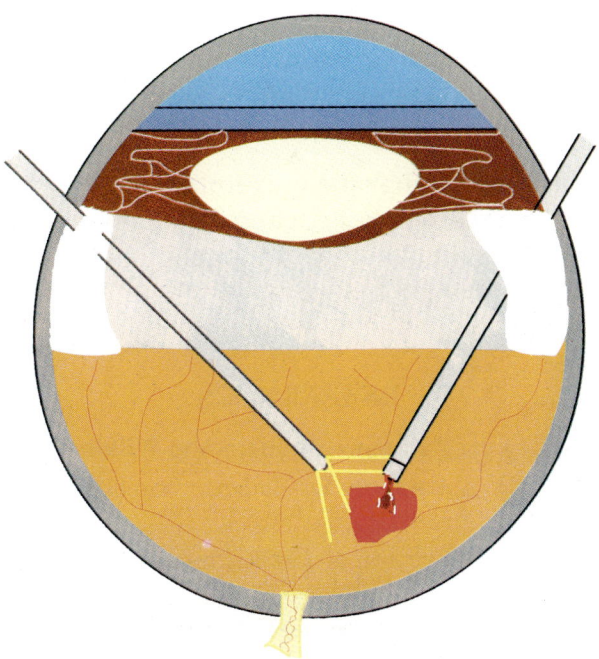

Fig. 9.28 *Vacuum needle with silicone tip allows gentle sweeping of the clotted blood*

During segmentation due to the pressure of the lower blade of the scissor as the retina cutting, slit retinal breaks may be created. In case of delamination iatrogenic breaks are more common and sometimes the existing hole gets enlarged (Fig. 9.29).

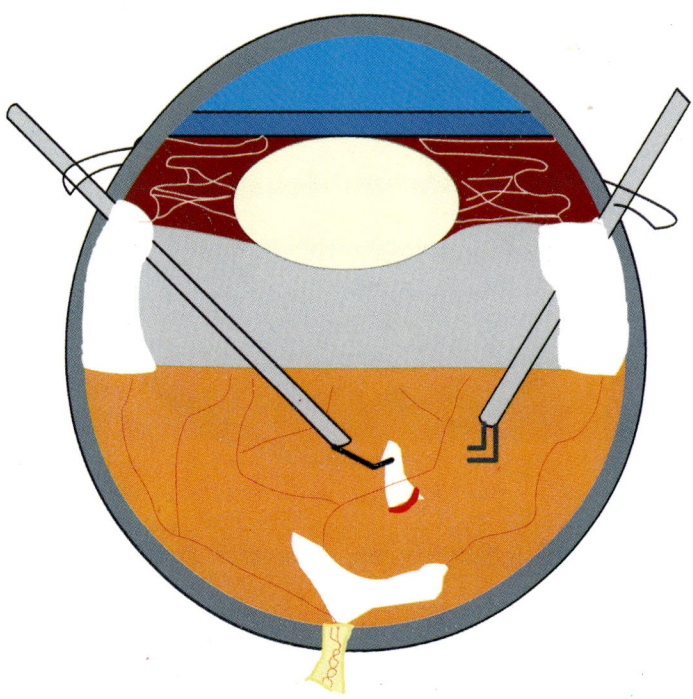

Fig. 9.29 *Iatrogenic breaks are common in delamination*

However, traction and retinal distortion must be relieved, otherwise the holes produced by segmentation, delamination and by retinotomy will remain open causing rhegmatogenous retinal detachment.

However, the anatomical results of diabetic vitrectomy is not poor by current technique, the functional results remain unsatisfactory. Among the causes for poor functional results, neovascular glaucoma (NVG) and renal anemia by diabetic nephropathy are important to consider in the indication for diabetic vitrectomy.[5]

REFERENCES

1. Charles S: *Vitreous Microsurgery*. Baltimore, William and Wilkins, 1981.
2. Michels RG: Rice TA, Rice EF: Vitrectomy for diabetic vitreous haemorrhage. *Am J Ophthalmol* 95:12, 1983.
3. Abrams GW, William GA: En bloc excision of diabetic membrane. *Am J Ophthalmol* 103:302, 1987.
4. Meredith TA, Kaplan HJ, Aaberg TM: Pars plana vitrectomy technique of relief of epiretinal traction by membrane segmentation. *Am J Ophthalmol* 89:408, 1980.
5. Meredith TA: Delamination of epiretinal membrane with a diamond knife. *Arch Ophthalmol* 115:1598, 1997.

Surgery for Proliferative Vitreoretinopathy

Introduction

The most important cause of failure of retinal detachment surgery is due to development of proliferative vitreoretinopathy (PVR). Due to better understanding of the pathobiology of this disease, there has been improved the visual outcome after vitrectomy surgery. Tractional retinal detachment in proliferative vitreoretinopathy (PVR) occur secondary to the dispersion, proliferation and migration of cells within the vitreous cavity and on both surfaces of the retina.[1]

The Boston Retina Society introduced the initial classification of proliferative vitreoretinopathy in 1983, but subsequently in 1991 Machemer and coworkers in their silicone study adopted a new classification.[2]

CLASSIFICATION

Proliferation vitreoretinopathy is classified into the following grades.

Grade A: Vitreous haze and   pigment clusters on interior retina.

Grade B: Wrinkling of the inner retinal surface, retina stiffness, vessels tortuosity rolled and Irregular edge of retina break, decreased mobility of vitreous.

Grade C: (P-1-12) Posterior to equator focal diffuse or circumferential full thickness fold, subretinal stands.

C A-1-12 Anterior to equator, focal diffuse or circumferential full thickness subretinal strands anterior displacement, condensed vitreous with strands.

Grade D: Fixed retinal folds in four quadrants.

Grade D1: Wide funnel.

Grade D2: Narrow funnel.

Grade D3: Closed funnel.

ANATOMIC PRESENTATION IN PROLIFERATIVE VITREORETINOPATHY

In proliferative vitreoretinopathy cellular membrane grow on the inner and sometimes the outer of surface of the retina (Fig. 10.1).

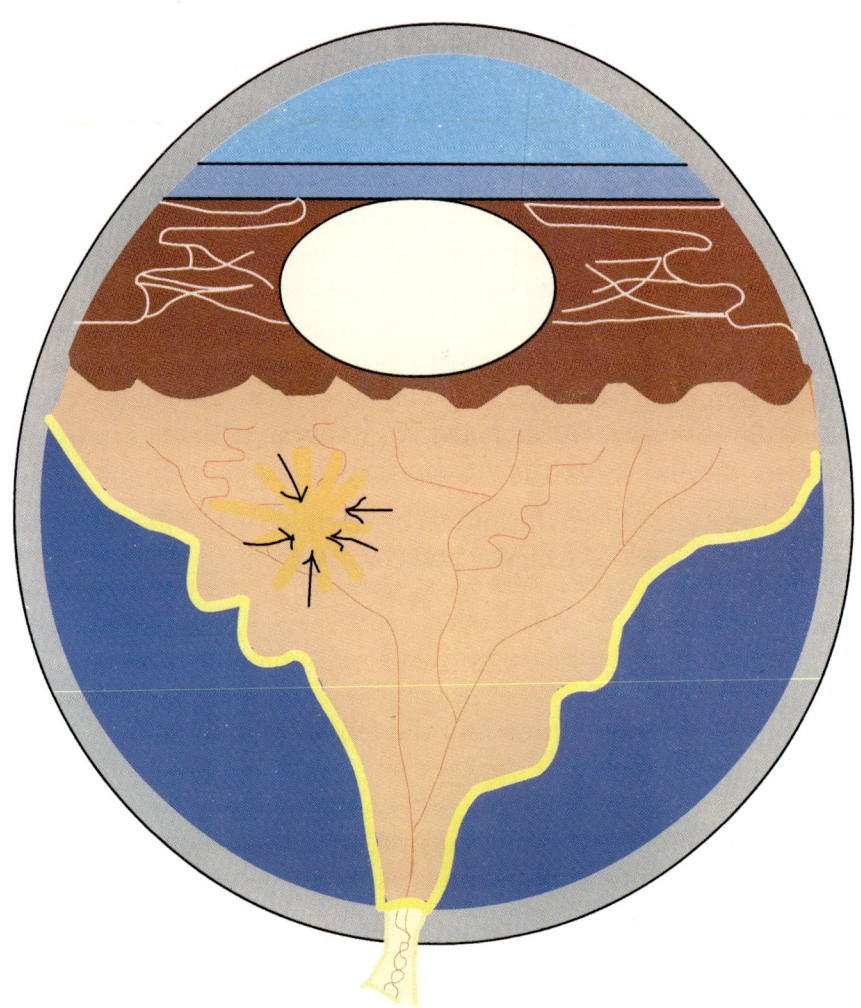

Fig. 10.1 *Growth of cellular membrane on the inner surface of retina*

At times there is contraction of membrane confined to the posterior pole, which has been called an exaggerated macular pucker (Fig. 10.2).

When the subretinal membrane produced contraction, it produced a ring that folds the retina just anterior to the disc, it has been termed as napkin ring configuration (Fig. 10.3).

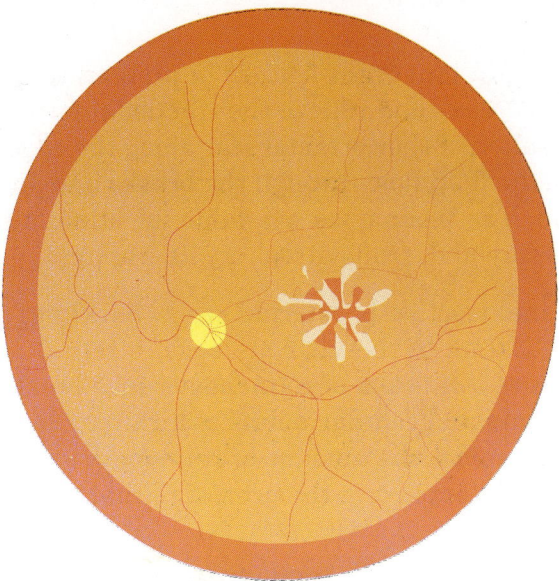

Fig. 10.2 Exaggerated macular pucker

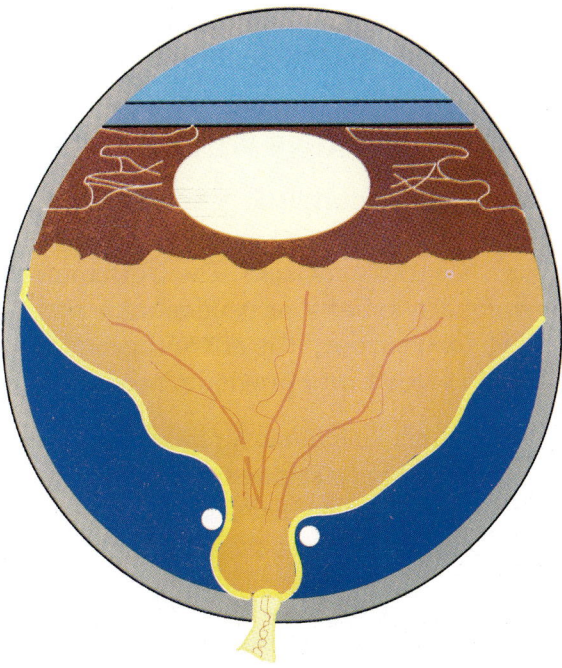

Fig. 10.3 Napkin ring configuration

Subretinal membrane may be difficult to detect because the overlying retina obscures them. In some cases membrane bridges the peripheral retina and the posterior surface of the iris creating iris retraction seen at the slit lamp.

PRINCIPLES OF TREATMENT OF PROLIFERATIVE VITREORETINOPATHY TO CLOSE ALL RETINAL BREAKS

Closer of the retinal breaks is an important feature in proliferative vitreoretinopathy surgery. The proper closure of all the breaks and relieve the tractional forces is generally consider necessary to stimulate the formation of chorioretinal scar along the edges of all retinal breaks. The purpose of closer is to block the fluid flow through the breaks and also produce strong adhesion between retina and choroid. The techniques available for stimulating localized chorioretinal scars are transcleral diathermy and, transvitreal cryotheraphy.

The ability to release retinal traction is external sclera buckling, peeling or segmentation of preretinal membrane, de-buckling of the vitreous base, internal tamponade, and relaxing retinectomies and retinotomies. All forms of retinopexy cause breakdown of the blood-ocular barrier and release of pigments and cellular debris, which may lead to development of proliferative vitreoretinopathy. Therefore the amount of retinopexy should be minimal and if cryotherapy is used, it should not be applied to the area of retinal pigment epithelium (RPE).

OPTIMAL TIME FOR OPERATION IN PROLIFERATIVE VITREORETINOPATHY

The timing of intervention should be performed after 4 to 6 weeks of developing proliferative vitreoretinopathy. Theoretically waiting for 4 to 6 weeks may jeopardize the health of the photoreceptors but it appears that preretinal membranes are easier to peel as a single sheet, thereby making the surgical procedure much easier to perform and possibly more effective.[3]

VITRECTOMY TECHNIQUE IN PROLIFERATIVE VITREORETINOPATHY

The routine 3-port vitrectomy instrumentation is preferred, with separable infusion cannula secured on the sclera by 6.0-vicryl sutures and the fiber optic light probe and the vitrectomy probe, each introduced through separable incision. The 3-circumferential pars plana incision is made 3 mm posterior to the limbus in aphakic or psudophakic and 4 mm posterior to the limbus in phakic eyes. If vitrectomy is done earlier, it is advantageous to make radial parsplana incision since these are less likely to extend into previous incision.

It is mandatory to remove crystalline lens in most phakic eyes, eventhough no significant lens opacities are present. This is done by phacofragmentation through the parsplana. There are advantages of removal of crystalline lens as visualization and tissue dissection in anterior peripheral part of the posterior segment and facilitates methods for fluid gas exchange become easier.

In cases where no retinal breaks are evident, in which traction from periretinal membrane appears to be the primary causes of the detachment or in cases where the location of retinal breaks is such that they cannot be sealed by scleral buckle alone, vitrectomy combined with scleral buckling are done.

The buckle 287 (explants) 7 mm wide is used and two mattress suture 5.0 (Alcon) are used in each quadrant to do intrascleral bites 3 mm apart (a total 10 mm apart) than the width of the silicone explants material. The broader scleral buckle is especially useful in large myopia eyes.

In eyes with pseudophakia, the intraocular lens is generally not removed because vitreous surgery can be performed without any difficulty. The vitrectomy probe is used to excise the central portion of the vitreous gel including the anterior vitreous surface in aphakic eyes. Attention is emphasised to dissect the peripheral anterior vitreous. It is easier to approach this region before relieving posterior traction, because the presence of posterior traction keeps the anterior fibrous tissue on stretch, allowing them to move easily for segmentation. The assistant and the contact lens in the other hand do either by cotton applicator or by scleral depressor in one hand the scleral depression. For a nice view of the periphery, the surgeon has to remove as much as vitreous possible in each quadrant. Care must be taken while removing the vitreous in vitreous base because excessive traction may lead to iatrogenic tears of the peripheral retina. Introduction of wide angle viewing system and vitreous shaver helps proper dissection of vitreous base and thereby expecting excellent results.

The posterior segment attention is given after removing anterior peripheral fibrous tissue. A vitreoretinal pick is used to identify and also it helps to separate the preretinal membrane on the retinal surface. The aim is to remove as much as the abnormal tissue as possible and to relieve tangential traction between retinal fold. The chance of iatrogenic tear is minimized if the retina pick is moved posterior to anterior manner. The rigid folded retina in the posterior pole thus becomes mobile allowing it to flatten more easily.

The peeling is best done from posterior to anterior direction, of course, the ability to remove the preretinal membrane varies from case to case. If the preretinal membrane is firmed with the retinal tissue, it can be separated with the help of intraocular scissor. As you know it is difficult to remove all preretinal tissue, particularly inferiorly a high, broad encircle buckle is used to offset the traction.

After completion of vitrectomy, all the retinal breaks are marked with diathermy because it is extremely difficult to identify many retinal tears after fluid-gas exchange. Before doing fluid-gas exchange, it is helpful to use blunt 20-gauge needle to aspirate subretinal fluid. If retinal breaks exist or existing retinal breaks are inaccessible because of anterior location, a posterior retinotomy is made. The retinotomy is positioned superior and usually nasal to the optic disc in an area of retina without residual traction. The retinotomy is marked with diathermy and this allows for easier penetration of a tapered, blunt needle at the time of retinotomy. The application of diathermy is also limits bleeding from the edge of the retinotomy.

MEMBRANE REMOVAL IN PROLIFERATIVE VITREORETINOPATHY

In a typical case of vitreoretinopathy, there is an anterior circumferential traction with multiple posterior star-fold in phakic eye (Fig. 10.4).

Once it is decided to remove the anterior portion of the vitreous tractional base, one has to remove the lens. After central vitreous is removed, the anterior vitreous (alone with any membrane attached to the ciliary's body is removed by using scleral depression (Fig.10.5).

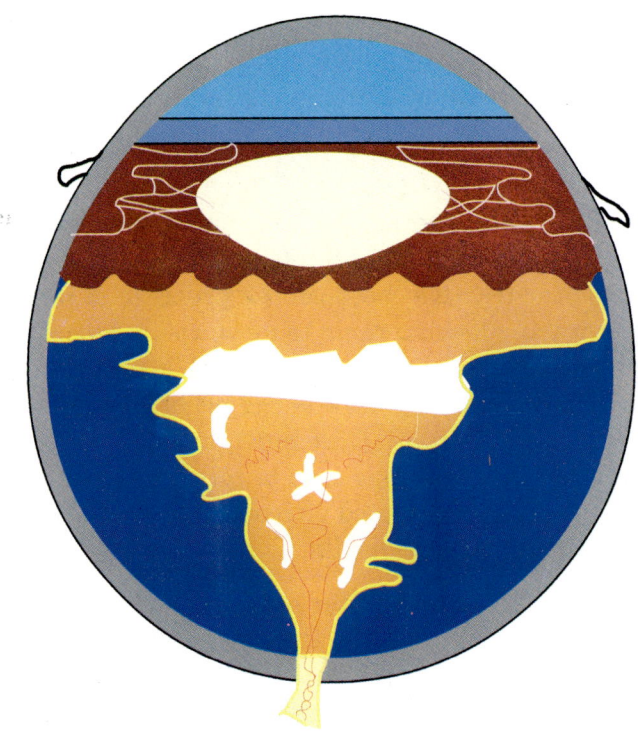

Fig. 10.4 *Multiple posterior star fold in phakic eye*

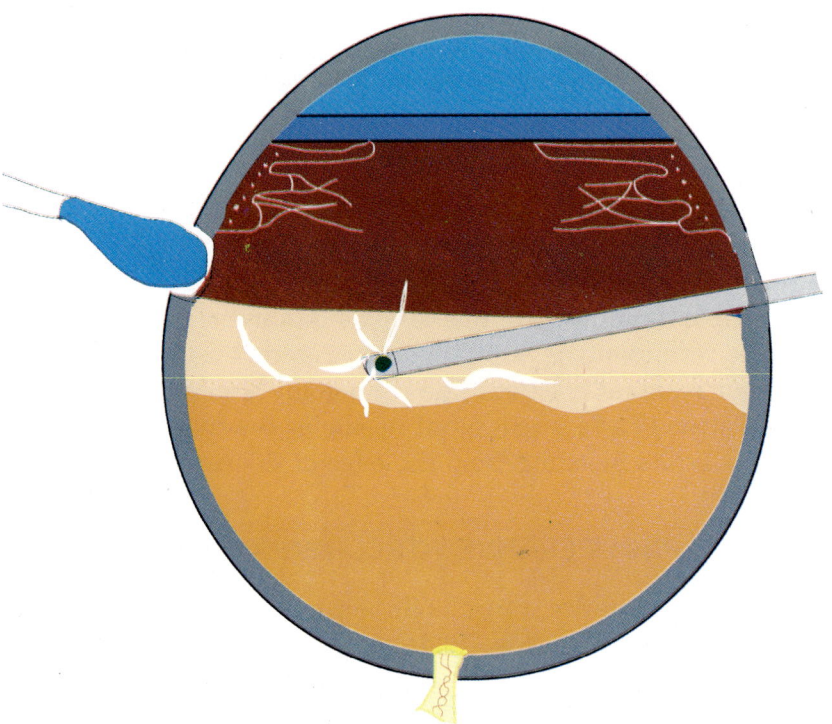

Fig. 10.5 *Lens is removed along with membrane attached to the ciliary body.*

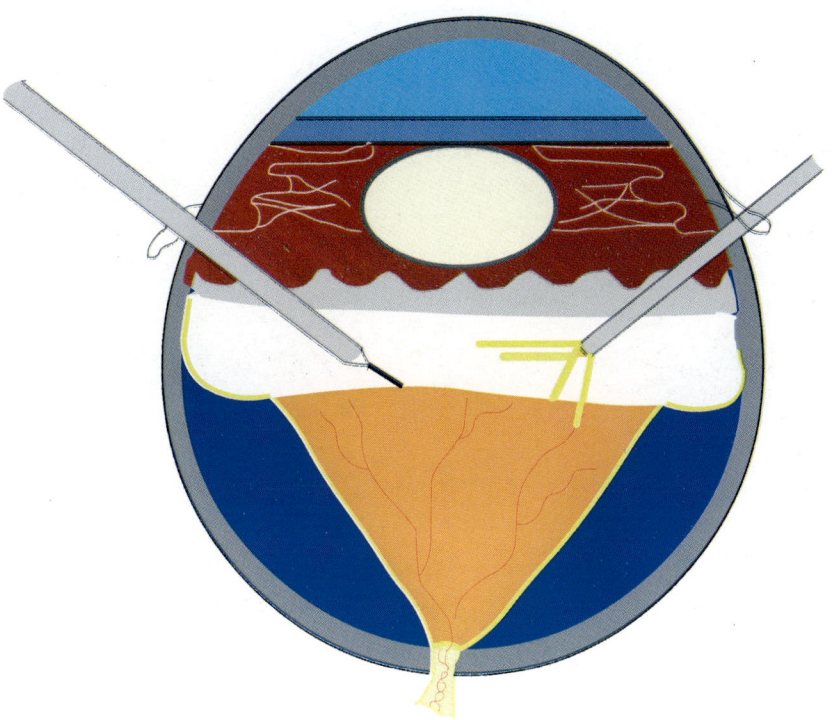

Fig. 10.6 *Membrane stripping from posterior to anterior direction*

The membrane stripping is done from posterior to anterior directions (Fig. 10.6).

This process stabilizes the anterior retina. In some cases a bimanual technique is helpful. In one hand the membrane is manipulate with a lighted pick, while the other approach the membrane with a pick, forceps or scissors. As membrane is peeled to the posterior vitreous base, it becomes so adherent to the retina that it cannot be separated any further. If traction remains, radial cuts may be made in fibrous component of the membrane when there is anterior loop traction exists, the vitreous base is pulled forward to create a taco-configuration. The opening of the taco may be covered with vitreous and membrane. The taco can be opened with the help of vertical scissor, allowing the retina to fall posteriorly.[4]

During manipulation, breaks may be created at the point of adherence of the retina and membrane. As described earlier, iatrogenic breaks may be marked with the internal diathermy, so they can be recognised, treated and after the retina is reattached.

In some advanced cases, in spite of meticulous dissection in the area of vitreous base, anterior–posterior or circumferential traction remains. This traction is sufficient to prevent reattachment. If this situation arises, retinectomy may be cosidered. The retina is treated with diathermy just posterior to the area of traction but as far as anterior is possible. With the help of vertical scissor a retinotomy is carried out as far as necessary to relieve traction on the posterior retina (Fig. 10.7).

In some cases, the residual anterior membrane is removed with cutting probe. Once the retina is flattened, the posterior edge of the retinotomy is treated high endolaser photocoagulation (Fig. 10.8).

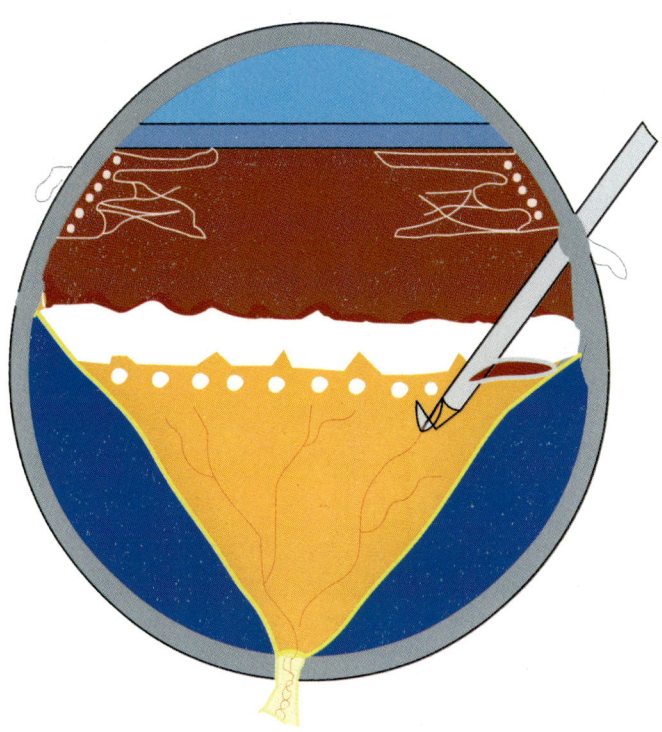

Fig. 10.7 *Diathermy followed by retinectomy*

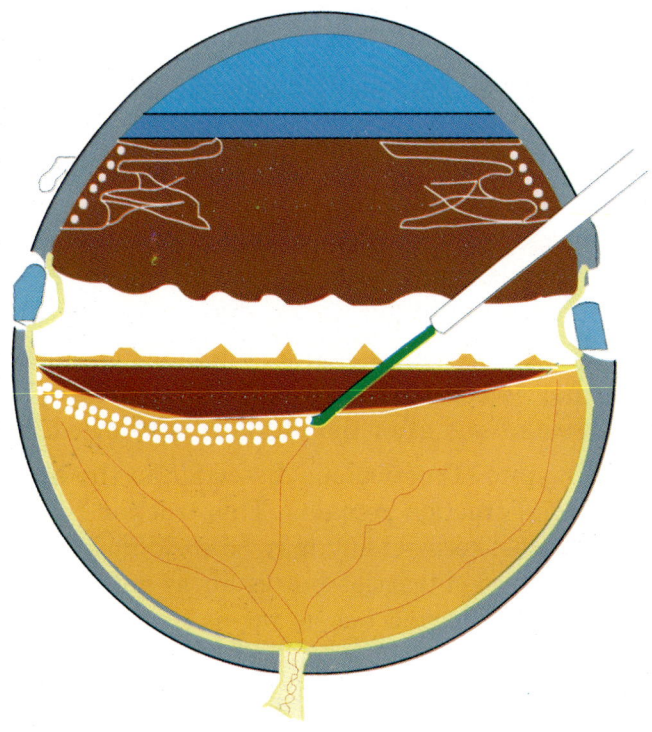

Fig. 10.8 *Retina is flattened and posterior edge treated with laser photocoagulation*

Posterior subretinal fibrosis is a tricky situation and it causes retinal redetachment. Diathermy is applied and retinotomy is performed over thick membrane area. Sometimes, the membrane is extensive and it is mandatory to remove. By the help of en-grapping forceps the membrane is pulled and it release the traction. During the membrane maneuver it may begin to create marked distortion of the retina and may lead to iatrogenic breaks. Giving lateral forces with less displacement of the retina can minimize this. In some of the cases side-to-side motion often will break membrane to retina attachment with less traction on the retina then with posterior to anterior force.

Lightened pick is used to separate the membrane and membrane is grasped with forceps to separate from the retina. When the membrane is separated from the retina it can be removed by the help of cutting probe under the membrane with the part up to protect the retina. In this situation the maximum cutting speed is desirable. When the membrane produces star folds, this membrane is engaged with the help of either pick or microvitreoretinal blade or are pulled lateral to the surface of the retina to release traction.

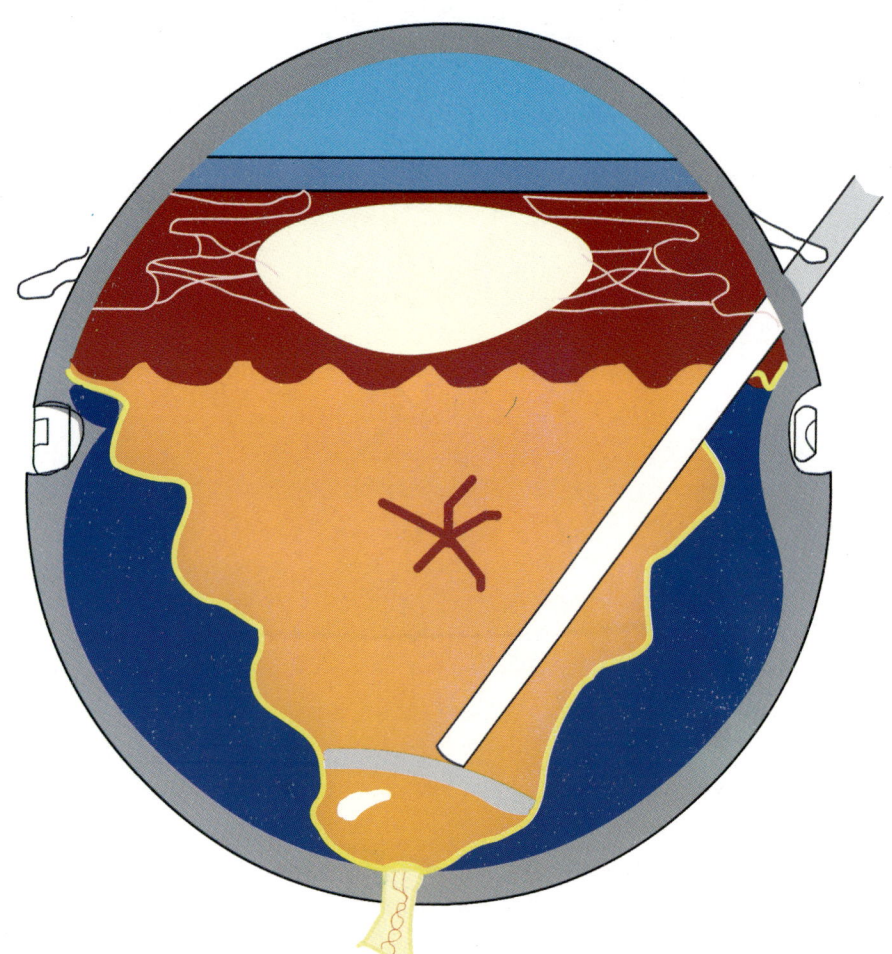

Fig. 10.9 *Perfluorocarbon injected over the optic disc to flatten retina*

MEMBRANE REMOVAL WITH PERFLUROCARBON TECHNIQUE IN PROLIFERATIVE VITREORETINOPATHY

In case of severe proliferative vitreoretinopathy, perfluorocarbon liquid can be used   to aid membrane dissection[5] (Fig. 10.9).

In this case, posterior membrane is dissected first and then perfluorocarbon is used to stabilize the posterior retina while anterior membrane is dissected. Small amount of perfluorocarbon is injected over the disk to flatten the retina, as it flattens, the tractional area is identified (Fig. 10.10).

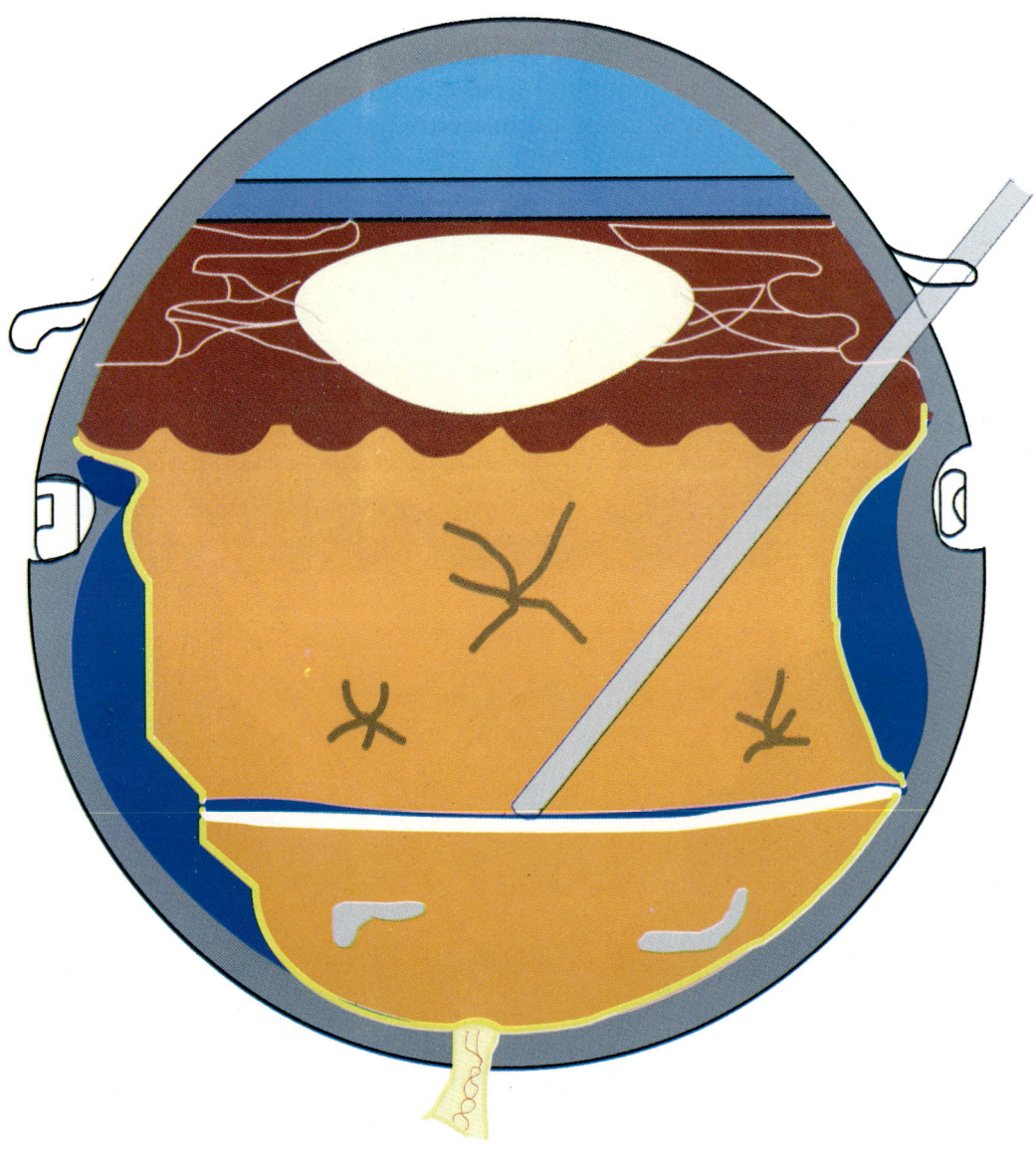

Fig. 10.10 *Retina is stabilized and flattened*

The star-fold are opened by engaging membrane in the center of the fold while anterior-membrane stripping is done and in this situation one can inject more perfluorocarbon to flatten greater area of the retina.

Once the retina is flattened, the help of wide-angle system up to the buckle area may visualize the whole retina. As the anterior-traction is relieved: the retina will be flattened posteriorly an on the buckle. While injecting perfluorocarbon one must be careful not to inject more than the level of the break, because it can migrate into the subretinal surface.[6] After drainage of the subretinal fluid, laser endophotocoagulation is done to treat the breaks (Fig. 10.11). Once this procedure is finished, the perfluorocarbon is removed by active or passive suction and is replaced by silicone oil as long-term tamponade.[7]

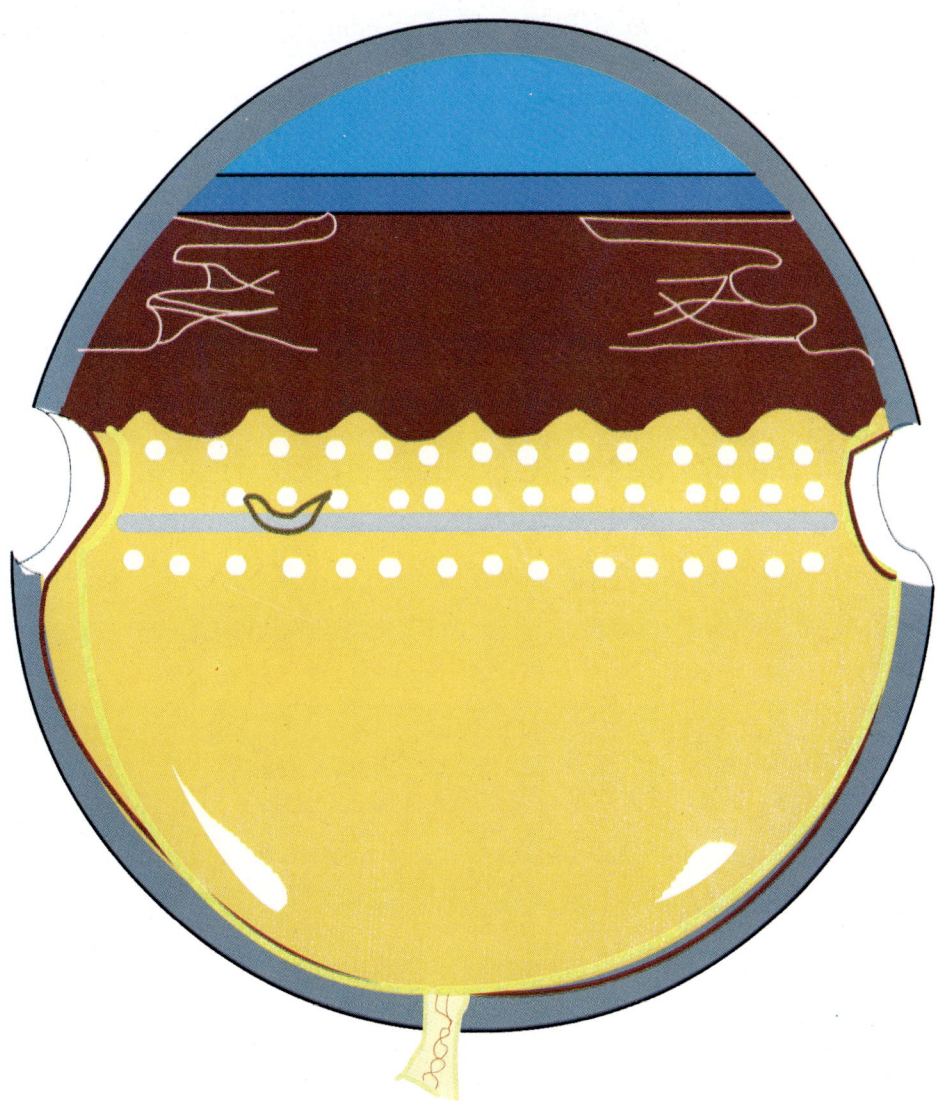

Fig. 10.11 *Laser photocoagulation is used to treat breaks after subretinal fluid drainage*

REFERENCES

1. Charles S: *Vitreous microsurgery* : Baltimore, Williams and Wilkins, 1981.

2. Machemer R, Aaberg Tm, Freeman HM et al.: An updated classification of retinal detachment with proliferative vitreoretinopathy. *Am J Ophthalmol* 112: 159-165, 1991.

3. Abrams GW et al: Vitrectomy with silicone oil or long acting gas in eyes with severe proliferative vitreoretinopathy. Results of additional and long term follow up. Silicone study Report 11. *Arch Ophthalmol* 115: 335, 1997.

4. Lean JS et al: Management of complex retinal detachments by vitrectomy and fluid/ silicone exchange. *Trans Ophthalmol Soc UK* 102: 204, 1982.

5. Chang S, Ozmert E, Zimmerman NJ: Intraoperative perfluorocarbon liquids in the management of proliferative vitreoretinopathy. *Am J Ophthalmol* 106: 668, 1988.

6. Peymom GA, Schulman JA, Sullivan B: Perfluorocarbon liquid in ophthalmology Survy. *Ophthalmol* 39: 375, 1995

7. Silicone study group: Vitrectomy with silicone oil or perfluoropropone gas in eyes with severe proliferative vitreoretinopathy results of randomized trial silicone study report. *Arch Ophthalmol* 110: 780, 1992.

Management of Ocular Trauma and Retained Intraocular Foreign Bodies

Introduction

In ocular trauma, the ophthalmologist must take an exact medical history first. The case history enables one to determine the position of intraocular foreign body for its contamination. Some time it may be helpful in determining the extent and degree of blunt injuries of the ocular tissues.

Careful examination should reveal the assessment of the visual function of the eye. Prognosis is better when there is good light projection. But it happens some time in cases where there in no light perception at all, the eye may recover with some visual function. It in better to repair and wait several days for chances of visual recovery.[1]

The eye should be examined with indirect ophthalmoscopy, and slit lamp. Difficulty arises in the presences of hazy media caused by a traumatic cornea, hyphaema, cataract or vitreous haemorrhage. In all such cases a plain x-ray orbit with posterior anterior and lateral views should be obtained. This test identifies retained intraocular foreign body as well as indicates multiple foreign bodies.

Ultrasonography (A+B Scan) plays an important role in the management of ocular trauma. It gives accurate information about the location of the foreign body as well as the presences of vitreous haemorrhage, posterior vitreous detachment or retinal detachment if any.

However, it has its limitations i.e. it should be used very cautiously in the presence of a large open wound or a recently repaired wound. Also it can miss a small foreign body. MRI is best avoided in the presence of a suspected metallic foreign body. But CT scan of higher resolution and smaller cuts should be done in difficult cases.

WOUND CLOSURE

Wound closure should be done under general anaesthesia using microsurgical control and techniques because the extent of wound plays a role in the prognosis. It is necessary to close the wound in the cornea and the sclera. If there is a scleral wound behind the insertion line of an extraocular muscle, an encircling band procedure is performed in order to reduce the risk of post-traumatic retinal detachment.

A perforating injury to the globe occurs when there is both an anterior entry site, created by missile or sharp object and a posterior exit site. The posterior exit site is usually obscured by haemorrhage, and finding a foreign body behind the globe by imaging studies makes the diagnosis. Initial management is to close the anterior wound but to allow the posterior wound to heal without closure because attempting to close very posterior wounds usually causes extrusion of intraocular contents.

TIMING OF SURGERY

In case of penetrating injury of the posterior segment with a vitreous haemorrhage, 2 step surgery should be undertaken. Repair of the wound closure should be done in first stage. If there is vitreous haemorrhage, posterior vitreous detachment will occur after 1st to 2 weeks. From the surgical point of view, the required vitreous surgery can be performed much more easily after 1 to 2 weeks.

The vitreous often remains adherent to the retina on the side of the eye closest to the exit so there is no separation between the exit site and the vitreous base.[2] From the technical point of view, the needed vitreous surgery can be performed much more easily when there is posterior detachment, which usually occurs after 7 to10 days duration. Attempting foreign body removed at the time of repair may have problem like incomplete work-up and absence of posterior vitreous detachment. Delaying surgery beyond 2 weeks might cause fibro ocular proliferation along the tract of the injury, which may further lead to tractional or combined retinal detachment.

THE ROLE OF INFECTION IN TIMING OF SURGERY

If an infection is suspected, one must carefully evaluate the clinical sign that help us to identify infection, such as patient's pain, red eye, and swollen conjunctiva. The foreign body must be removed if an infection is suspected, and vitrectomy must be performed with injection of antibiotics in the vitreous cavity during the same surgical session. But if infection can be excluded, it is much easier to remove the attached vitreous from the retina after one to two weeks. Removing the attached vitreous earlier is very difficult even for an experienced surgeon and can cause additional retinal damaged. The vitreous base is often damaged and contraction later may cause detachment from anterior breaks, a prophylactic buckle is recommended.

RISK OF INTRAOPERATIVE HAEMORRHAGE

The risk of intraoperative intraocular haemorrhage is as much as three times higher in the first week than in the second week of penetrating injury. Therefore, it is easier to perform wound closure and vitrectomy as two step procedure.

In cases of severe posterior segment trauma, the successful surgery requires that the vitreous be removed from retina and from the wound. If fibroplastic ingrowth occurs, it can lead later to proliferative vitreoretinopathy (PVR) and also anterior segments cicatrisation. Shrinkage of the anterior segment can especially be observed after severe concussion injuries of the eye such as after an explosion.

One should not perform primary anterior segment surgery with intraocular implantation before the opinion of posterior segment surgeon. This may impede subsequent vitreoretinal surgery. Only if the posterior segment is not involved and if larger retinal wounds can be excluded primary implantation of an intraocular lens may be indicated.

In cases where both the anterior and posterior segments are injured, it is preferable, if possible, for an experienced anterior segment surgeon to work together. What can be achieved when two surgeons from these specialties cooperate is amazing.

VITRECTOMY ENDOLASER SILICONE OIL TAMPONADE

Visualizing the retina is the primary objective for performing vitrectomy in cases in which there is a vitreous hemorrhage or to expose a large foreign body or large retinal injury. Removal of the vitreous haemorrhage is essential to reduce the postoperative risk of proliferative vitreoretinopathy (PVR). Retinal injury must be treated at the end of the surgery by endolaser, which is less traumatic than cryosurgery. If the injury is not too large and without any traction, air-injection into the vitreous may be sufficient. In hopeless cases primary vitrectomy and silicone oil injection should be tried as it reduces the circulation of proliferative vitreoretinopathy stimulating factors like, blood, platelets, etc. After the blood ocular barrier is stabilized, severe hypotony is avoided and good view of the fundus is possible.[3] Eye filled with silicone oil is now accepted worldwide for these severe cases.

REMOVAL OF FOREIGN BODIES

In general, all intraocular foreign bodies should be removed, especially the reactive one. Even a non-reactive foreign body carries the risk of infection and mechanical damage, so it must be removed. In the past year the authors had to remove an iron foreign body using strong magnets. It is no more used as it produces more retinal damage than the injury. The removal of small foreign body with an external magnet still requires, the skill of an experienced surgeon since it can be difficult to determine in what precise location to remove the foreign body. The safest way now is over the pars plana route.

THE ROLE OF VITRECTOMY

All iron (ferromagnetic) foreign bodies longer than 2 mm in diameter in which there is vitreous haemorrhage and the posterior retina cannot be visualized should be removed by vitrectomy.

The advantages of this procedure in that removal of the foreign body in under precise control in all phases.

Moreover, intraocular blood, which we have previously emphasized stimulates proliferative vitreoretinopathy (PVR), can also be removed as well as vitreous strands that can act as a scaffold for subsequent fibrosis. This fibrosis may cause subsequent tract ional retinal detachment.

TECHNIQUES OF INTRAOCULAR FOREIGN BODY REMOVAL

Currently almost all intraocular foreign bodies are removed by pars plana vitrectomy technique. A standard three port pars plana vitrectomy is performed (Step 1) The foreign body is lifted from the retina using an intraocular electromagnet and transferred to a foreign body forceps for a firm grip. It is then taken out of the eye. This technique needs several modifications like enlargement of port size with micro vitreoretinopathy (MVR) blade to facilitate the introduction of foreign body forceps. All the steps involved in the procedure (Step 1 to 7) are depicted and explained in Figs 11.1 to 11.7.

STEP 1

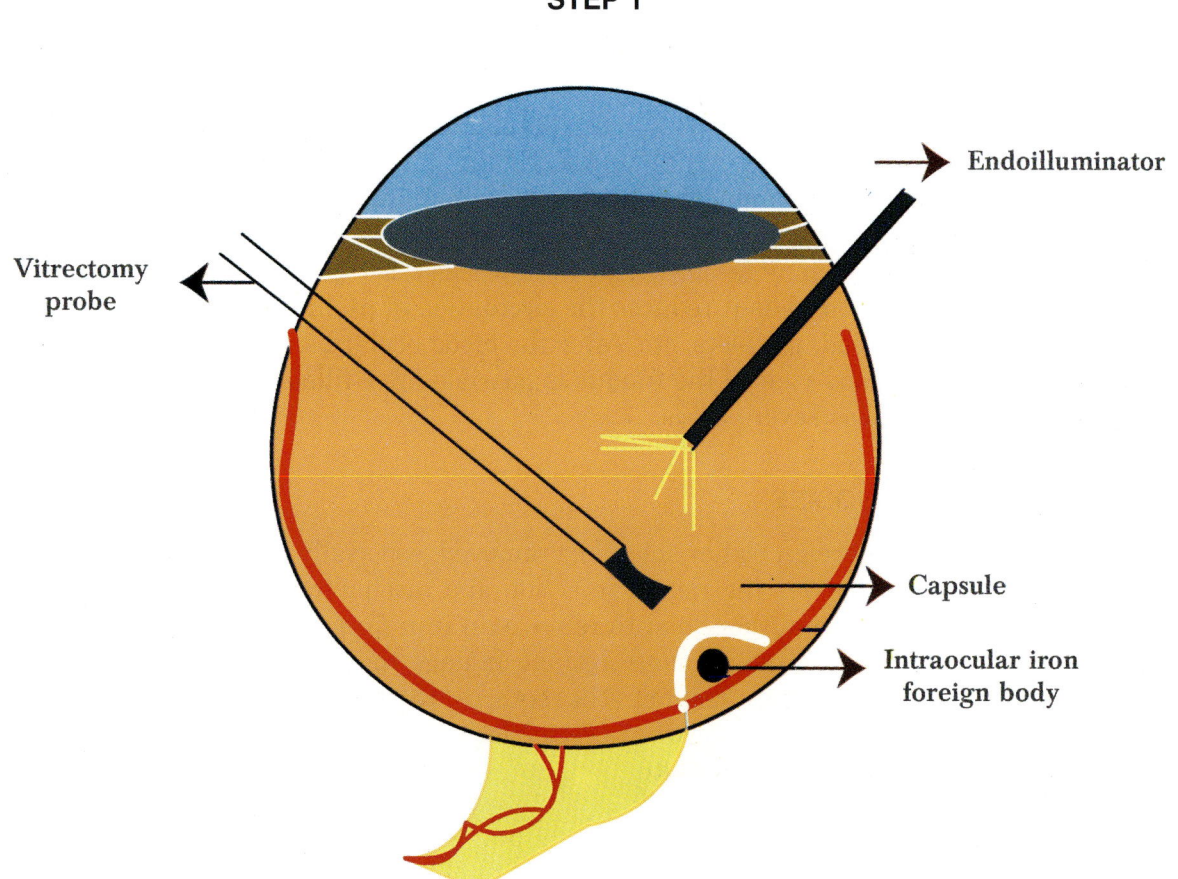

Fig. 11.1 Three ports standard vitrectomy

STEP 2

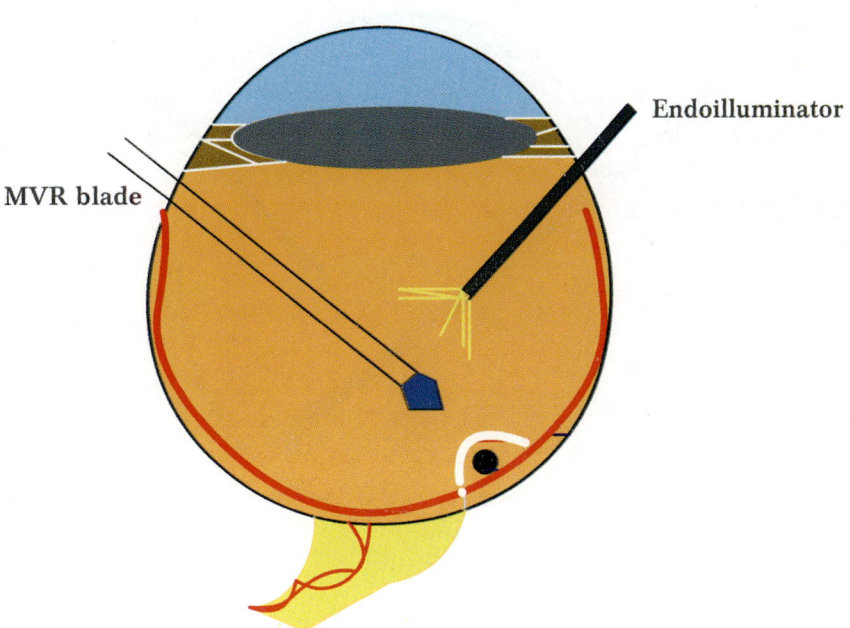

Fig. 11.2 *Cutting of the capsule by MVR blade*

STEP 3

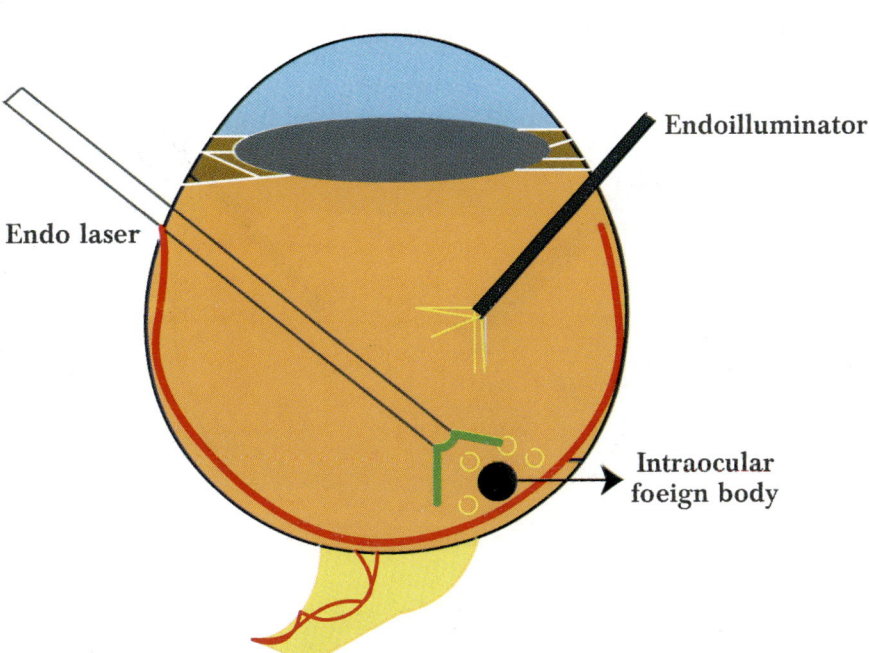

Fig. 11.3 *Endolaser to prevent detachment*

STEP 4

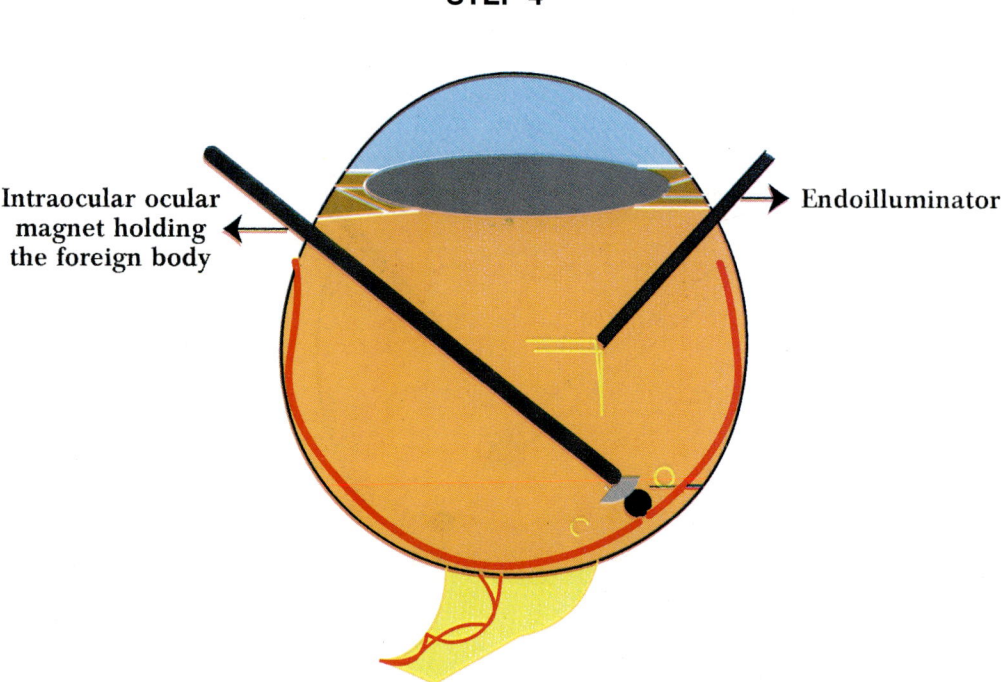

Intraocular ocular
magnet holding
the foreign body

Endoilluminator

Fig. 11.4 *Use of intraocular magnet to remove intraocular foreign body*

STEP 5

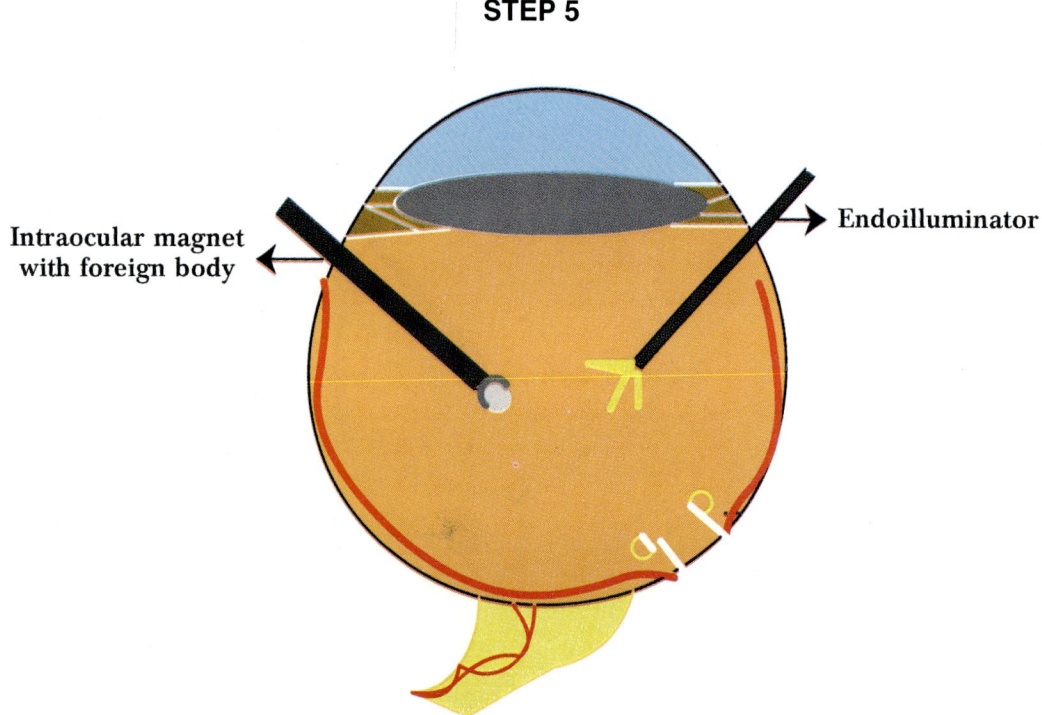

Intraocular magnet
with foreign body

Endoilluminator

Fig.11.5 *Intraocular iron foreign body removed through pars plana*

STEP 6

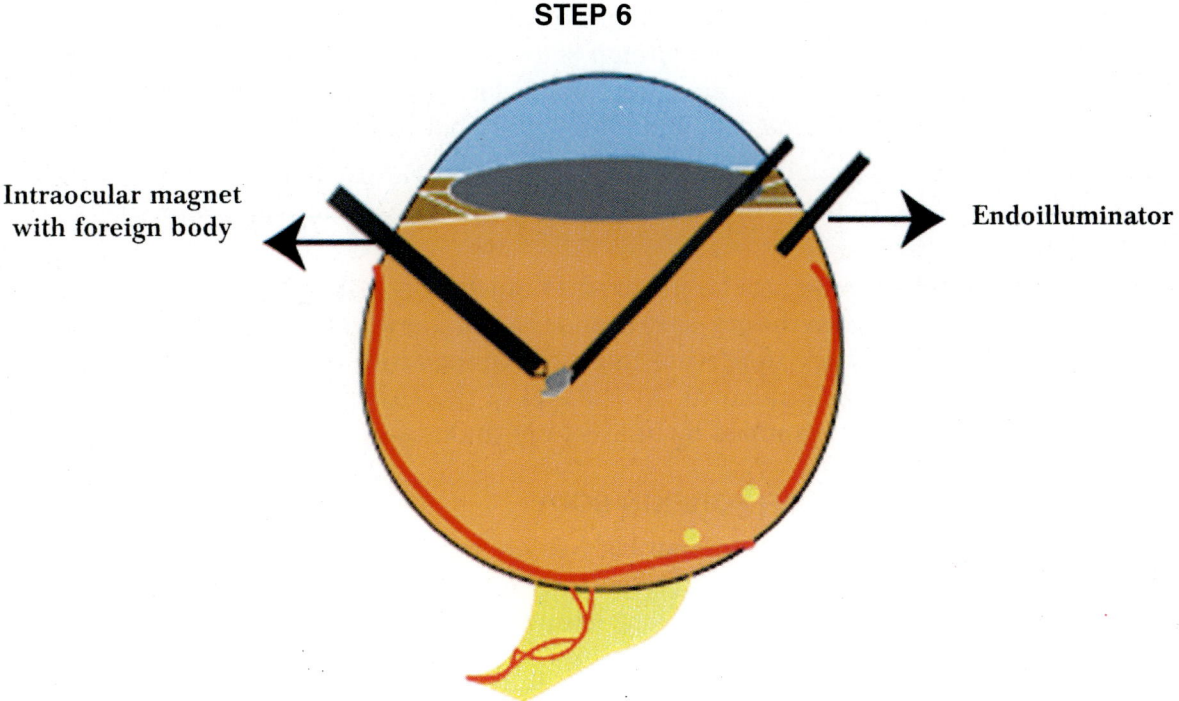

Fig. 11.6 *Bigger iron body removed by gripping technique*

STEP 7

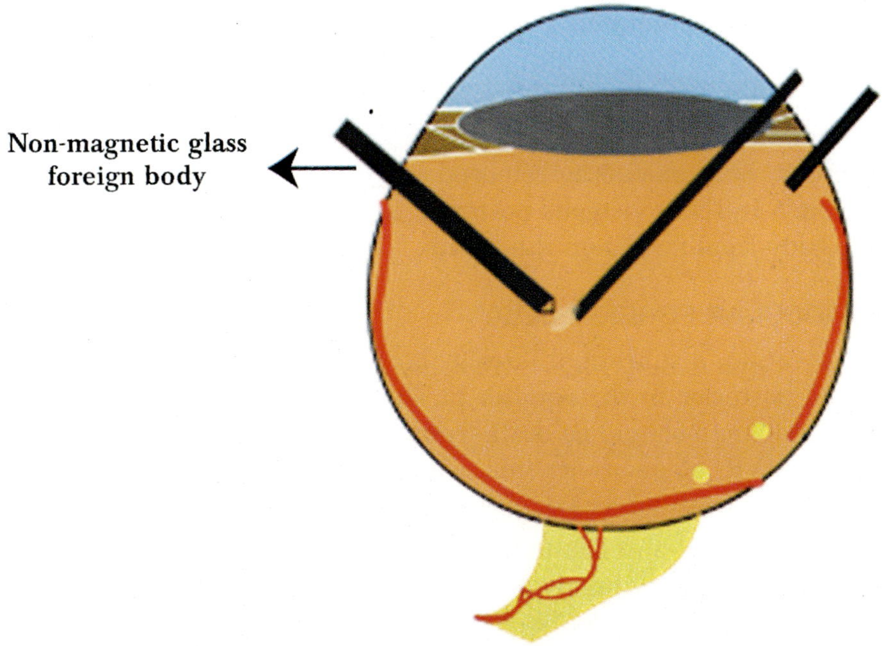

Fig. 11.7 *Non-magnet foreign body grasped directly by foreign body forceps.*

In case of non-magnetic foreign body, it might have to be grasped directly with a foreign body forceps (Fig. 11.7). After the removal of foreign body, the ports need to be spurred with an 8.0-vicryl sutures to bring back to its original 20G size before proceeding further. It is now mandatory to create a posterior vitreous detachment if it dose not exist.

This is achieved by using high suction or a pick. This procedure helps in completing removal of vitreous by which it prevents epiretinal membrane formation and proliferative vitreoretinopathy.

The anterior vitreous should also be removed as much as possible. It is always preferable to use an encircling band between the ora serrate and the equator to give a support. Perfluorocarbon (PFCL) is some time necessary to prevent macular damage in the event of an accidental slippage of the foreign body while removal. At the end of the surgery, the sclera needs to be indented 360° with band and examined by indirect ophthalmoscopy to rule out any dialysis.

LARGE RETINAL INTRAOCULAR FOREIGN BODY

One can try to extract up to 5 mm foreign body safely through the pars plana route. A limbal approach should be used in the case a foreign body measuring more than 5 mm in size, in an aphakic patient. In phakic patient with clear lens, the pars plana approach should be used for a foreign body up to 7 mm in size. If the foreign body is bigger than 7 mm, then the lens need to be scarified, and the foreign body extracted through the limbal route.

ENCAPSULATED RIOFB

In case of encapsulated intraocular foreign body it should be first surrounded by multiple rows of endophotocoagulation. The capsule usually opened up by using a microvitreoretinal (MVR) blade. Intraocular magnet may be required to lift it out and later it can be transferred to the foreign body forceps (griping technique).

RETAINED IOFB - IN THE VITREOUS CAVITY

In this situation, standard pars plana three-port vitrectomy should be performed anterior to the foreign body. Foreign body should be removed with the help of foreign body forceps after completion of vitrectomy. Initially vitreous posterior to the foreign body acts as a cushion and prevents the foreign body from falling on the retina.

SUBRETINAL INTRAOCULAR FOREIGN BODY

In the presence of flat retina, a subretinal intraocular foreign body will be found at the site of impact. If it is located posterior to the equator, it should be surrounded by multiple rows of endophotocoagulation. The site should be diathermized using endo-diathermy and by the help of a microvitreoretinal (MVR) blade or vitreous scissors is used to remove the overlying retina. The foreign body is grasped with forceps or lifted out with intraocular magnet.

If the foreign body is located anterior to the equator, then an external approach should be used .By the help of indirect ophthalmoscope one should localize the foreign body and sclerotomy should be made after using external diathermy. The under lying choroids should also be diathermized before using foreign body forceps or an external magnet. 8 0 vicryl should suture sclerotomy , and a scleral buckle should be applied.[4]

In presence of retinal detachment, an iatrogenic retinal break (retinotomy) should be created. The foreign body should be grasped with forceps and taken out. Fluid air exchange should be performed to flatten the retina. Some cases might need silicone oil injection or long-acting gases for internal tamponade. Retinopexy is mandatory for retina breaks.

GLASS AND OTHER FOREIGN BODIES

Nonmagnetic and non-copper containing intraocular foreign bodies, the surgeon must be individualizing the treatment plan. If aluminium, one can often wait. Glass foreign bodies if not contaminated, that may well tolerate, as glass is an inert material, which usually tolerated by the eye.[5]

Some time it is difficult to remove glass foreign bodies, especially in eyes with vitreous hemorrhage in which good view of the fundus impossible.

However, it is noticed that glass foreign bodies with sharp edges can cause delayed retinal detachment. Glass foreign bodies with attached retina, patient can remain under observation.

Before the introduction of vitrectomy, the ophthalmologist had to remove the foreign body through external route and wait, hoping that no retinal detachment would occur. Removing of the vitreous haemorrhage could not be performed but after introduction of vitrectomy it provides better approach to managing intraocular penetrating trauma. After primary repair, surgeon can expose retinal injuries and foreign bodies and remove them under microscopic control, as performs prophylactic measures to prevent post-traumatic retinal detachment.

REPAIR OF SCLERAL LACERATION, RUPTURES AND PROGNOSIS

The most important step in repairing scleral laceration and identification of scleral ruptures of the injured site. The conjunctiva is dissected: taking care not to put pressure on the globe. The majority of lacerations occur at the limbus; the next most common area is in between the muscle insertions. More than 75% of ruptures occur superiorly. Due to edematous of conjunctiva it should be is retracted for proper visualization. It is evident that most rupture does not extrude the vitreous, because the choroid is more elastic than the sclera. When the vitreous is protruding through the wound it should not be pulled from the eye because anterior rupture and lacerations are close to the vitreous base and traction may tear the retina.

LOCATIONS AND EXTENT OF PENETRATING INJURIES RELATED TO PROGNOSIS

It has been seen that injury limited to the cornea have the best prognosis and better than non-extensive cornea-scleral involvement. When there is cornea-scleral injury and it extend posteriorly, the prognoses is worse. However when the injury involved the sclera and limited to the anterior to the rectus muscle insertion have better prognosis than injury extending further posterior. Posterior extension involving equator have less favorable prognosis. The worst prognosis when there is double perforation.

The danger zone is the area extends between the limbus and the equator. Secondary complication occurs in penetrating injury with incarceration of the vitreous, which subsequently develops cyclitic membrane with fibrenous tissue and causes tangential retina traction on the peripheral retina and sometimes-proliferative vitreoretinopathy.

PROLIFERATIVE VITREORETINOPATHY (PVR) IN OCULAR TRAUMA

Proliferation vitreoretinopathy presents a challenge to the vitreoretinal surgeon. The risk of proliferation of vitreoretinopathy depends upon the breakdown of the blood ocular barrier, inflammatory reactions, blood inside the eye, an extended wound and incarceration of vitreous in the wound.

Results are usually satisfactory when there is planned surgery by performing microsurgical wound closure followed by vitrectomy and intraocular tamponade as previously described. The risk of proliferative vitreoretinopathy is greatest in young patients who are precisely the most frequent patients with severe trauma.[6]

SURGERY OF PVR IN PENETRATING TRAUMA

Proliferative vitreoretinopathy is usually tackled by modern vitrectomy techniques. The most important area is the vitreous base. Vitreous base incarceration and contraction may lead to redetachment. It is mandatory, during vitrectomy the periphery of the fundus must be indented by scleral depressors and visualized and all tractions and proliferations must be removed from the peripheral retina.

Fibrovascular proliferation may occur due to injury to the choroids and the pigment epithelium where subretinal strands may develop. The best way to remove subretinal stands by performing a peripheral retinotomy large enough to visualize the posterior surface of the retina. In this kind of advanced surgery, the temporary use of intraoperative perfluorocarbon (PFCL) is very helpful.

Moreover, incarcerated retina must be severed from the incarcerated wound even by means of extended retinotomy, if necessary. Whenever there is proliferative vitreoretinopathy (PVR), the surgeon must emphasize to the patient that at least two procedures are necessary. First the surgery and then silicone oil removal as second procedure later on. In modern era vitrectomy has provided a dramatically different and better approach to managing intraocular penetrating trauma. Overall microsurgical approaches are necessary for precise recognition and saving the vital tissues. It allows better closure of lacerated wound by use of fine stitching materials.

Vitrectomy has given the capability to clear up the mess created by ocular trauma. The mixture of blood, vitreous, lens matter, uveal pigments and contaminants introduced by perforating object is capable of causing endophthalmitis. It can be more easily removed by use of vitrectomy cutters through pars plana route.

REFERENCES

1. Coleman DJ, Lucas BE, Randeau MJ, and changes : management of IOFB. *Ophthalmology* 94: 1647, 1987.
2. Williams DF Miller Wf, Abrams GW, and Lewis H: Results and prognostic factors in penetrating ocular injuries with retained intraocular foreign bodies. *Ophthalmoscopy*, 95: 911, 1988.
3. Michels, RG: Vitrectomy methods in penetrating ocular trauma. *Ophthalmology* 87: 629, 1980.
4. Slushar, MM, Sarin LK, and Federman JL management of intra retinal foreign bodies. *Am J. Ophthalmol* 80: 838, 1975.
5. Hutton, WH, Sunder, WB and Vaiser, a surgical removal of non-magnetic foreign bodies. *Am. J. Ophthalmol* 80: 838, 1975.
6. Peyman GA et al: Vitrectomy in the management of intraocular foreign bodies and their complications. *Br J Ophthalmol* 64: 476, 1980.

Retinopathy of Prematurity (ROP)

Introduction

Retinopathy of prematurity is an abnormal proliferative retinopathy, which affects pre-term infants exposed to high oxygen concentration. Improved neonatal care offered to premature infants with low birth weight. Now survival chances are more than in the past. Prematurity, low birth weight and oxygen administration have been identified as some of the major risk factor associated with retinopathy of prematurity (ROP).

PATHOGENESIS

The retina is unique among the tissue in that it has no blood vessels until the fourth month of gestation, at which time vascular complexes come from the hyaloid vessels at the optic disc, which grow towards the periphery. Some of these vessels reach the nasal periphery after 8 months of gestation, although they do not reach the temporal periphery until about 4 weeks after delivery. This incomplete vascularized temporal retina is susceptible to high concentration oxygen damage, especially in the pre-term infant.

CLASSIFICATION

The international classification for retinopathy of prematurity (ROP) (ICROP) and cryotheraphy for retinopathy of prematurity (ROP) trial (CRYO-ROP trial) have enabled setting up of guide lines to decide on treatment of retinopathy of prematurity.[1]

Retinopathy of prematurity is classified by the zone of the eye involved and by the extend of disease (Fig. 12.1).

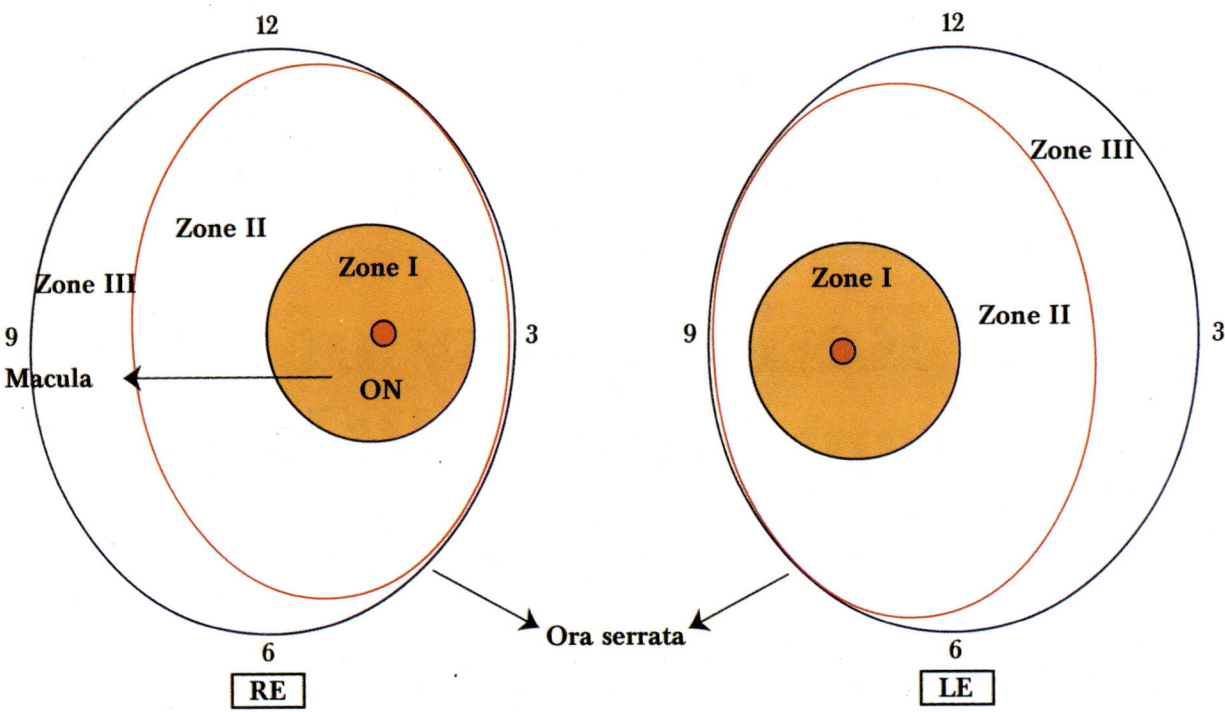

Fig. 12.1 *Borders of zones and clock hours to describe location and extent of ROP*

Zone I   It is bound by a circle whose radius is twice the distance from the disc to the macula.

Zone II   It extends from the boarder of zone I peripherally to a point tangential to the nasal oraserrata and includes a circular area centered on the disc bounded temporally near equator.

Zone III It is the residual crescent of the retina anterior to zone II.

The extend is determined by the number of clock hours involved.

STAGING

Staging is as follows:

Stage 1: Demarcation line

There is a thin structure that separates vascularised retina posteriorly from avascular retina anteriorly. This is the first path gnomonic of a thin, tortuous, grayish-white line, which runs roughly parallel with the ora-serrata (Fig.12.2).

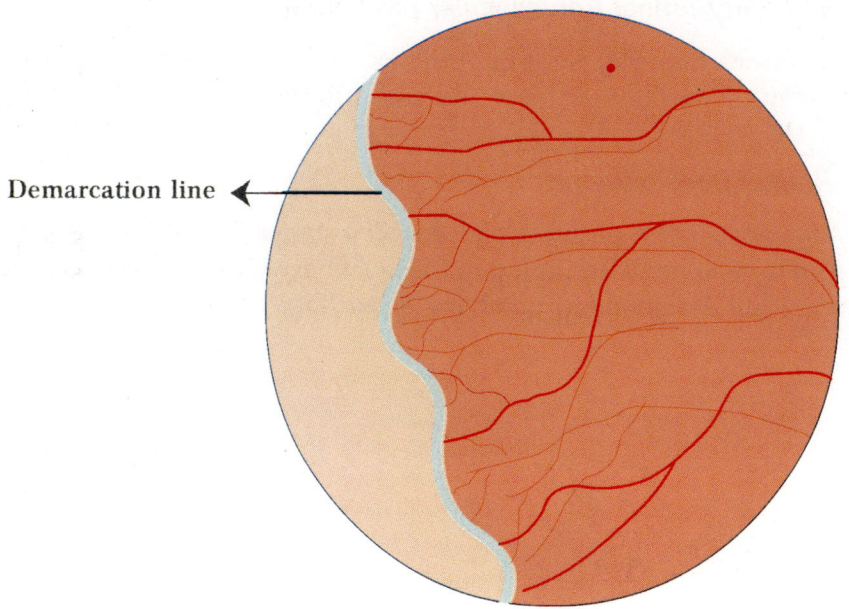

Fig. 12.2 *Diagrammatic representation showing demarcation line*

Stage 2: Ridge

If retinopathy of prematurity (ROP) progresses, the demarcation line develops into ridge of tissue which extant out of the plane of the retina. Blood vessels enter the ridge and small isolated neovascular tufts may be seen posterior to it (Fig 12.3).

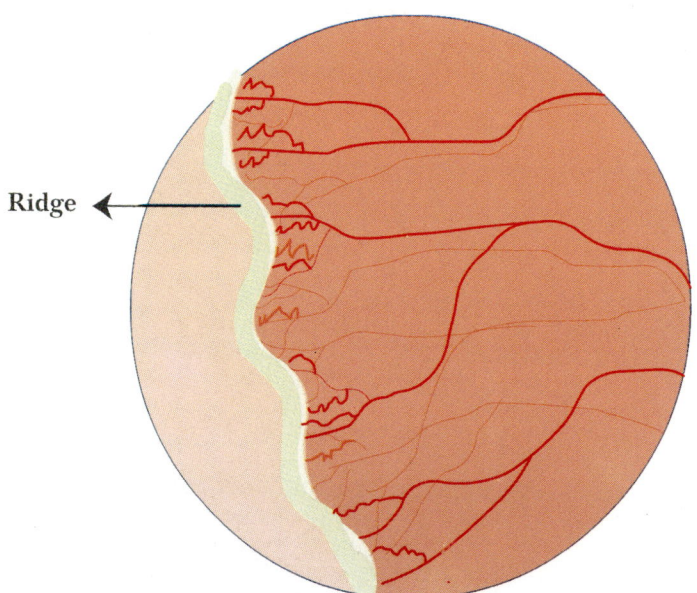

Fig. 12.3 *Diagrammatic representation showing ridge*

Stage 3: Ridge with Extra-retinal fibrovascular proliferation

As the disease progresses the ridge becomes pink as a result of the development of fibrovascular proliferation along the surface of the retina and into the vitreous (Fig. 12.4).

Stage 4: Partial Retinal Development

Unequivocal development of the retina is added to 3rd stage. This stage is subdivided into 4 A, a concave tractional development occurring in the periphery without involvement of the macula and 4 B, a partial retina development involving fovea (Fig. 12.5).

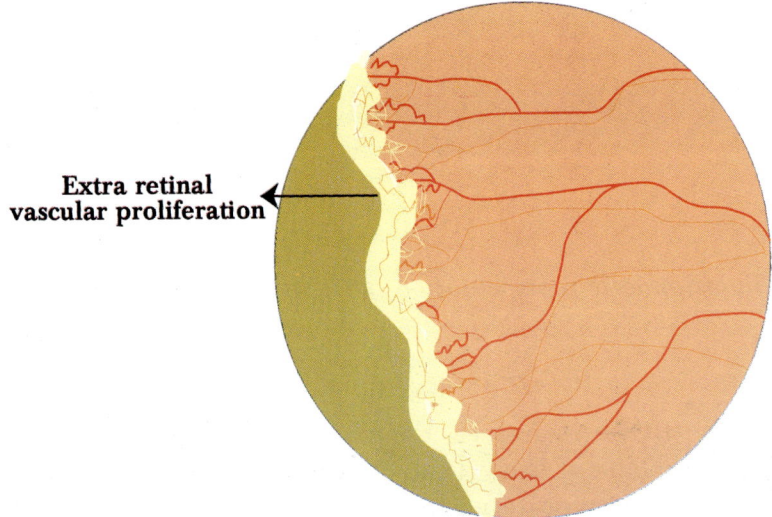

Extra retinal vascular proliferation

Fig. 12.4 *Diagrammatic representation showing extraretinal fibrovascular proliferation*

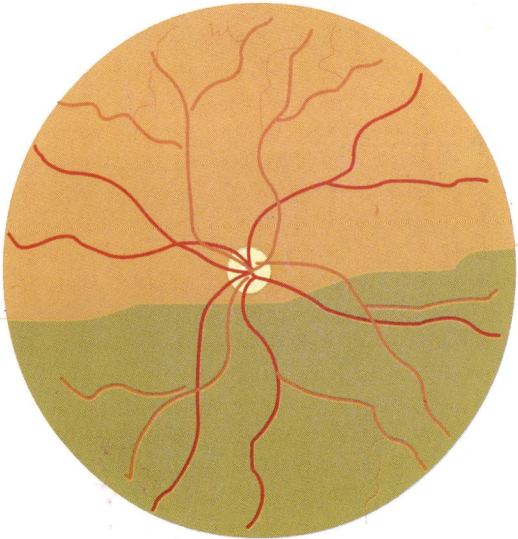

Fig. 12.5 *Diagrammatic representation showing retinal detachment*

Stage 5: Total Retinal Detachment

Total retinal detachment that is funnel-shaped. This may be characterized additionally by dividing the funnel into anterior and posterior portions and describing whether each section is open or closed.

PLUS DISEASE

Plus disease is characterized by dilatation of the veins and tortuosity of the arterioles in the posterior fundus. When these changes are present, a plus sign is added to the stage number.

THRESHOLD DISEASE

Stage 3 with more than 5 cumulative clock hour for more than 8 interrupted clocks hours involvement with plus sing is known as threshold disease. More then 70 to 80% of retinopathy of prematurity infants will regress spontaneously[3], leaving few if any residue. Retinal detachment is rare, but sometime its development in frequently preceded by the following signs:

   a. Progression of 'plus' disease

   b. Development of fresh vitreous haze

   c. Increasing preretinal and vitreous haemorrhage

   d. Gross vascular engorgement of the iris and failure of the pupil to dilate

SCREENING

The eyes of all infants born less than 36 weeks or weighing less than 1500 gm, who have received supplemental oxygen, should be screened for retinopathy of prematurity (ROP). Those bodies having intraventricular haemorrhages are at increased risk of developing retinopathy of prematurity. As pupil are difficult to dilate before 31 weeks, visualization of fundus very difficult and also impaired by tunica vasculosa lentils. The most appropriate time to screen an infant is between the postconceptual age of 32 and 36 weeks. Retinopathy of prematurity rarely appears for the first time after 36 weeks, and retinal detachment seldom develops before that time. The pupils in a pre-term infant should be dilated with 0.5% Cyclopentolate with or without 2.5% phenylephrine.

Eyes with threshold diseases are considered as semi-emergency and should be treated as early as possible. The treatment options are transconjunctival /transcleral cryo or laser photocoagulation of the entire avascular retina anterior to the ridge, preferable up to oraserrata.

CRYO ROP study has shown a 50% reduction in the unfavorable outcome of treated versus untreated groups of threshold retinopathy of prematurity (ROP). Argon and diode laser photocoagulation have shown to be as effective as cryo in the management of threshold retinopathy of prematurity. Several advantages have been cited for laser photocoagulation vis-a-vis cryo, particularly with the advent of indirect delivery system. The advantages of laser photocoagulation as it produce less manipulation of the globe and less anaesthesia. The eyes treated with laser develop less myopia than cryotheraphy.

LASER/CRYO TREATMENT IN RETINOPATHY OF PREMATURITY

In retinopathy of prematurity there is a distinct demarcation between vascularised and avascular zones. A ridge may develop at this junction, followed by neovascularisation. The zone of involvement describes the location of the neovascularisation. When five or more clock hours of the periphery are involved by neovascularisation and there is dilation of the posterior vessels, cryotherapy has been shown to be beneficial in reducing the risk of posterior retinal abnormalities. Laser photocoagulation has become popular substitute for cryotherapy. Laser is applied using indirect ophthalmoscopic attachment, with the target area being the same as for cryotherapy; burns are placed a half-burn width apart (as for diabetic scatter photocoagulation) but also can be placed more cofluently (Fig. 12.6).

Successful treatment has been reported with either argon or diode laser. Laser photocoagulation requires less manipulation of the globe and less anaesthesia and it produces less external hyperemia.

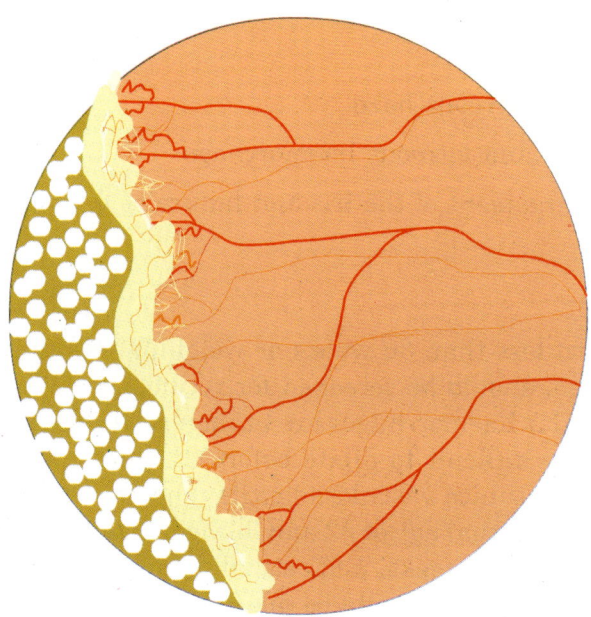

Fig. 12.6 *Laser burns are placed over the avascular retina*

SURGICAL MANAGEMENT OF RETINOPATHY OF PREMATURITY

With improved neonatal care that enables low weight infants to survive, the incidence of retinopathy of prematurity (ROP) has increased throughout the world. Threshold disease responds to cryotherapy and laser photocoagulation and can prevent progression to retinal detachment in a majority of cases. However, zone I disease (especially rush disease) can progress to retinal detachment despite treatment. Unrecognised zone II diseases can also lead to retinal detachment. Surgical treatment is required at this stage. Scleral buckling has been recommended and is successful in stage - 4 and some cases of stage 5 diseases.

The basic goals of surgical procedure are to improve vision but the surgical procedure differs from case to case. The surgery is done under general anesthesia and by standard 3-port vitrectomy. If necessary, lens is sacrificed and the sclerotomies are made 0.5 mm from the limbus, usually through or just behind the iris root (Fig. 12.7).

Bimanual surgery is done using the curved vitreous scissors (DORC, Holland) and pick forceps after fill up the eye with viscoelastic substance.

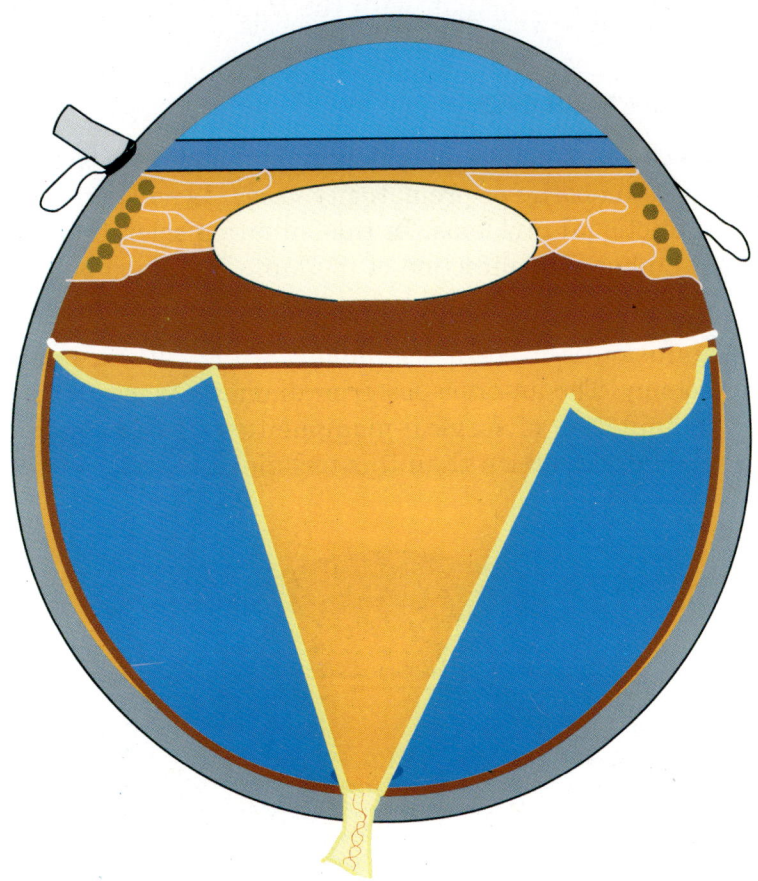

Fig. 12.7 *Infusion placed through the limbus as pars plana in infants is very short*

MANAGEMENT OF PUPIL

To keep the pupil widely dilated throughout operation, adrenaline (0.1 ml of 1:1000 dilution) is added to the 500 ml of infusion fluid. However, in most of the cases the pupil is bound down at one or more places and did not permit adequate dilatation. In an attempt to get maximum dilatation, temporary iris retractors (Greishaber, Switzerland) are used.[4] In most cases, however, iris is sacrificed in the meridian of the sclerotomies and this not only offered good visualization of the periphery but avoided the iris prolapse that tended to occur frequently through the sclerotomy

SURGICAL OPTIONS

    A. *Scleral buckling*: If the retinopathy of prematurity develops stage 4 A, where is necessary retinal detachment (RD) extends 3 times the width of ridge or in case where retinopathy of prematurity develops stage 4 B.

    B. *Lens sparing vitrectomy*: This is done of traction limited to posterior pole retinopathy of prematurity only.

    C. *Lensectomy + Vitrectomy*: When retinopathy of prematurity progresses to stage v, this procedure has some value with guarded prognosis.

POSTERIOR TRACTIONAL PROBLEMS

Posterior tractional detachments causal by posterior development of neovascularisation are being seen very often in retinopathy of prematurity cases. Lens sparing vitrectomy has been successful for posterior tractional problems. In this situation sclerotomy is usually performed 0.5 mm posterior to the limbus. The direction of the knife is carried out towards the posterior pole passing through the iris root to avoid the peripheral lens (Fig. 12.8).

Normally a lighted infusion is used in sclerotomy, while cutting instruments are passed through the other sclerotomy. The anterior posterior diameter is greater in case of infant than adult therefore there is limitation of surgical manipulation. If retinopathy of prematurity infant associated with peripheral traction than this technique is not advisable.

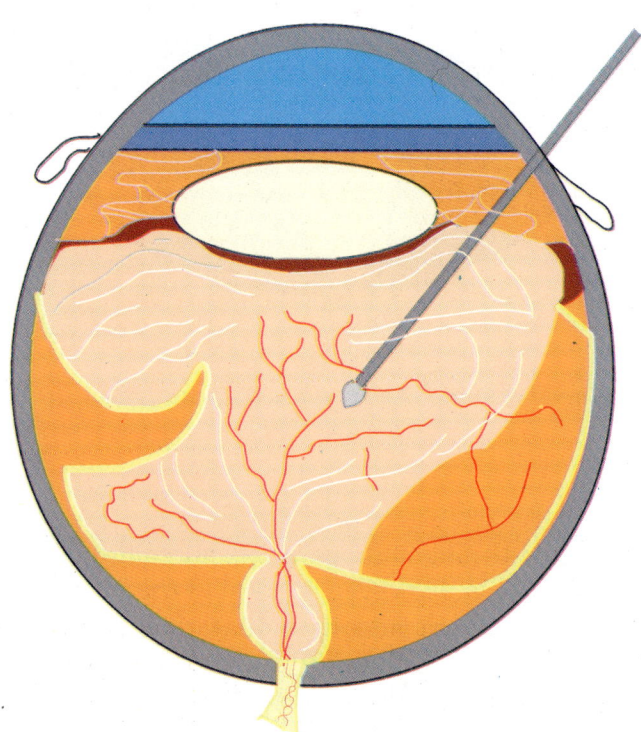

Fig. 12.8 *Lens pairing vitrectomy direction of knife directed towards posterior pole*

PERIPHERAL TRACTION PROBLEMS

In peripheral traction in case of retinopathy of prematurity, fibrous tissues originate from the areas of neovascularisation and draw the retina anteriorly and inwardly. The temporal detachment may be trough. In most cases the area behind the lens is a dense sheet of fibrous tissue obscuring detail of the underlying retina. The anterior of the eye can be accessed surgically only with very anterior sclerotomy and lens removal. Behind the lens there will always be a sheet of grayish white membrane and the infusion is usually placed through the limbus because the parsplana in infants is very short and the retina is drawn up. The microvitreoretinal blade is passed 0.5 mm behind the limbus, lensectomy is usually done first so that there is access to the proliferative tissue and one can avoid peripheral breaks if the retina is removed with the vitreo cutting probe. Once the lens material is removed, the capsular remnants are also removed meticulously to avoid residual traction later on.

After lensectomy, a slit is made in the center of the membrane initially with microvitreoretinal blade and star-shaped cuts are carried towards the periphery with scissors, which should be carefully kept anterior to the retina. The membrane can be removed by delaminating technique facilities this phase while light is provided by the operating microscope. Once periphery is reached, the line of dissection is carried out circumferentially so that sheet of membrane can be separated. The vitrectomy cutter may be used to remove the sheets of delaminated membrane. Careful evaluation of the peripheral membrane is important. The membrane usually can be dissected from the ridge of retina that is closer to the center of the vitreous cavity. When the trough is tight the help of scissors and forceps may cut the membrane, an attempt is made to remove the membrane deep within the funnel (Fig. 12.9).

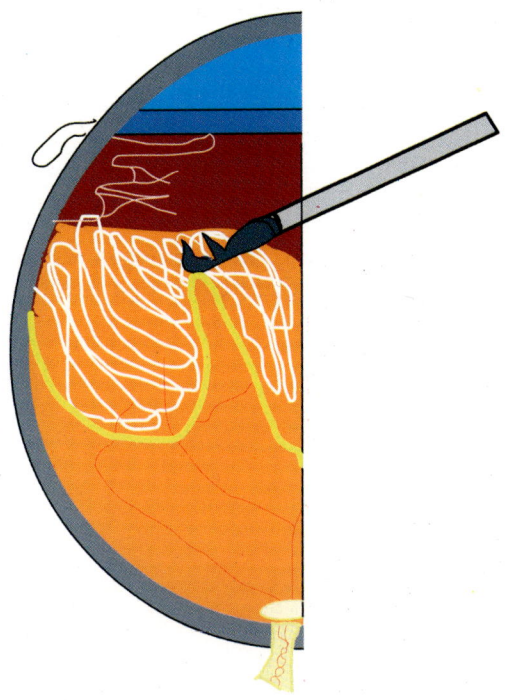

Fig. 12.9 *Tight membranes cut with scissors*

The wide-angle illumination is very helpful in this stage. One should be after that the cutting probe is dangerous and unnecessary in most instances because there is little residual formed vitreous. Viscoelastic injection into the funnel is some times helpful to define the area of traction, but viscoelastic should be removed at the end of the operation. Most authority in the world does not drain subretinal fluid because the retina will reattach at the end of the procedure, as no retinal breaks exist. Scleral buckle is not advisable because the residual traction is usually too anterior to be affected and buckle may interfere with subsequent growth of the eye. A small air bubble may be left in the end of the operation.

COMPLICATIONS

Retinal dialysis, bleeding during operation and posterior retinal breaks usually encounter during operation. Secondary glaucoma during retinopathy of prematurity frustrating, invasive procedures are best avoided due to high risk of staphyloma.

The improved anatomical success rates have been confounded by disappointingly poor visual function forever, surgery should be performed when indicated as even visual improvement with hand movement allows many patients to remain ambulatory.

REFERENCES

1. Cryotheraphy for retinopathy of prematurity cooperative group-multi center trial of cryotheraphy for retinopathy of prematurity. Preliminary results *Arch Ophthalmol* 106: 47-79, 1988.

2. Retinopathy of prematurity–Internal classification. *Arch Ophthalmol.* 102 : 1130–34, 1984.

3. Cryotheraphy for retinopathy of pre maturity cooperative group-multicenter trial of cryotherapy for retinopathy of prematurity, one year outcome—structure and function. *Arch Ophthalmol*: 108: 1408-16, 1990.

4. Copal L, Sharma T.: Periphery to center dissection for stage 5th retinopathy of prematurity added by temporary iris retractor a pilot study Hong Kong *J Ophthalmol*: 1: 41-44, 1997.

5. Orellana J: Scleral buckling in acute ROP stages in treatment of ROP. In Eichenbaum JW Mamolok A, Mittikn, Orellana J, editor year book. Chicago: Medical Publisher Inc pp 194-211, 1990.

6. Surgery for stage - 5 retinopathy of prematuring. The learning curve and evolving technique. Lingam Copal, Tarun Sharma et al *Indian Journal of Ophthalmology* 101-106, 2000.

Rhegmatogenous Retinal Detachment

Introduction

A tear or a hole in the retina causes Rhegmatogenous retinal detachments. Retinal detachment does not result from a single, specific disease rather it is the end result of numerous disease processes in which subretinal fluid is present.

There are three types of retinal detachment:

- Rhegmatogenous
- Exudative
- Tractional.

Both exudative and tractional detachments are sometimes referred to as secondary or non-rhegmatogenous retinal detachments. The pathogenesis of retinal breaks which cause rhegmatogenous retinal detachment include the development of posterior vitreous detachment (PVD) which may cause retinal break by traction on the retina, or by ocular trauma. The break can be usually identified preoperatively, but occasionally the presence of minute unseen break must be assumed.

DIAGNOSIS

The diagnosis of retinal detachment is made on the basic patient's history and detailed ocular examination. Retinal detachments are more common in myopia, aphakia, trauma and lattice degeneration. The usual symptoms among the patients are floaters and flashes, decrease in vision and constriction of visual field. The key to successful retinal reattachment surgery needs detailed and careful fundus evaluation by binocular indirect ophthalmoscope with scleral depression and 3-mirror examination of periphery retina.[1] During retinal evaluation attention should be paid to number, size and location of retinal breaks and extent of detachment. One should look for peripheral retinal degeneration, particularly lattice and also any proliferative vitreoretinopathy changes.

SURGICAL ANATOMY OF CONJUNCTIVA, TENON'S CAPSULE AND MUSCLES ISOLATION

Conjunctival opening can be performed either at the limbus or 2 to 3 mm posterior to the limbus. Sometimes radial relaxation incisions are necessary to prevent tearing of the conjunctiva.

In patients with filtering blebs or recent limbal wound, the peritomy can be extended posteriorly to the area of previous surgery.

Conjunctival opening at the limbus can be facilitated by spreading with scissors beneath tenon's capsule just posterior to the limbus (Fig.13.1).

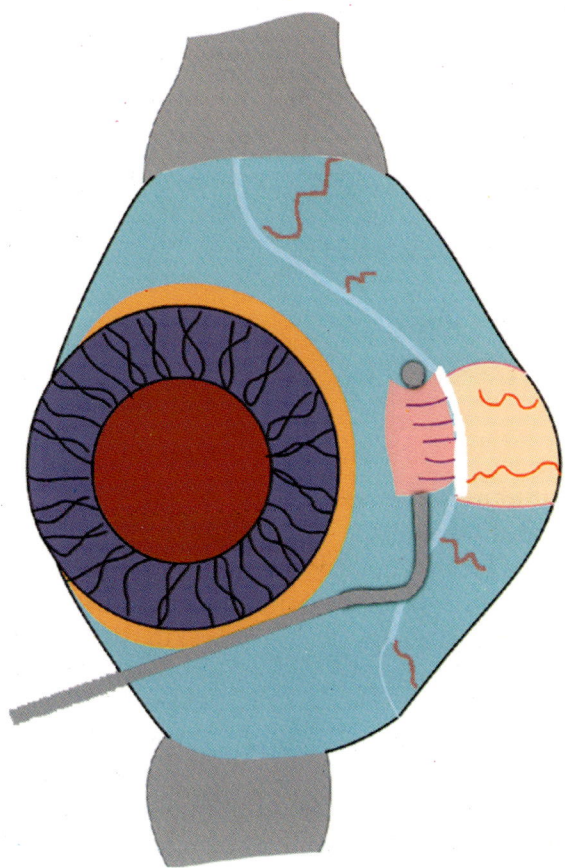

Fig. 13.1 *Rectus muscles are isolated with muscle hook*

The tenon's capsule fuses anteriorly with the conjunctiva and posteriorly it ends at the optic nerve sheath. Tenon's capsule reflects posteriorly around the muscle for 10 to 12 mm. With the help of blunt scissors the tenon's capsule and episcleral tissue separated to improve exposure. Significant resistance to passage usually means the muscle hook is not on the scleral surface and should be repositioned. The muscle is best engaged by staying anterior to the equator and prevents injury to the vortex vein. Once the muscle insertion is engaged, the connection to tenon's capsule can be identified and separated from the muscle. The rectus muscles are initially isolated with simple muscle hook, taking care the entire insertion. A perforated muscle hook with a 2-0 black-silk suture is then passed through the muscle in reverse direction (Fig 13.2).

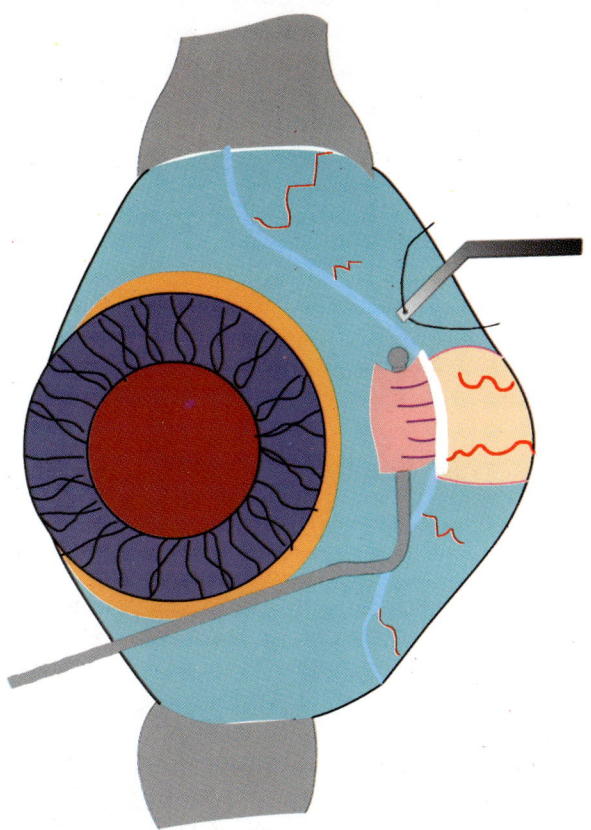

Fig. 13.2 *Muscle hook passed in reverse direction*

Some surgeons prefer 4-0 silk for these traction surface sutures. When the vertical rectus muscles are isolated, care should be taken not to strip too posteriorly to avoid damaging the levator palpebrae superioris muscle (LPS) superiorly or the inferior oblique muscle and lockwood's ligament inferiorly.

The superior rectus muscle requires additional care to avoid the superior oblique muscle tendon, which inserts 3 to 4 mm posterior to the lateral margin of the superior rectus insertion.

Passing the muscle hook from the nasal side anterior to the oblique muscle insertion best avoids engaging the superior oblique muscle tendon insertion.

After all rectus muscles are isolated, the surface of the sclera is inspected in each quadrant for evidence of thinning, staphyloma or anomalous vortex vein. Scleral thinning may appear as a gray and blue area and are very common super temporally.

Isolation of the four rectus muscles usually allows adequate access to all areas of scleral necessary to perform scleral buckling. The scleral in each quadrant is examined retracting the conjunctiva and tenon's capsule with a retinal retractor.

LOCALISATION AND TREATMENT OF RETINAL BREAKS

Precise and meticulous localisation of retinal break on the scleral surface is very critical and important for successful of retinal detachment surgery. Approximately 85 to 90% of cases can be cured with a single operation.[3] Using an indirect lens; the periphery is examined with scleral depressor for 360° to confirm the finding recorded on the drawing that was made at the preoperative examination (Fig. 13.3).

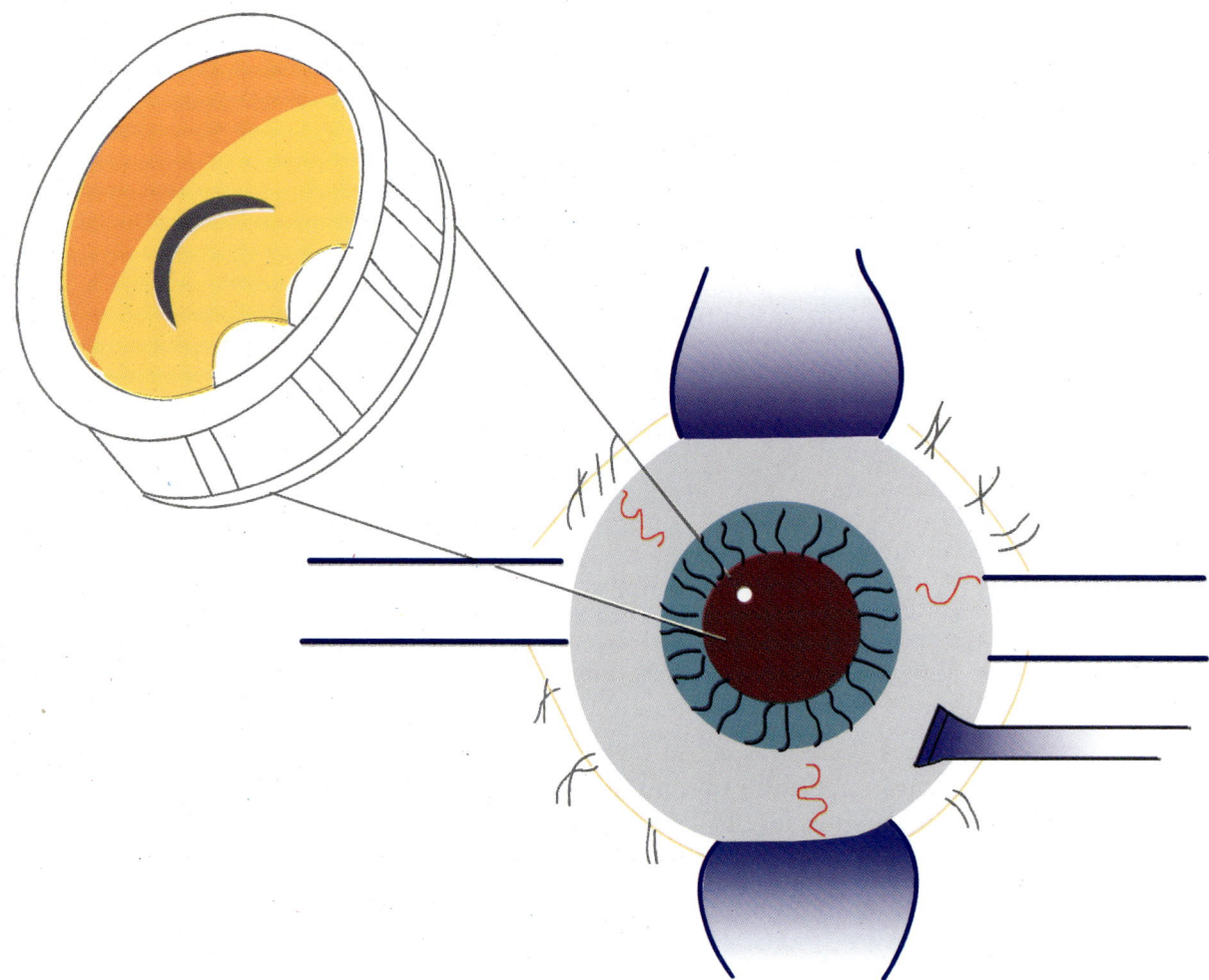

Fig. 13.3 *Periphery of retina is examined with scleral depression by indirect lens*

Several instruments for localization and for marking the sclera have been described. When the sharper sclera marker is used for localization, it is important to accurately inspect the sclera. While indentation within the eye is being observed, the most posterior location of the break is marked on the sclera with a small instrument that has rounded raised circle on it's end (O'Connor marker localizing) which place one mm circular mark on the sclera with mild indentation. When the tear is large the two-end may also be marked so its extent is indicated on the sclera surface. The marker leaves a transit round indentation on the sclera. Some surgeon prefers diathermy for this localisation.

The indentation is marked with ink taking care to first dry the sclera to prevent running or smearing of the ink. A cautery or diathermy tip is applied to the ink mark to tatton it into the sclera. For small flap tears or atrophic holes, a single mark or the posterior edge is sufficient. Large flap tear and non-radial tear requires localisation of both the anterior and posterior extent of the break. Anterior posterior orientation is particularly important when radial buckle is employed. Marking the most posterior extent and the circumferential extent of the break is adequate. This approach is also sufficient for marking a retinal dialysis, which is marked anteriorly at the edges of the dialysis, and then most posterior extent is marked.

The problem arises when the retina is bullously detached. Accurate localisaton of retinal breaks is difficult. Bullously elevated breaks appear to lay more posteriorly then their true location because of parallax. Rarely, it may be necessary to drain subretinal fluid to flatten the retina before localisation. It sometimes softens the eye and makes further drainage difficult due to choroidal swelling secondary to hypotony.

The treatment of retinal break is to create an adhesion between the retinal pigment epithelium and the retina. This is induced by thermal injury with one of the three energy sources, diathermy, cryotherapy, and laser. The morphologic and cellular responses of the retina and pigment epithelium to each of these energies are essentially similar. After two weeks of application, all three modalities show comparable effects on retinal adhesive force. Photocoagulation adhesion occurs within twenty four hours of application. Cryopexy reduces retinal adhesion for one week after application.

The goal of the treatment is to do transsclera cryotherapy surrounding the retinal break. One or two rows of continuous treatment are used. Treatment usually is carried to the oraserrata. The end-point of treatment is when a white lesion first becomes visible in the retina. Longer application of the freezing lesion promotes pigment dispersion in the subretinal space and into the vitreous cavity.

BASIC SURGICAL TECHNIQUE

The rhegmatogenous retinal detachment can be performed either by local or general anaesthesia. The operative field is prepared for surgery by applying 0.5% betadine solution. Careful use of antisepsis can minimize the risk of postoperative infections. The major sources of infections are the lashes and the lid-margins so care should be taken to scrub the lash margins with povidone-iodine solution, which is a non-toxic to the cornea and conjunctiva.

After scrubbing, the skin surface is dried with sterile gauge. This is particularly important when disposable adhesive drape is used. The goal of the surgical draping is to isolate and protect the surgical field from contamination. The oral and nasal cavities are the common sources of contamination. By properly applying adhesive draper, one can effectively seal off these areas from operative field.

BASIC REQUIREMENTS OF RETINAL DETACHMENT SURGERY

There are four basic requirements in repairing rhegmatogenous retinal detachment with a scleral buckle. These are:

1. Precise localisation of all the retinal breaks.
2. Creation of a chorioretinal adhesion around the retinal break.
3. Placement of scleral buckle to relieve vitreoretinal traction on the break.
4. Drainage of subretinal fluid externally or internally.

In rhegmatogenous retinal detachment, scleral buckling is an effective surgical technique. The scleral indentation is achieved with scleral buckling. Alternative technique of detachment repair like vitrectomy, pneumatic retinopexy and temporary infallible balloon elements are also done with good success results.[2]

METHODS OF BUCKLING

Scleral buckling or indentation (explant technique) allows the surgeon to place accurately over retina tear or hole, which represents a traditional gold standard. The ability to treat retinal pathologs without scleral dissection has resultant in explants surgery become the of choice for most retinal surgeon.

When an encircling element is used, suture usually preplaced to retain it. With the help of calipers, the width of the proposed is marked on sclera (Fig 13.4).

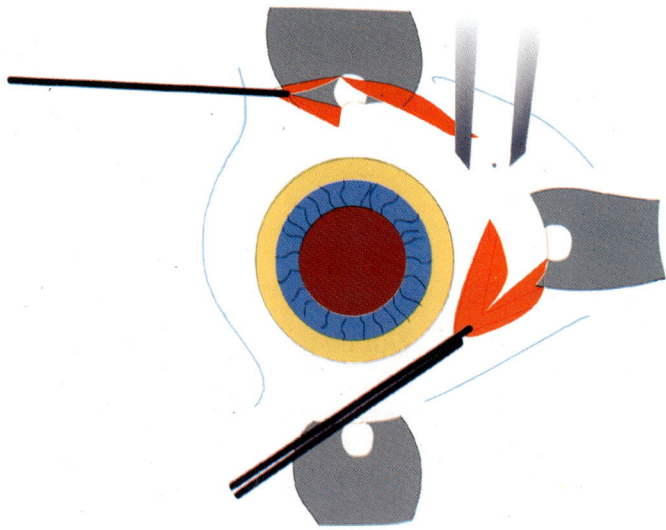

Fig. 13.4 *Width of buckle is measured with calipers*

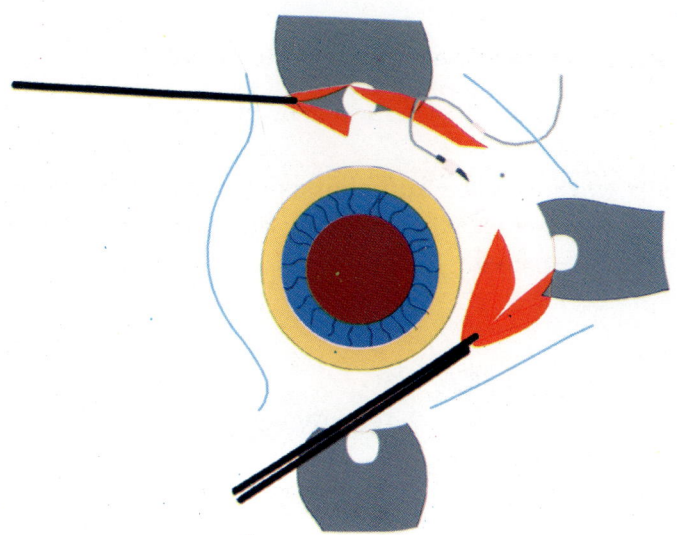

Fig. 13.5 *Posterior bite 3 mm behind the proposed mark*

The posterior bite of the suture should be placed at least two to 3 mm behind the proposed mark (Fig 13.5).

The suture bites are taken at a depth of half the scleral thickness and should be 5 mm to 6 mm in length. Nylon, siliconized silk, Dacron are favoured as suture materials by most surgeon. One suture per quadrant is sufficient to secure the buckle elements and the suture is typically centered in mid-quadrant. When one is suturing posteriorly, the vortex vein and their tributaries must be avoided. Thin sclera also creates problems, and sometimes long suture passes are not possible. In this case several short bites in areas of thicker sclera may be effective.

Once the sutures are in position, the silicone elements are pass under the muscles and sutures. The ends of the tires and bands are grasped simultaneously and pulled beneath the muscle The ends of the band can be cut to produce a tapper, which help to identify whether twisting has occurred during the passage under muscle. When the leading edge of the tire is passed out of the last quadrant in which it will be used to support, it is advanced without being passed under the suture in the next quadrant until the trailing edge reaches a position under a rectus muscles, depending on the number of the quadrants to be supported by the tire.

The tire now is cut so that its end will fall under the rectus muscle belly. Support of 1 or 2 quadrants by the tire is recommended. Use of broad elements in three quadrants increases the likelihood of choroidal detachment.

Encircling procedure is particularly indicated in the following conditions.

1. Cases with multiple breaks in different quadrant.

2. Aphakic

3. Pseudophakic

4. Myopia

5. Diffuse vitreoretinal pathology condition

6. Proliferative vitreoretinopathy of Grade B or greater.[4]

For buckling procedure various sizes and shapes of buckle are available. A wide variety of silicone plates, tires, and sponges exist (Fig. 13.6). Some popular approaches for use of these elements as exoplants are illustrated.

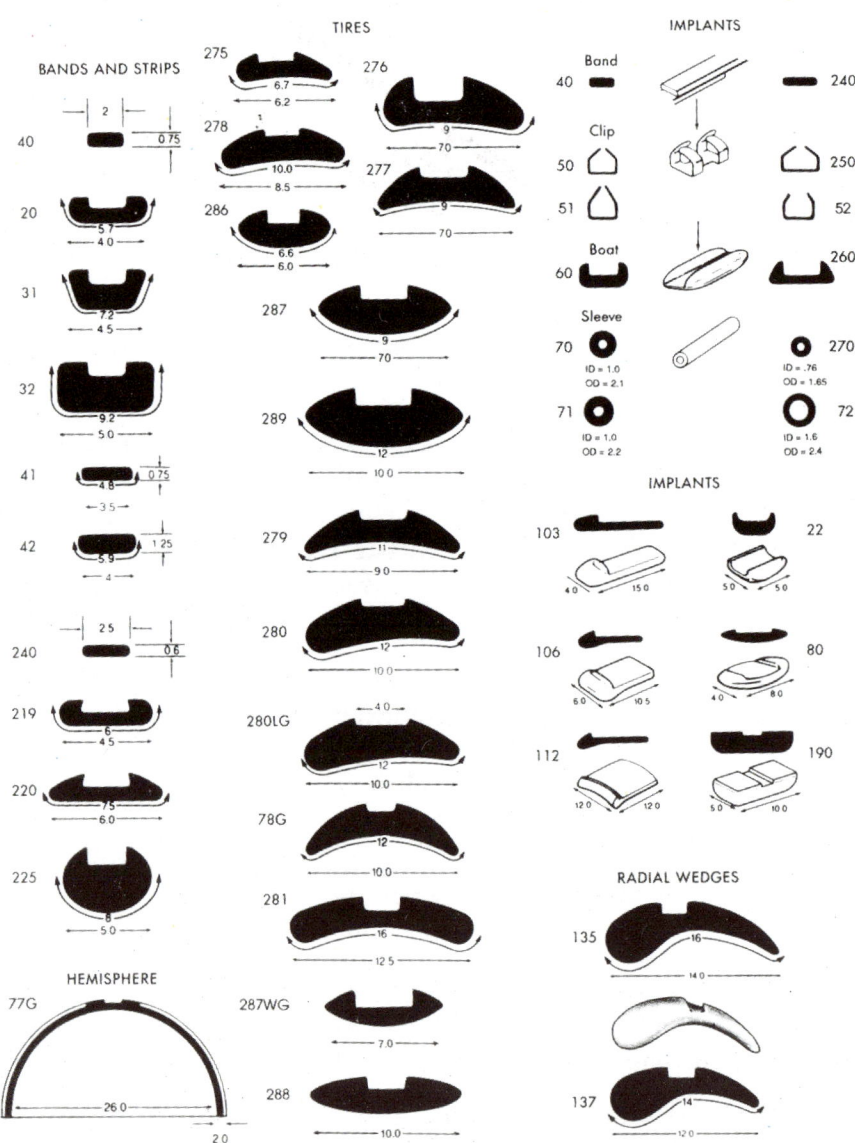

Fig. 13.6 *Cross-sectional diagram of various solid silicone rubber scleral buckling elements and materials for securing together the ends of an encircling band (Courtesy: MIRA, Inc., Waltham, MA).*

Either sponges or solid silicone rubber can be used as encircling elements. When retina is associated with traction, the buckle should be positioned such that the posterior edge of the break lies on the posterior crest of the buckle. The buckling effect should extend for 30-degrees on either side of the tear and extend anteriorly to the oraserrata.

A solid silicone band (240) 2.5 mm wide is often used to support the base. The vitreous base approximately lie 3 mm posteriorly to the oraserrata nasally and 2 mm posterior to the oraserrata temporally. This encircling band fits into the group of the buckle. The advantage of the encircling 240 bands are relieved traction at equator permanently, thus a false oraserrata posterior to the actual anatomical ora is created.

SECURING THE ENDS OF THE BAND

The encircle band is secured to the sclera with either mattress sutures or through scleral funnels to prevent migration of the band once it is shortened. The ends of the band can be secured with non-absorbable suture, tantalum clip or silicone-sleeve.

As the band is pulled down on each side of the sleeve to stretch it slightly, the other end of the band is passed through the sleeve in opposite direction. The two ends may be tapered to facilitate passage. The end of the band to pull opposite directions to shorten the band. A tantalum clip also may be used to fasten the band, but it is not easily adjusted once applied. 5.0 alcon suture also may be used to fasten the ends. A second tie adds greater security.

MANAGEMENT OF SUBRETINAL FLUID DRAINAGE

The rational for drainage of subretinal fluid is to diminish intraocular volume so that the tire and band may be pulled up to give proper indentation and allow the break(s) to settle close to or on to the buckle. Although some retinal detachments can be effectively managed without drainage, it is preferred to drain in conditions like.

1. Bullous detachment.

2. Inferior breaks.

3. Proliferative vitreoretinopathy.

4. High myopia.

5. Chronic detachment.

6. Poor retinal pigment epithelium function.

The selection of drainage site is important. Both internal and external anatomy guides the choice of drainage site. When large breaks are present a site, two clock hours from the drainage site is preferred. Externally the vortex veins usually are found in the mid quadrant and must be avoided. The long posterior ciliary vessels at the 3 O'clock and 9 O'clock positions are potential sites of haemorrhage if incised accidentally.

DRAINAGE OF SUB RETINAL FLUID

Subretinal fluid drainage is done where the detachment is highest and it should be close to the recti muscles (Fig. 13.7).

There are relatively avascular zones. Drainage along horizontal recti is preferred to vertical recti and nasal quadrant is preferred over temporal zone as it is distant from macula. It should be done slowly to avoid incarceration of the retina in the sclerotomy.

If the location of the external site is questionable, an area of sufficient retinal elevation is marked on the sclera with a marker used for guidance. Externally, the vortex veins usually are found in the mid-quadrant and must be avoided (Fig. 13.8).

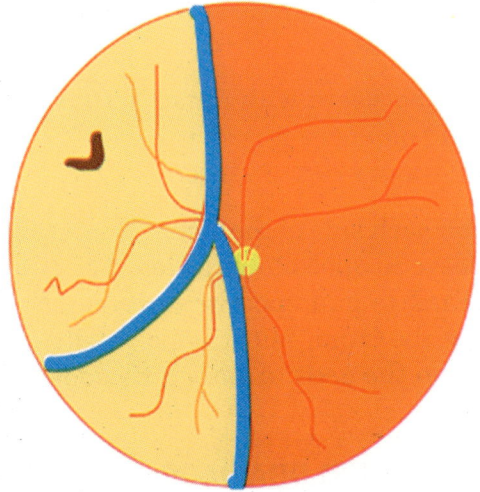

Fig. 13.7 *Drainage in bullous retinal detachment with break*

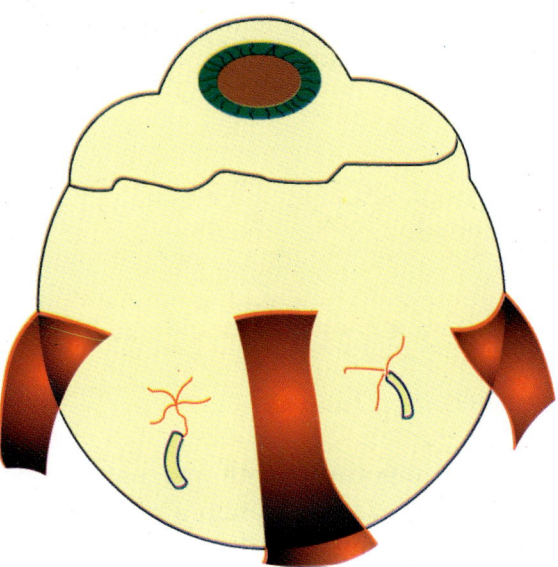

Fig. 13.8 *Vortex found mid-quadrant must be avoided*

Before drainage of fluid the pressure is checked manually. The suture, buckle, and speculum are adjusted to ensure the lowest possible intraocular pressure. Entering into the subretinal space may be made with a diathermy tip, 26 or 27 size needle or other sharp needle. The diathermy tip enters until a slight trickle of fluid is apparent; it is then is pulled slightly anterioly to create an oval shaped hole in the choroid. Ideally, fluid should drain slowly from the incision site. No pressure is applied initially to the eye and fluid is allowed to drain until it slows or stop spontaneously. At the end of the drainage, gentle pressure is applied to drain if same amount of fluid still remain. Pressure should be applied safely anterior to the drainage site approximately mid-way between the site and limbus. When the intraocular pressure appears low, pressure may be maintained by placing cotton tipped swab in the quadrants away from the drainage site. By this maneuver pressure rises and displaces fluid towards the drainage site.

If the drainage site is not beneath a tire, it should be closed with a suture and this suture usually placed before drainage.

Once drainage appears to be completed, the mattress suture over the drainage site is pulled up to close the site, and a temporary tie is made, the band is pulled upwards from the globe to pull the slack out of all quadrants. The two ends than are pulled in opposite directions to tighten the band.

The most serious complications are more frequently associated with drainage of subretinal fluid than with any other steps in buckling procedure, because it converts an extraocular to an intraocular procedure. Drainage produces accidental perforation of the globe intraocular haemorrhage, iatrogenic retinal breaks, vitreous loss, hypotony retina, fish mouth, meridional folds, and intraocular infection.[4]

There are also disadvantages of non-drainage operation that might result in failure to close the retinal breaks and reattach the retina, thus necessitating additional surgery.

BUCKLE POSITION, SUTURE FINALISATION AND ADJUSTMENTS

The encircling band is secured to the sclera with mattress suture. To make sutures permanent, the loop first is cut and the short end of the suture is removed, and an additional throw is placed to secure the knot (Fig. 13.9).

The knots are rotated posteriorly by grasping each limb of the suture with a tying forceps and adjusting them simultaneously (Fig. 13.10).

This reduces the tendency of the intrascleral portion to cut through the sclera during adjustment. In the final buckle position, the ends of the tire should be beneath muscle bellies and the knots should be rotated posteriorly (Fig. 13.11).

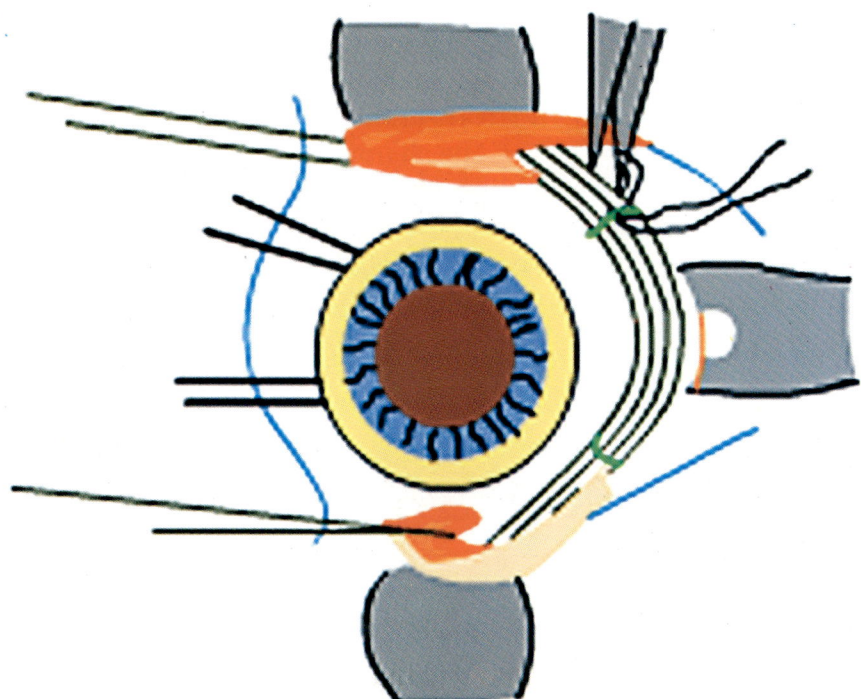

Fig. 13.9 *Loop is cut to make the suture permanent*

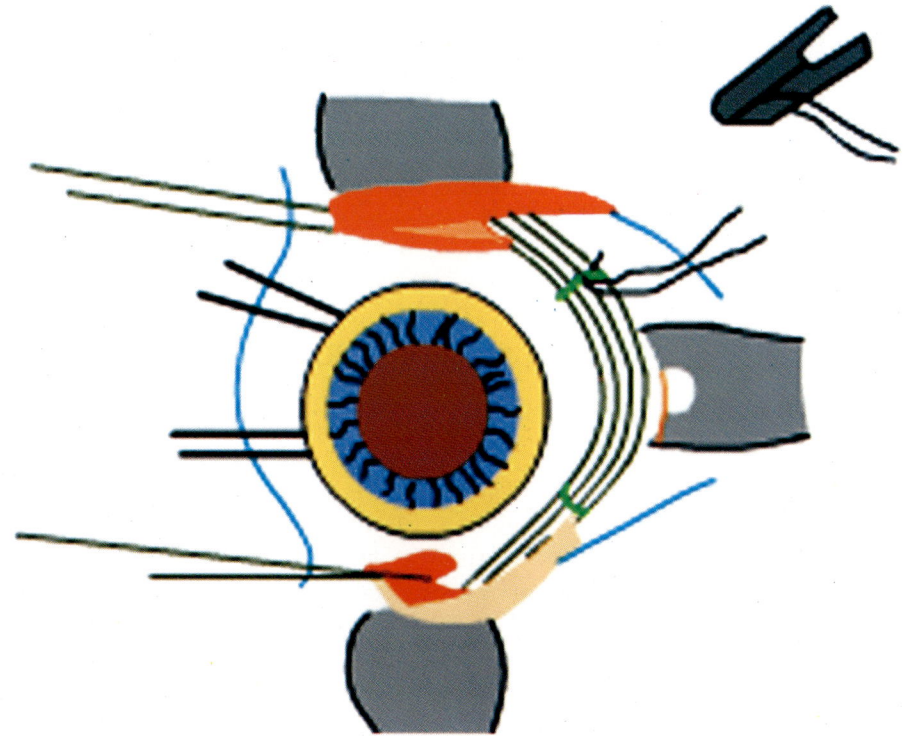

Fig. 13.10 *Short end of the suture removed*

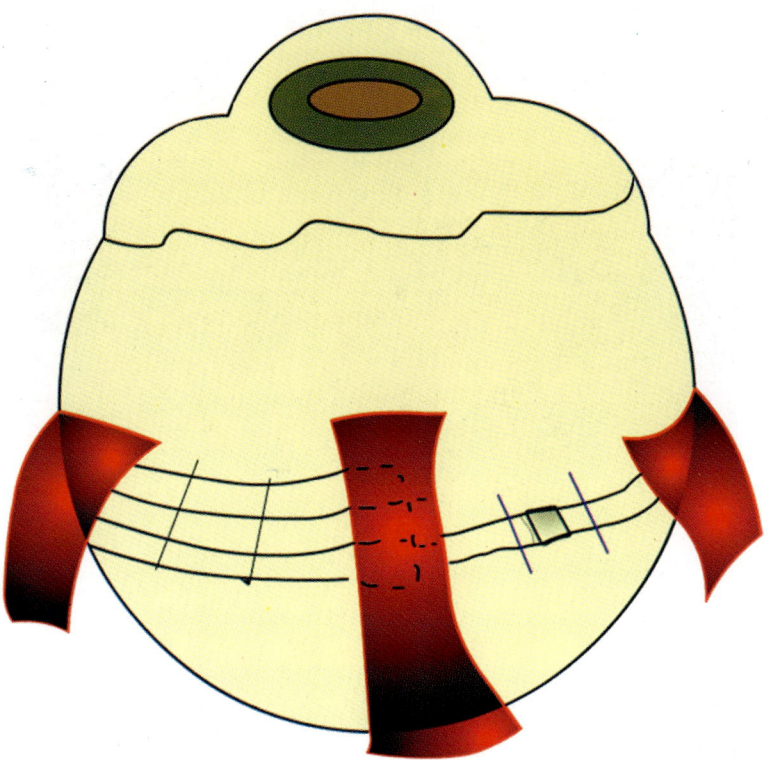

Fig. 13.11 *Ends of the tire beneath muscle bellies*

For adjustments of buckle there should be at least 1 mm between the posterior edge of the retinal breaks and the posterior crest of the buckle. If the posterior edge of the one buckle needs additional posterior extension or additional height, radial silicone may be added under the tire. Several pieces with different widths provide an additional three mm of posterior extension. A suture bite is taken 3 mm behind the initial posterior bite, which then is removed. The radial piece of silicone is positioned beneath the tire. The suture is then pulled up tied, and the knot rotated posteriorly in standard fashion.

Occasionally the eye may remain too soft after fluid drainage is completed and buckle has been adjusted. An injection of air, long acting gas, or saline may be used to bring the pressure to normal. This is done by holding the two horizontal recti muscles by their sutures for stabilisation and the superior rectus muscle by its insertion with a forceps, a 27-gauge needle is inserted through the parsplana 3.5 mm posterior to the limbus and slow injection is completed. Pressing on the eye may monitor the pressure with an instrument or cotton tipped swab. The 6 O' clock position may be chosen if the retina is highly elevated superiorly or if 12 O' clock position is unsuitable. A bubble of gas or air may offer the additional benefit of providing internal tamponade for superior breaks. At the end of the procedure, the intraocular tension is checked with Schiotz's tonometer but one should be in mind because tonometer sometimes gives false reading when gas has been injected into the eye.

STEPS OF OPERATION

STEP 1

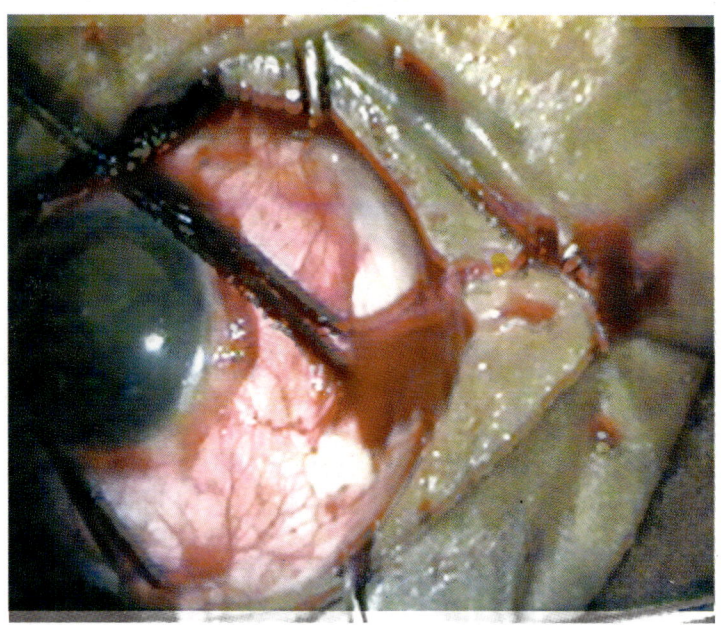

Step 1. *Silicone band passed through the muscle*

STEP 2

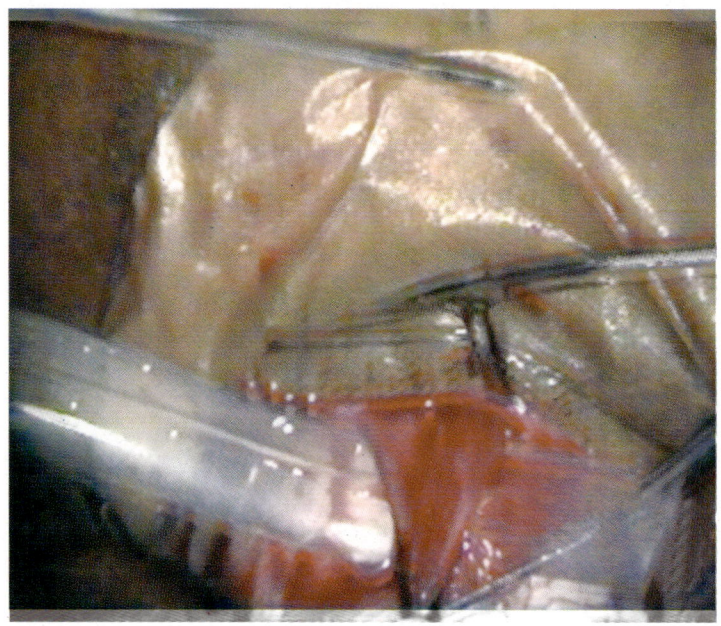

Step 2. *Once the sutures are in position, the silicone band passed under the muscle and suture*

STEP 3

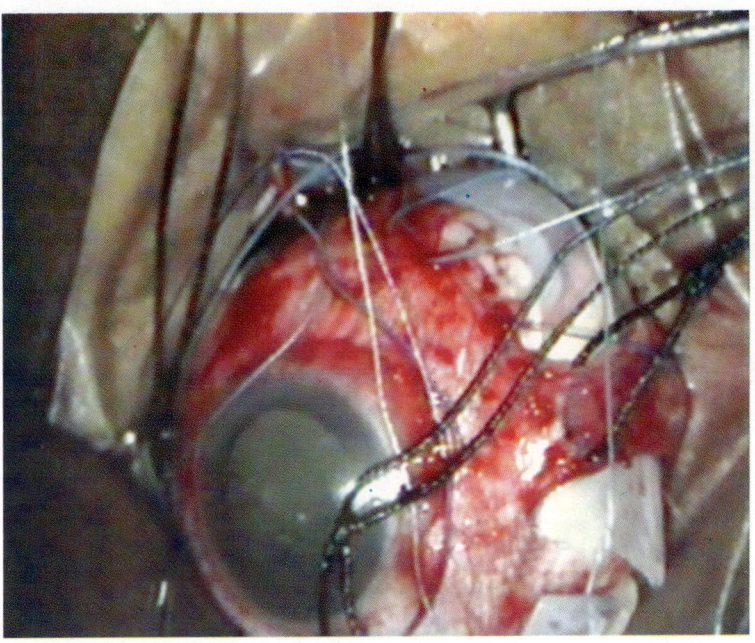

Step 3. The tire and bands are pulled together

STEP 4

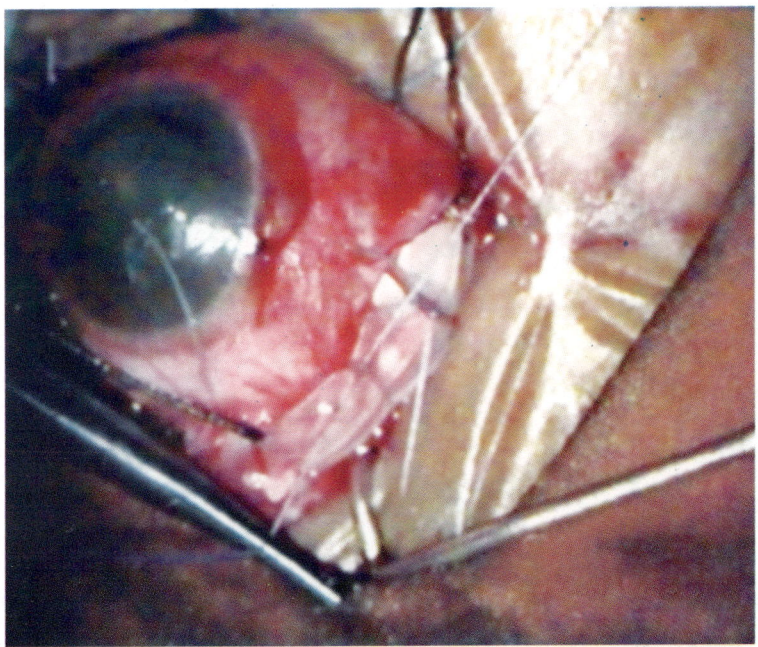

Step 4. *The tire and bands are pulled together sequentially from one quadrant to the next passing through the sutures*

STEP 5

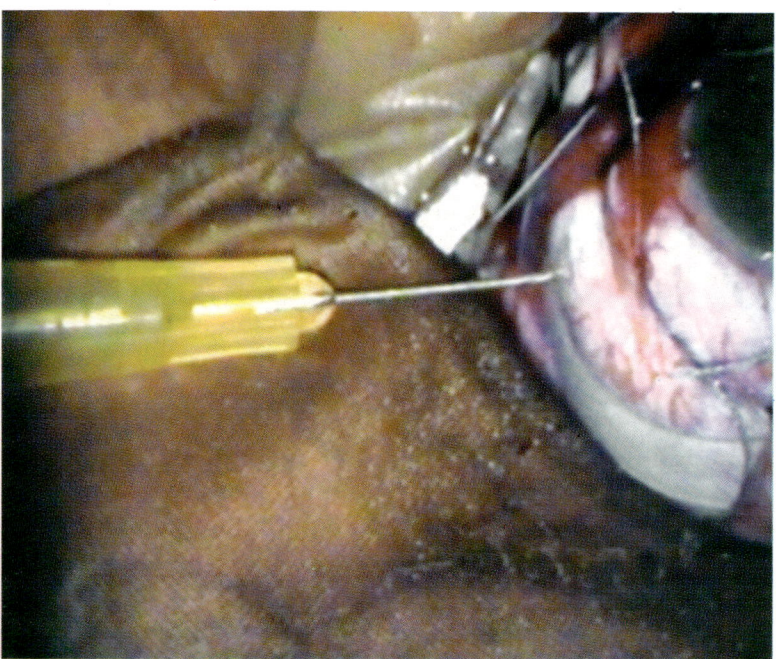

Step 5. *Drainage of subretinal fluid with 27-gauze needles*

STEP 6

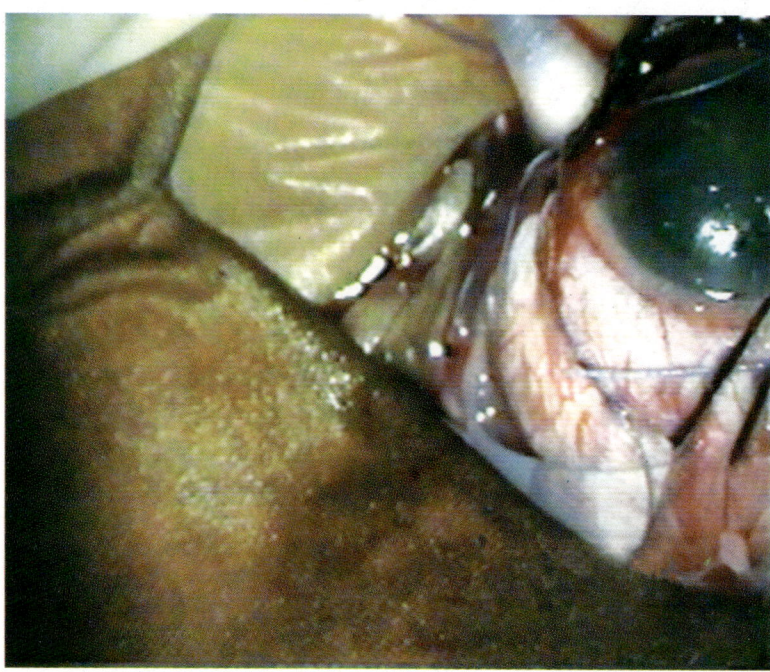

Step 6. *Subretinal fluid drained by pressing the swab stick to get maximum result*

STEP 7

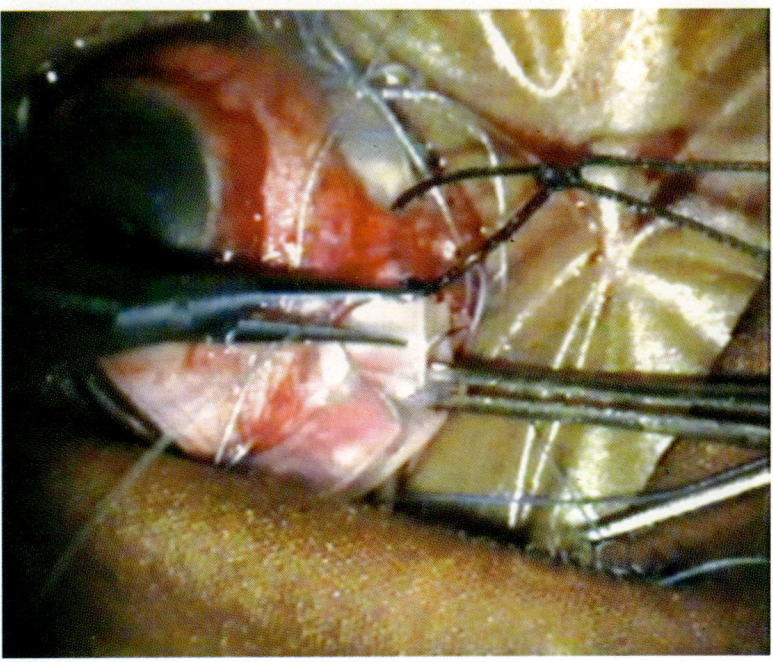

Step 7. *The tire is cut so that its end fall under rectus muscle securing the ends of the band*

CUSTODIS TECHNIQUE

It is now well established that whenever there is one break, it can be treated with meridian buckle without subretinal fluid drainage. The retina hole is marked by diathermy over the scleral by indirect opthalmoscopy and two vertical mattress sutures are placed using double arm 5.0 alcon sutures.

The anterior suture is placed 0.5 mm from the scleral mark. Each bite is taken in an anterior to posterior direction. Suture is spacing typically two mm wider than the width of the buckle. Such wider spacing creates a higher indentation. The second suture is placed symmentically behind the first, again taking both bites in an anterior to posterior direction with a double-needle suture.

The buckle is placed beneath the sutures and spread slightly with forcep as the suture is tightened.

It is important to tighten the posterior suture first to ensure adequate indentation of the posterior buckle. The anterior suture is tightening after assessing the intraocular pressure and buckle position. The buckle may be cut close to suture leaving enough buckle be left in position to ensure that it does not slip out from under the suture. It is essential to check the intraocular pressure and central retinal artery. If the artery is closed or if the intraocular pressure is very high after acceptable time, a paracentesis may be performed. This is done by the help of a twenty 7-gauge needle with a tuberculin syringe without plunger and is inserted into the anterior chamber at the limbus and held in position over the iris. The fluid is removed slowly and the intraocular pressure is reduced. The procedure may be repeated after sometime if the pressure still remains high. The closer of the limbal incision is not necessary.

INTRAOPERATIVE COMPLICATION OF SCLERAL BUCKLING

Corneal Clouding

Adequate visualization is necessary for the success of the operation. Corneal clouding is a common intraoperative problem. This is usually caused by the epithelial oedema from increased intraocular pressure (IOP), which occur during scleral depression. Mild amounts of oedema may be resolved with topical glycerine or by rolling the epithelium with dry cotton tip application. Extensive epithelial oedema usually requires debriment with a rounded iris repositer. The cornea is scraped centripetally starting about 2 to 3 mm from the limbus. The epithelial cells are removed with swab stick to prevent dispersion otherwise it may result epithellial inclusion cysts.

Scleral Perforations

If a suture is placed too deeply, intraocular penetration may occur. Such penetration may be recognized externally by the drainage of subretinal fluid, blood, pigments or combination through the suture. When perforation is recognized, the retina should be inspected immediately with indirect ophthalmoscope to determine the depth of the perforation. When suture placement is too deep over the attached retina, both subretinal haemorrhage and an iatrogenic retinal break can occur. The iatrogenic break should be treated with cryotherapy or indirect laser photocoagulation.

When there is scleral perforation, which some times results subretinal haemorrhage immediate pressure over the perforation site should be applied and the eye positioned to prevent gravitation of the blood beneath the fovea. If massive subretinal bleeding occurs, immediate vitrectomy with internal drainage of subretinal fluid and removed of subretinal blood should be considered.

Miosis

Miosis sometimes results despite adequate preoperative dilation. It may result from hypotony at the time of drainage or from surgical inflammation secondary to cryotherapy or paracentesis. If intraoperative miosis occur, 0.2 ml of (1:10.000) adrenaline dilution preservative free may be consider for aphakic or pseudophakic eyes. Photocoagulation with endolaser may be obtained by treating the iris stromal midway between the pupil and the angle directed through the cornea. This will dilate the pupil but postoperative inflammation does occur.

Drainage Complications

Drainage complication can occur despite the use of proper technique. Sometime dry tap is due to failure to completely perforate the choroid. Steady advancing the needle until fluid is present around the needle can do this. Retinal perforation does occur if the needle strikes the retina because of shallow subretinal fluid or excessive entry of the needle. If the drainage is in the bed of the buckle, usually no treatment is required with possible exception of cryotherapy. If the perforation occurs outside the bed of the buckle, a new unsupported retina break has been created and this require cryotherapy and adjustment of the buckle for adequate support.

Choroidal haemorrhage occasionally occurs during drainage. This complication may be recognised during drainage if the flow stops abruptly before the expected amount of drainage has occurred. A subtle grey change may be seen plugging.

When the incarceration is severe, it may become a retinal break or may distort the retina so that the break remains elevated. If this situation occurs, the sclera should be closed initially with a mattress suture taking care not to include the retina in the suture. The site is now treated with cryotherapy like new retinal break.

If the drainage site is temporal, the eye should be positioned to place the drainage site as inferiorly possible to prevent the subretinal blood from gravitating to the fovea. Drainage in nasal sites is advantage that the haemorrhage if occurs less likely to reach into the fovea. If a large amount of blood is in the subretinal space and beneath the fovea, a vitrectomy with internal drainage of subretinal blood should be considered.

Late complication like subchoroidal neovascularisation can occur months to year after drainage at the drainage site. Treatment of the vascular mass with photocoagulation or cryotherapy may include resolution of the neovascularisation.

The most serious complications associated with drainage of subretinal fluid because it converts an extra ocular to an intraocular procedure.

POSTOPERATIVE COMPLICATION

Glaucoma

Scleral buckling may result secondary glaucoma. The diagnosis may obscure in first few days due to inflammation or discomfort unless intraocular pressure (IOP) is measured.

Angle closure glaucoma does occur after scleral buckling with or without pupillary block. When angle closure occurs without pupillary block there is high intraocular tension (IOP), corneal oedema, shall owe of the peripheral and sometimes central angle. When pupillary block is present, there is accompanying iris bombe. Initial management consists of medical therapy to control the intraocular pressure (IOP) and hourly topical corticosteroid to decrease inflammation and minimise formation of synechia. If medical treatment is unsuccessful in opening the angle, surgery is necessary. When there is pupillary block glaucoma, yag-laser iridectomy is performed along with the medical treatment. A patient iridectomy that fails to deeper the angle and lower intraocular pressure (IOP) confirms that mechanism other than pupillary block are operative. When it occurs, Dio green laser burn 200 mm and 0.2 duration are placed on the iris as close as possible to the angle. This causes iris to contract and pull away the iris from the angle. If laser surgery is unsuccessful in spite of all intraocular pressure (IOP) not reduces excessive height of the buckle should be considered and the possibility of loosening or cutting the encircling band entertained.

Anterior Segment Ischemia

Anterior segment is chemia is suspected after encircling procedure. This is more common if more than one rectus muscle is disinserted. The initial clinical findings are stromal corneal oedema, fibrinous anterior chamber reaction and raised intraocular pressure with shallow anterior chamber. Late postoperative complication may be anterior or posterior synechial, cataract and corneal vascularisation. Sometimes angle closer glaucoma and anterior segment ischemia is difficult to diagnosis. Mild case of anterior segment ischemia responds to medical treatment with topical steroid or systematic steroid. In severe cases, it is necessary to cut the encircle band.

Extrusions and Buckle Infection

Scleral buckling as it is a foreign bodies and therefore at risk for extrusion and infection. Infection after diathermy manifest as acute pain, vitrifies and scleral abscess and usually occurring first three to eight days after surgery. The scleral necrosis facilitates scleral formation and intraocular inflammation.

Infection after cryotherapy and scleral explants appear less acute condition which manifest as irritable eye with Conjunctival swelling. This appears after 2 weeks to 2 months after surgery. Clinically it shows fistula formation, glaucoma formation and purulent discharge and sub conjunctival haemorrhage.

Effective management of infected scleral buckling material usually requires removal of the buckle elements. Topical broad-spectrum antibiotic may improve the situation. If the buckle is extrused, it may be removed and infection gets cured after removal of scleral buckling material. Placement of photocoagulation around the retinal breaks or sites of vitreoretinal traction 2 weeks before removal may be essential when possible.

Choroidal Detachment

Choroidal detachments or choroidal oedema is common after scleral buckling procedure due to accumulation of serious fluid in the supra-choroidal space. It is occurred both diathermy and as well as cryo therapy procedures. Vortex vein obstruction is the main factor for development of choroidal oedema. The security of choroidal detachment depends upon the involvent of quadrant buckle and obstruction of vortex vein. More the number of quadrants buckled more vortex veins are involved. There is more chance of choroidal detachments if placement of scleral sutures further posterior than 14.0 mm from the limbus. Drainage of the subretinal fluid enhances the choroidal detachment.

Although the incidence of choroidal detachment is relatively high, the overall effect on vision is minimal. Choroidal detachment usually appears two to four days after surgery. There may be associated vitreous base, which is presumably is an inflammatory vitritis. Systematic and local corticosteroid has been used to treat choroidal detachment. But incase of massive choroidal detachments, whether haemorrhagic or serous are best managed with prompt surgical drainage.

In aphakic or pseudophakic eyes the choroidal detachment are drained with a transcleral cut down into the suprachoroidal space while infusing air with an air pump through the limbus or anterior parsplana. In phakic eyes, the A/C is deepened with a balanced saline solution injection through a limbal step incision before choroidal drainage.

Cystoid Macular Oedema

The cause of cystoids macular oedema is not known though some authors believe that it is due to prostaglandin mediated inflammation. However, cystoids macular oedema occurs as a response to ocular inflammation. The surgical trauma of scleral buckling, subretinal fluid drainage, cryotherapy or diathermy results in significant ocular inflammation or the therapeutic rational for the treatment of the macular oedema is to suppress ocular inflammation.

Macular Pucker

The major causes of decreased vision after scleral buckling is due to macular pucker. Preretinal membrane occurs due to release pigment epithelial cells and retinal glial cell after scleral buckling. Risk factors identified for the development of macular pucker include preoperative proliferative vitreoretinopathy of grade B or greater, old retinal detachment and vitreous loss during drainage. It has been seen that myopic patient have a lower risk of macular pucker than emmetropic patients.

Postoperative Diplopia

Postoperative diplopia is a serious problem after scleral buckling. Fortunately the incidences vary 3 to 4 % and it increases after re-operation. The cause of diplopia is unknown, perhaps it may be due to placement of large buckle beneath the rectus muscles or may be due to formation of adhesion between the buckle and the muscles or may be traumatic damage to the rectus muscles during buckling may also play a role.

Postoperative diplopia may resolve spontataneously and completely. Surgical management can be difficult because of the anatomic alternations that occur after scleral buckling. This diplopia after scleral buckling may be treated with prisms. If muscle surgery is necessary an adjustable suture technique should be considered.

Changes in Refractive Error after Scleral Buckling

Refractive changes after scleral buckling depends upon the surgical technique. Segmental buckle have little effect on refractive error. However, large radial elements if it extends anteriorly beyond the oraserrata may induce an irregular astigmatism because of changes in corneal curvature. Encircling procedure induce the greatest change in refractive error. This change greater for phakic than aphakic eyes because of anterior displacement of the lens, resulting in an increased myopic shift. However, the refractive error after scleral buckling usually stabilizes within 2 to 3 months after surgery.

MAIN CAUSE OF FAILURE OF RETINA DETACHMENT (RD) SURGERY

The goal of retina detachment (RD) surgery is to re-attach the retina to the pigment epithelium. The failure of surgery depends upon the inadequate closer or localisation of the hole or has reopened due to inadequate cryotherapy, failure of sub-retinal fluid to absorb or preretinal organisation Sometimes retinal holes are missed during initial examination that subsequently caused the redetachment. It is therefore necessary to do an extensive search for missed or additional breaks taking special care to search areas of poor visibility such as within retinal folds. The new breaks may be due to vitreous traction or excessive inflammatory fibrin reaction.

The most common cause of surgical failure is proliferative vitreoretinopathy (PVR), which accounts for 90% of all permanent surgical failures. It is best to recognise the signs early to improve the likelihood of final anatomic and visual success. When presented with a primary failure, look for proliferative vitreoretinopathy (PVR) with either residual or recurrent vitreoretinal traction changes, which are usually evident about six weeks after scleral buckle surgery, can keep breaks open. If proliferative vitreoretinopathy (PVR) is present, re operation should be considered.

FAILURE OF PRIMARY RETINAL DETACHMENT—PITFALLS

Although most rhegmatogenous retinal detachments can be cured with scleral buckling. Much failure in retinal detachment (RD) surgery result from error in technique during surgery. These intraoperative errors can begin with anaesthesia.

Retro bulbar anesthesia may produce an ocular perforation or anaesthetic injected into nerve sheath may produce profound complication. General anaesthesia can also alter the surgical success by creating hyperperfused ocular tissue or with inadequately controlled hypertension, may produce intraoperative bleeding.

Adequate exposer is essential for proper placement of buckle. Care of the vortex vein while expose the posterior scleral is must to avoid intraocular haemorrhage. With a posterior buckle the vortex vein could be compressed resulting glaucoma. If all vortex veins are closed the result can be multiple choroidal haemorrhage with or without choroidal detachment, oedema of iris, and exudates in the anterior chamber with posterior and peripheral anterior synechia.

Sometimes irregularities in the scleral thickness may be noticed with age. The scleral may become thinner at the equator, dehiscenses can form that can later develop into staphyloma, with eventually ectasia and necrosis.

Adequate fundus visualisation is necessary for successful treatment of retinal breaks. Pre-operative examination during surgery, can reduce the chances of anatomic and visual success if there is inadequate visualisation of the fundus due to corneal opacity, lens opacification miosis or vitreous haemorrhage all can lead to failure retinal detachment surgery.

The most important factor of poor localisation of retinal breaks and missed breaks could prevent properly sealing all the retina breaks and possible failure to reattach the retina. The modality of choice for sealing of the retina breaks is cryotherapy. Other modality are indirect laser, pneumatic retinopexy or diathermy are performed in selective cases.

PRECAUTION WITH CRYOTHERAPY

Chorioretinal adhesion with cryotherapy is applied all around the breaks. It is essential to be able properly visualise the formation of the ice ball in order to achieve adequate treatment as well as to eliminate excessive treatment. Excessive treatment produce tear in the posterior edge. Rupture of the globe could occur if the cryprobe is not properly thawed beam fore removal. Cryotherapy may contribute to cellular proliferation vitreoretinopathy (PVR) as well as liberate pigment cells to pass through the retina break and into vitreous cavity.

PRECAUTION WITH SCLERAL BUCKLING

The correct choice of the scleral buckling element and its placement are important. Proper sterilisation of the buckle elements and proper placement of the buckle is essential for all the success of all operation. Scleral perforation while placement of the suture leads to vitreous incarceration and increased risk of proliferative vitreoretinopathy (PVR) and thereby leads to failure of reattachment surgery. Suture of insufficient depth may prematurely loosen the intended buckling effect, with resultant failure of the operation. The ocular pressure at the end of the procedure must be such that the central retinal artery is open and there is no threat of glaucoma.

If retinal breaks does not seal due to surgical error of the buckle then other methods are applied for proper closer of the breaks with pigment epithelium. These surgical procedure are drainage of the subretinal fluid vitrectomy, pneumatic retinopexy or injection of silicone oil or perfluoro carbon may be necessary to achieve anatomic success.

PREVENTIVE STEPS TO AVOID PRIMARY FAILURE

A successful primary reattachment surgery depends upon through evaluation of the cause of the detachment and selection of proper surgical plans. To get best surgical results, proper surgical approach and procedure are utmost important. Most of cases simple sealing the retinal breaks results excellent anatomic and functional success. When simple sealing is not sufficient a decision must be made as to which additional procedures might be necessary to achieve success. These could include pneumatic retinopexy, scleral buckling, cryotherapy, and vitrectomy with drainage and fluid–gas exchange.

The patient general health status must be considered when planning the operation. Patient willingness and physical ability to follow postoperative instruction is important. Without patient cooperation what might otherwise have been successful reattachment can result failure, However, the proper judgment to surgical approach plus being prepared to alter the surgical plan at any time throughout the procedure will continue to a final, anatomical and function success.

PNEUMATIC RETINOPEXY

Introduction

Pneumatic retinopexy is first reported by Hilton and Grizzard first report pneumatic retinopexy in the year 1986. There after it has become a popular alternative to traditional scleral buckling method. It is usually done as an outpatient, simple procedure. Candidate for pneumatic retinopexy should have tears in the superior quadrant between the 8 O' clock and 4 O'clock position.

A single tear or a group of tears should not occupy more than 1 O'clock hour. This procedure entails cryo over the break and gas injection as a single bubble which acts by two mechanisms:

  i. Surface tension effect of the gas bubble (scotch tape effect).
  ii. Buoyancy effect.

These two characteristics account for their efficacy in reattaching the retina. The choice of type and amount of gas depends on two factors:

  a. What size gas bubble is needed?
  b. What length of time the bubble should stay in the eye?

The air, SF_6 and C_3F_8 gas for their average duration maximum size and average expansion showed (Table 13.1)

<table>
<tr><td colspan="4" align="center">TABLE 13.1
Intravitreal Gas Duration and Expansion</td></tr>
<tr><td>Gas</td><td>Average Duration</td><td>Largest Size</td><td>Average expansion</td></tr>
<tr><td>Air</td><td>3 days</td><td>Immediate</td><td>No expansion</td></tr>
<tr><td>SF_6</td><td>12 days</td><td>36 hours</td><td>Doubles</td></tr>
<tr><td>C_3F_8</td><td>38 days</td><td>3 days</td><td>Quadruples</td></tr>
</table>

Preoperative Evaluation

Pneumatic retinopexy has become a popular alternative to traditional scleral buckling method.

Candidates for pneumatic Retinopexy should have tears in the superior quadrant between the 8 O'clock and 4 O'clock position (Fig. 13.12).

Good preoperative evaluation is vital to the success of pneumatic retinopexy. The patient should physically capable of maintaining positioning, as needed, especially with regards neck and the back problems. Travel by air pose a hazard because the intraocular gas bubbles will expand at high altitudes and markedly increase the intraocular pressure.

Through pneumatic retinopexy is a simple, out patient procedure certain characteristics were excluded:

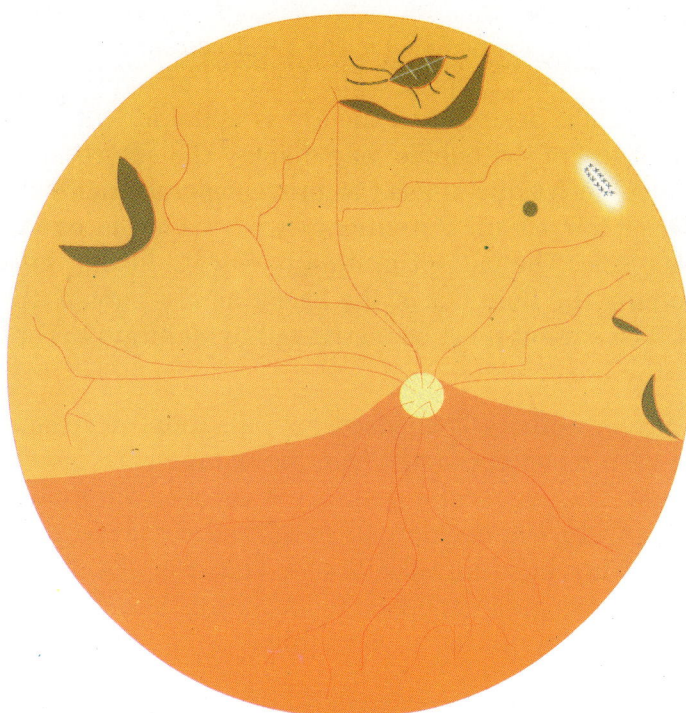

Fig. 13.12 *Ideal case for tear in superior quadrants between 8 O'clock position and 4 O'clock position*

1. Breaks larger than 1 O'clock hour or multiple breaks extending over more than 1 O'clock hour of the retina.
2. Breaks in the in the inferior 4 O'clock hours of the retina.
3. Presence of proliferative vitreoretinopathy grades C or D.
4. Cloddy media precluding full assessment of the retina.
5. Physical disability or mental incompetence precluding maintenance of the required positioning.
6. Severe or uncontrolled glaucoma.

Procedure

Treatment is begun by preoperative topical antibiotic with, maximal dilatation of pupil, reduce intraocular pressure (IOP) by intravenous monitor or global message by super pinky as it facilate gas injection. Procedure is done under topical/retrobulbar (optional as its helps to prevent vagal stimulation). After applications of beta dine over conjunctiva, cryotherapy is placed around the retinal break trans conjunctively. When the break is too far posteriorly for cryotherapy, it may be settled initially by gas injection and treated sub sequentially by laser. It is sometime difficult to locate break beneath the gas bubble. SF_6 or C_3F_8 amount 0.3 to 0.6 ml is drawn into tuberculin syringe attached to millipore filter and then inject the gas briskly into the globe with 27 gauge needle after needle tip has been visualised and slightly withdrawn (to obtain single gas bubble).[5] A slow injection of gas into the vitreous cavity is made to achieve an initial bubble size of 0.3 ml. Pure sulfur hexa fluoride (SF_6) is the most common choice so that the bubble will expand over the next twenty four to forty eight hours. Pure perfluorocarbon (C_3F_8) may be chosen if a longer tamponade is desired and the eye is aphakic. When the macula is attached, the upward flotation pressure of the bubble may display the sub-retinal fluid down under the macula. The "steam roller" technique is used to prevent detachment of the macula.[6] Immediately after the gas injection the patient is positioned with his/her face to the floor to displace the bubble into the posterior pole. The patient gradually elevate his/her head over approximately 30-minutes, thereby forcing the fluid out of the break as the bubble assumes a progressively more superior position. The patient must be instructed to maintain his or her head in a position so the gas will support the break.[7]

The central retinal artery activity is checked for pulsation, if present paracentesis is performed. Prone position with tear upper-most (can mark tape with arrow upper most, this is a paramount for the success. The intraocular pressure is checked after 6 to 8 hours Initial success result around 80%, with subsequent buckling 95 to 98% success reported.[8] This patient must be instructed to maintain his/her head in a position so that the gas will support the break, gas beneath the retina is a troublesome complication. Gas in this location rises, pushing the peripheral retina anteriorly. This complication is more likely to occur with large breaks and small bubbles 'fish eggs' (Fig. 13.13).

The most common serious complication of pneumatic retinopexy is the formation of new breaks, probably through the mechanism of changing the pattern of vitreous traction. Complication is reported in around 25% of cases (Fig. 13.14).

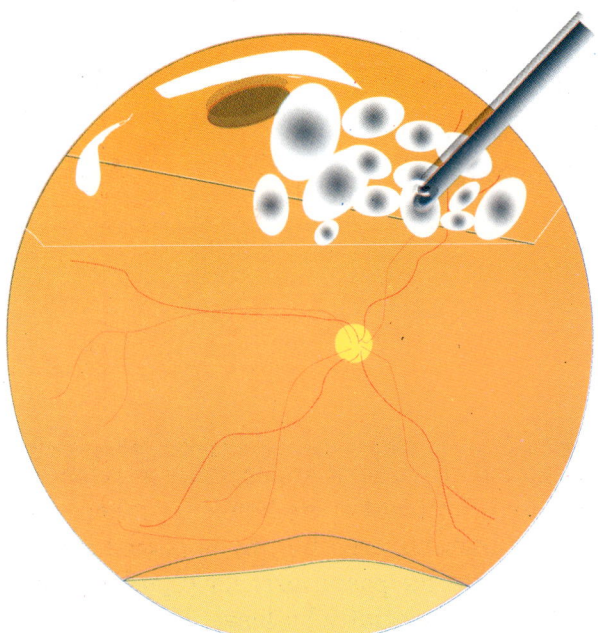 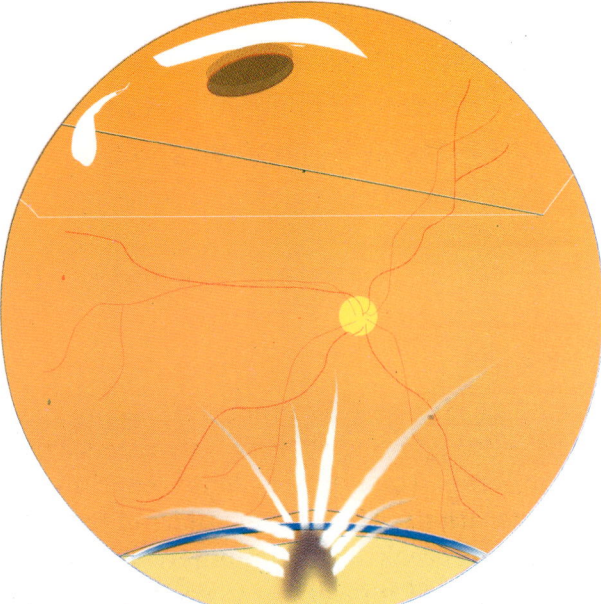

Fig. 13.13 *Complications occurs with large breaks and small bubbles (fish eggs)*   *Fig. 13.14* *Formation of a new break is a serious complication due to vitreous traction*

RHEGMAGETONOUS RETINAL DETACHMENT
(FLOW CHART)

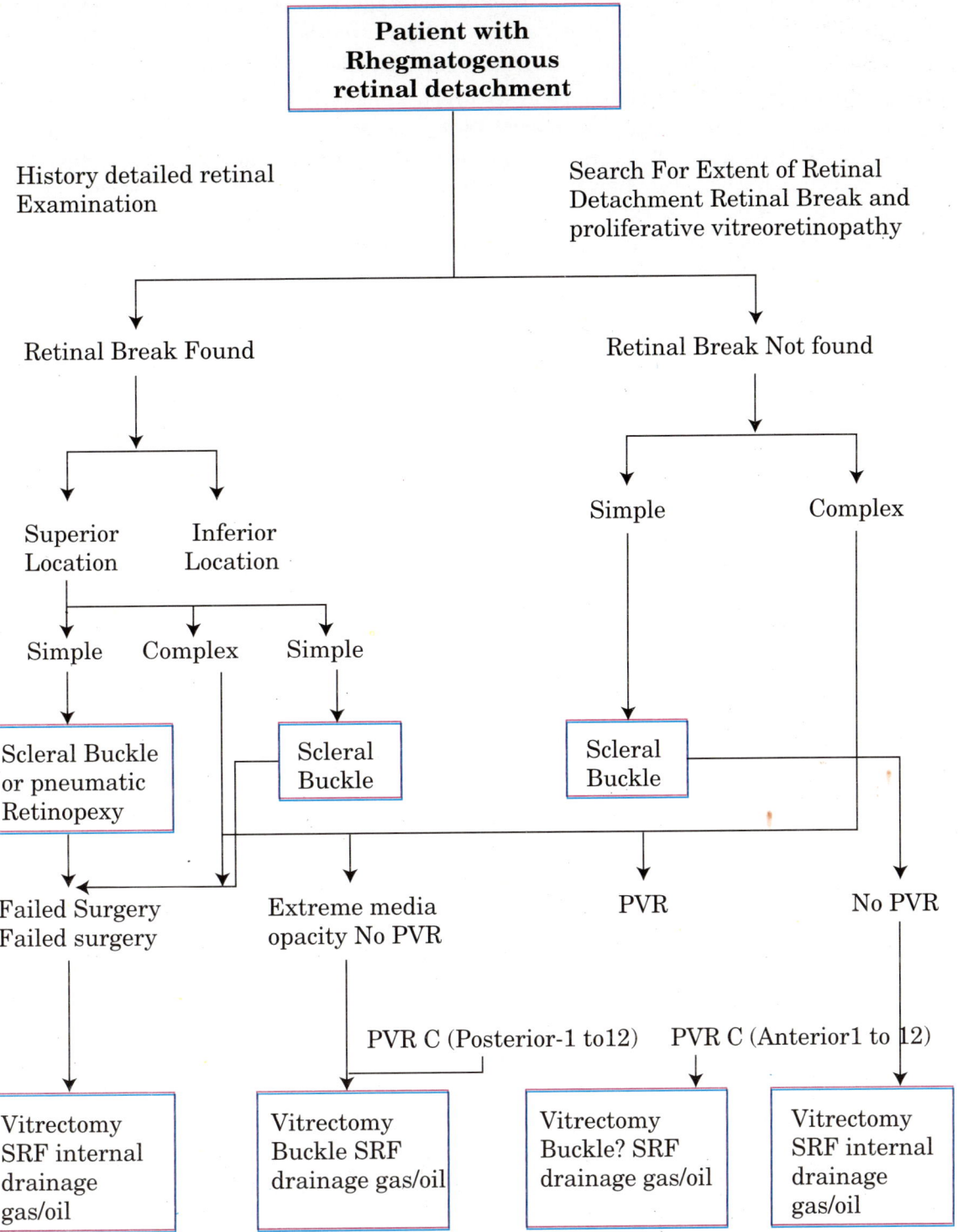

Patient with Rhegmatogenous retinal detachment

History detailed retinal Examination

Search For Extent of Retinal Detachment Retinal Break and proliferative vitreoretinopathy

Retinal Break Found

Retinal Break Not found

Superior Location

Inferior Location

Simple

Complex

Simple

Simple

Complex

Scleral Buckle or pneumatic Retinopexy

Scleral Buckle

Scleral Buckle

Failed Surgery Failed surgery

Extreme media opacity No PVR

PVR

No PVR

PVR C (Posterior-1 to12)

PVR C (Anterior1 to 12)

Vitrectomy SRF internal drainage gas/oil

Vitrectomy Buckle SRF drainage gas/oil

Vitrectomy Buckle? SRF drainage gas/oil

Vitrectomy SRF internal drainage gas/oil

REFERENCES

1. Benson WE: *Retinal Detachment: diagnosis and management*, Comb ridge, Harper and Row, 1980.

2. Hilton GF, Mc Lean EB, Brinton DA: Retinal detachment: principle and practice, *Ophthalmology Monographs*, ed 2, San Francisco, American Academy of Ophthalmology, 1995.

3. Wilkinson CP, Rice TA: *Michel's Retinal Detachment*, St. Louis, Mosby-Year-Book 1997.

4. Willians GA, Aaberg TM, Sr: Technique in scleral buckling In Ryan SJ, editor: *Retina, vol 3, Surgical Retina*, ed 2 St. Louis, Mosey-Year-Book, 1994.

5. Tornambe PE, Hilton GF: The retinal detachment study group. Pneumatic retinopexy, A multi center randomized controlled clinical trail comparing pneumatic retinopexy with scleral buckling *Ophthalmology* 96: 772-784, 1989.

6. Tornambe PE, Hilton GF: DA, et al: Pneumatic retinopexy. A two-year follow up study of the multicenter trial comparing pneumatic retinopexy with scleral buckling. *Ophthalmology*, 98: 1115-23, 1991.

7. Hilton GF, Fornambe PE: Pneumatic retinopexy, an analysis of intraoperative and postoperative complications. *Retinal*: 11: 285-94, 1991.

8. Lincoff H, Mardirossian J, Lincoff A, et al: Intraviteral longevity of three perfluorocarbon gases. *Arch Ophthalmol* 98 : 1610-1611, 1980.

Role of Vitreous Surgery in Primary Rhegmatogenous Retinal Detachment

Introduction

Rhegmatogenous retinal detachment occurs due to the entry of vitreous through the retinal break into the subretinal space and due to the traction from vitreous on the surface of the retina. In conventional surgeries the vitreous traction is relieved by a scleral buckle, cryo, diathermy or laser and SRF is drained. But when the traction on the retina is permanent and progressive, removal of traction by pars plana vitrectomy will be the best remedy for keeping the retina reattached permanently.[1]

Vitrectomy not only helps in relieving traction on the retina but also enables the surgeon to use intravitreal substances to tamponade the retina. Removal of foreign bodies, dislocated lens, dislocated IOL, etc. also can be performed alone with retinal detachment surgery if necessary. Retinotomies, retinectomy, preretinal and subretinal membrane removal, etc. are possible only by the vitreous surgery in rhegmatogenous retinal detachment complicated with proliferative vitreoretinopathy (PVR). When the retinal detachment is associated with giant tear, vitrectomy along with the use of perfluorocarbon liquid helps the retina to unfold and get reattached.

Vitrectomy can be indicated in certain cases of failure to detect retinal breaks.[2] If the retinal detachment is restricted posterior to buckle and if even scleral depression fails to show any fluid on the buckle, it is most likely that there is a break posterior to the buckle, only such "difficult to see break" best identified during vitrectomy.[3]

A prospective examination can direct our suspicion to some area but definite identification may not be possible. The high magnification of the operating microscope coupled with improved visualization by wide angle viewing system (EIBOS) helps in locating the break or by removing the opacities and membrane.

In primary vitrectomy there could be complacency in identifying preoperatively all retinal breaks in the belief that the breaks can be identified during vitrectomy.[4] It is important to realize that treatment of all retinal breaks are must for the success of the surgery irrespective of whether it is a primary buckling or primary vitreous surgery. The breaks located in the vitreous base and oraserrata should be given extra care. The wide-angle system with scleral depressor is a great help for panoramic view. There is no doubt that diligent preoperative examination and identification of these breaks will make the job easier during surgery. However, when there is extensive proliferative vitreoretinal lesion, it is wiser to do a thorough cleaning of the entire retina.

INDICATION FOR VITRECTOMY IN RHEGMATOGENOUS RETINAL DETACHMENT

1. Retinal detachment with especially grade C-focal, diffuse, full thickness of sub-retinal strand and grade-D fixed retinal fold in four quadrants.

2. Retinal detachment associated with vitreous haemorrhage.

3. Retinal detachment associated with vitreous foreign bodies.

4. Retinal detachment with giant tear and macular hole.

5. Retinal detachment with multiple horseshoe breaks and/or posterior breaks.

6. Psudophakic and aphakic and thick after cataract retinal detachment with vitreous disturbance.

7. Re operation.

8. Retinal detachment associated with retinoschisis.

9. Retinal detachment associated with choroidal coloboma.

10. Retinal detachment with large posterior tear.

But retinal surgeons do not strictly follow these indications. Indications vary from surgeon to surgeon and is only a guidance in decision-making regarding the procedure to be adopted in a given situation for getting the retina permanently reattached. Vitrectomy has become a less risky procedure and there is a tendency to perform vitrectomy, internal tamponade, even in uncomplicated rhegmatogenous retinal detachment as a substitute for conventional buckling, cryo and external subretinal fluid drainage.

With the development of modern materials like expandable gases and perfluorocarbon liquid, pars plana surgery can be a very predictable and safe surgical modality to reattach the retina and may even substitute and replace conventional retinal detachment surgery very soon (Fig. 14.1).

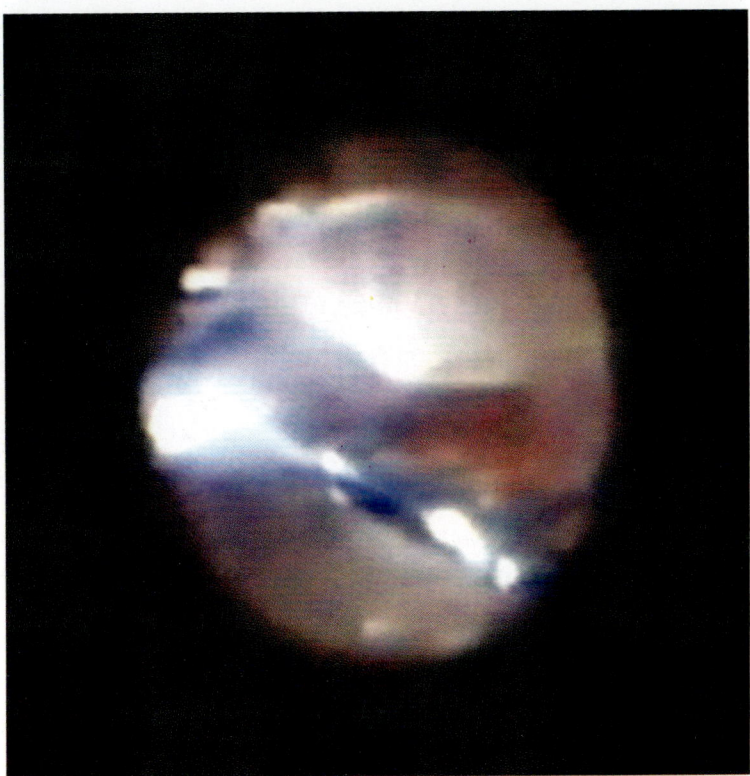

Fig. 14.1 *Vitrectomy in primary rhegmatogenous detachment*

The procedure is less traumatizing to the eye and postoperative inflammation and pain are much reduced when compared to the conventional surgery. Beside this, muscle related problems like postoperative diplopia, squint, etc could be almost eliminated if internal retinal reattachment surgery is performed. In conventional retinal detachment surgery, the sclera is penalized, occasionally leading to necrosis, even though the disease is not in the sclera but in the retina and vitreous. It is only rational thinking that when we treat a disease we should treat a diseased part of the organ rather than healthy part. It is still more deplorable to make a healthy part diseased in the process of treating an unhealthy part.

PARS PLANA VITRECTOMY FOR RETINAL DETACHMENTS

Advantages

1. Here is a minimal change in refractive error in the majority of patients with pars plana vitrectomy.
2. Capsule opacities can be removed intraoperatively to improve visualization of the fundus.
3. The retinal tear can usually be found with scleral depression using the microscope for proper visualization attached and stereopsis with wide angle viewing systems.

Disadvantages

1. Postoperative positioning is necessary, if air/gas injected.

2. Travel by air is restricted for 4 to 6 weeks (gass).

3. There may be iatrogenic complications (retina breaks, vitreous haemorrhage, etc).

4. Endophthalmitis risk (both oil and gas filled eyes).

5. Secondary glaucoma (especially in oil filled eyes).

6. In silicone IOL, with an open posterior capsule, oil come to back-surface of silicone IOL hence reduce the visual acuity.

PRIMARY VITRECTOMY IN RETINAL DETACHMENT CAUSED BY MACULAR HOLE

In high myopia, retinal detachment is very often seen due to macular hole.[5] the presence of a staphyloma causes the retina to be under traction as a result of the posterior bowing of the sclera and choroid (Fig. 14.2).

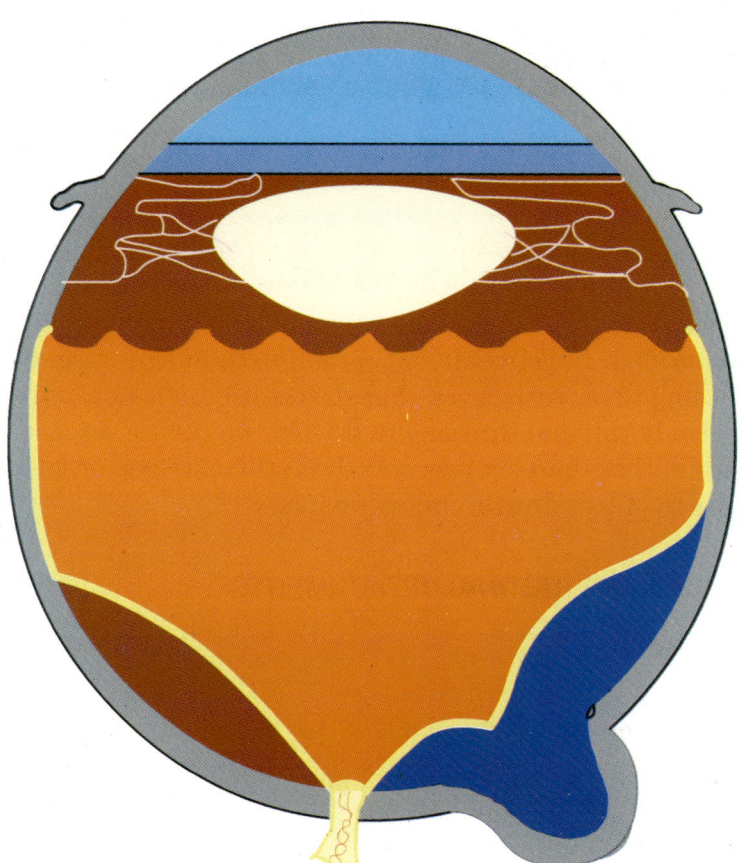

Fig. 14.2 *Rhegmatogenous retinal detachment with macular hole in high myopia patient*

In a few cases epiretinal membrane is also responsible for retinal traction. This problem may be tackled after vitrectomy, careful exploration of the retinal surface near the hole with the help of diamond and epiretinal scraper, it can be removed. A soft tipped cannula may be applied for gentle suction near the macula for residual vitreous or membrane.[6, 7]

The retina is flattened with an air–fluid exchange as the subretinal fluid is drained through the macular hole. The hole is sometimes treated with endolaser photocoagulation if the central vision is no good prior to development of detachment. Silicone oil tamponade is preferred by some surgeon and postoperatively; the patient is positioned facedown for week or longer.

PRIMARY VITRECTOMY IN RETINAL DETACHMENT CAUSED BY POSTERIOR   BREAKS

Posterior retinals breaks or beaks well extend posterior to the equator are difficult to treat with scleral buckling procedure. These breaks are well and good candidates for treatment with primary vitrectomy. The initial step in vitrectomy is to remove as much as the central vitreous possible. The most important factor to remove vitreous from the flap is to relieve traction. The flap should be left intact so that when the retina is flattened, the pigment epithelium is covered (Fig.14.3).

The residual attachment of vitreous is removed carefully so that fresh breaks are not caused. Traction should not be applied on the original break to avoid extending it.

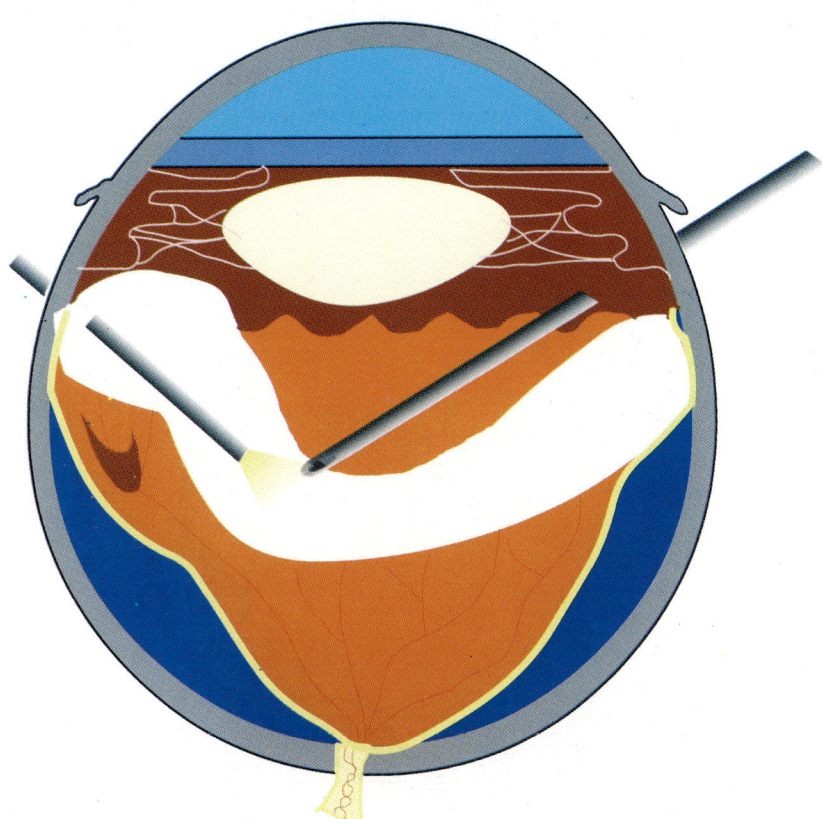

Fig. 14.3 *Retinal break posterior to the equator, good candidate for primary vitrectomy*

Before proceeding air-fluid exchange, the retinal break is treated with internal diathermy so it can be identified once the retina is flattened (Fig. 14.4).

The subretinal fluid is drained through the break (Fig. 14.5). It is easier to treat the break with endolaser photocoagulation or cryotherapy (Fig. 14.6).

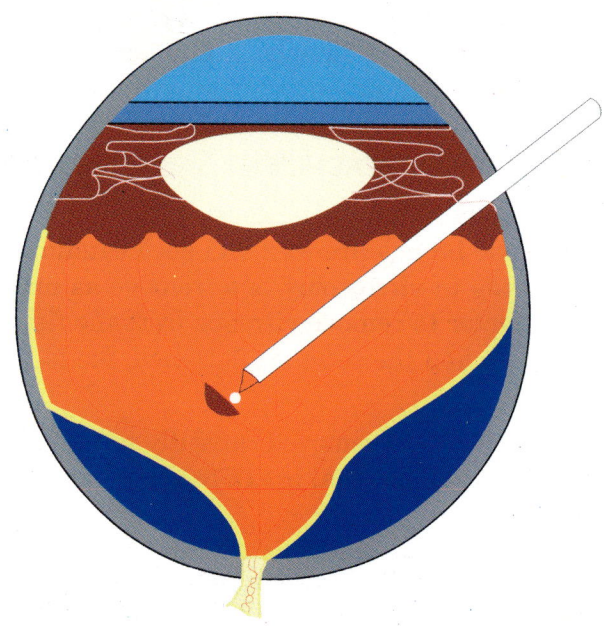

Fig. 14.4 *Retinal break is marked with internal diathermy*

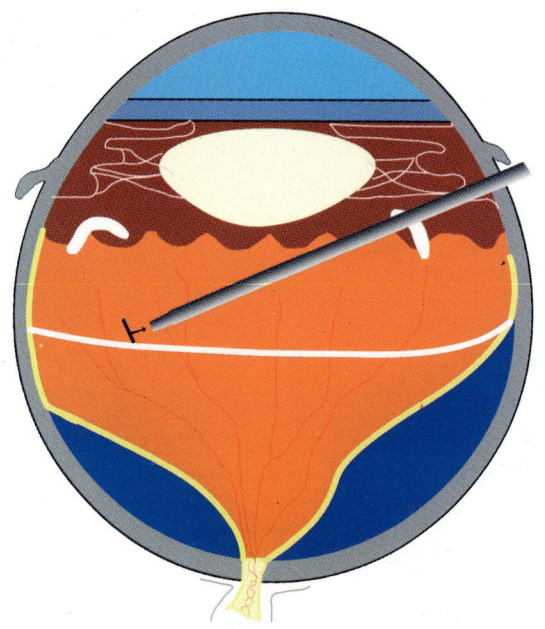

Fig. 14 .5 *Subretinal fluid drain through the posterior break*

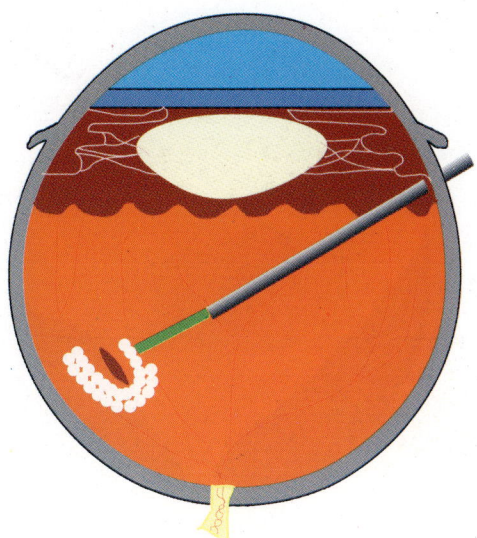

Fig. 14.6 *Posterior break treated with laser photocoagulation*

After surgery, short-acting SF_6 or long acting gas like C_3F_8 may be selected for most of the breaks. The patient is positioned in prone position to avoid cataract formation. A buckle may be added to support the vitreous base to relieve traction. It may not help the posterior break if vitreous traction has been relieved.

PRIMARY VITRECTOMY IN RETINAL DETACHMENT CAUSED BY PERIPHERAL BREAKS

Conventional peripheral breaks scleral buckling is the procedure of choice. In aphakic and pseudophakic eyes, more peripheral breaks may be accessed with the vitreous cutting probe (Fig. 14.7).

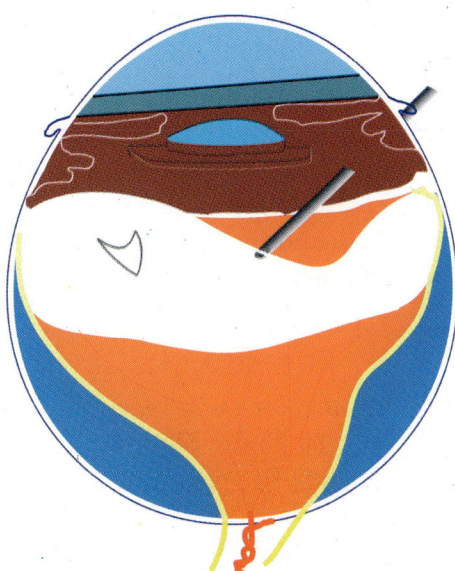

Fig. 14.7 *Psudophakic peripheral break treated with vitrectomy*

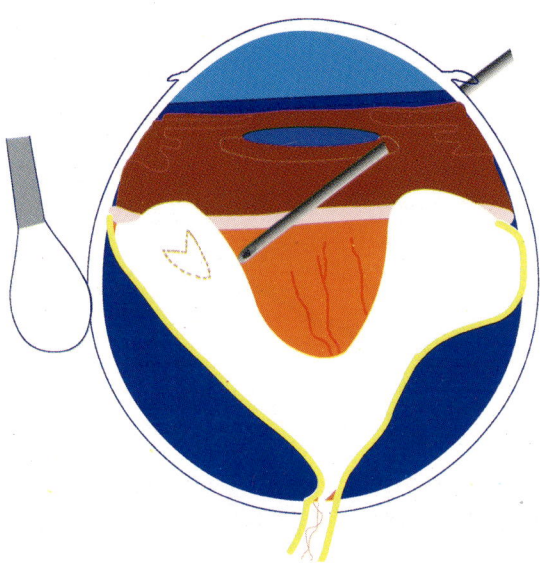

Fig. 14.8 *Vitreous base depressed by cotton applicator to expose ora serrata for better cutting vitreous traction*

The help of vitreous cutting probe or vitreous shaver can expose the peripheral break and oraserrata, so that the vitreous is thoroughly relieved (Fig. 14.8).

Before doing the air fluid exchange, the posterior edge of the break is marked with diathermy. Once the vitreous removal is completed. The break is treated with cryotherapy before or after vitrectomy. It is always nice to seal the break by endolaser photocoagulation after help to locate the break. Air–fluid exchange after the retina is reattached.

When the break is located more anteriorly, it is closed early before the air-fluid exchange, as trapping the fluid occur posteriorly. The cannulated extrusion needle can be inserted through the break for the initial phases of the exchange: so that the posterior fluid can be drained more effectively.

Small retinotomy can be done superiorly and drainage of the fluid is done and the patient is asked to lie in prone position, which is supported by the gas bubble. The site for retinotomy should be located superiorly close to the break or breaks so that both the breaks and retinotomy will supported by the gas bubble with the patient in a comfortable postoperative position. The buckle should support the posterior vitreous base and the posterior edge of the break. The patient position postoperatively is such that the break is supported on the buckle and by the gas bubble.

REFERENCES

1. Hilton Gf, Mc Lean JB, Brinton Da: *Retinal Detachment Principles and Practice.* San Franciser, American Academy of Ophthalmology, pp 65-67, 1989.
2. Gonin J: Treatment of detachment retina by searching retina tears. *Arch Ophthalmol* 4: 621-25, 1930.
3. Escoffery RF et al: Vitrectomy without scleral buckling for primary rhegmatogenous retinal detachment. *Am J Ophthalmol* 99: 275, 1985.
4. Leaver P.K: Role of vitrectomy in the management of retinal detachment. *JR Socmed* 83: 779, 1990.

Management of Giant Retinal Tear

Introduction

A giant retinal tear is a retinal break that extends circumferentially 90 degree or more in the periphery. Most retinal breaks can be re-opposed to the retinal pigment epithelium (RPE) by vitrectomy and prone fluid–gas exchange. The vitreous base produced traction on the anterior retina (anterior flap), so that the posterior retina is no longer fixed anteriorly and can slide, fold or scroll into the posterior segment. If left untreated, this produces adhesion and proliferative vitreoretinopathy. Once proliferative vitreoretinopathy (PVR) has developed, the success rate is reduced. Proper planning of giant retinal tear is essential. The elements in treating a giant retinal tear involve vitrectomy, repositioning the tear by air, silicone oil, or perflurocarbon liquid, and treating the tear by laser photocoagulation, or cryotherapy. Tamponade by gas, silicone oil, and scleral buckling may be required.

DIAGNOSIS AND PRE-OPERATIVE EVALUATION

The diagnosis of a giant retinal tear is easy. Most cases present with a history of sudden painless diminution of vision with symptoms of photopsia and floaters. The condition may occur following blunt trauma to the eye[1] Intravitreal surgical procedure [2] associated with other congenital anomalies (i.e. Marfan's syndrome) or may be idiopathic.[3] It has been observed that incidence of non-traumatic giant retinal tear is important since the fellow eye has high risk for the occurrence of a giant retinal tear. Indirect ophthalmoscopy usually reveals the presence of giant retinal tear. In rare cases where retina tears to the extent of 360° with severe proliferative vitreoretinopathy, the retina may be reduced to a stalk attached to disc. In such situation, it is possible for a surgeon to misdiagnose the bare choroid as perfectly attached retina. Some times, similar mistake has been known to be made in-patient with a completely inverted folded, over retinal flap. In these cases, the area of bare choroids may be misdiagnosed as attached retina. This mistake can be avoided by looking carefully for the presence of retinal vessels, which are obviously looking over an area of bare choroids. Careful evaluation of the folded flap will reveal that the retinal vessels are hazily seen and the normal pearly gray retinal sheen is missing. The important facts to be noted during the examination of a patient with a giant retinal tear are location of tear; extend of the tear, mobility of flap and extent of proliferative vitreoretinopathy. Evaluation of this parameter is important to determine not only the prognosis but also necessary decision-making regarding the surgical technique.

LOCATION OF GIANT RETINAL TEAR

The location of giant retinal tear could be superior, inferior or it may be located in the temporal or the nasal quadrant or partly in both. Inferior giant retinal tear are more difficult to tamponade postoperatively since both silicone oil and intraocular gases are lighter than water and tends to raise post operatively. This problem of inadequate tamponade dose not arises in superior tear, up to 180° lying in the temporal or nasal quadrant.

MOBILITY OF POSTERIOR RETINAL FLAP

Retinal tears occur as a consequence of traction by the vitreous on the retina.[4] This traction is directed towards the vitreous base, which is the area straddling the ora-serrata and is also the area of the firmest attachment of the vitreous to the retina. As a consequence, the traction on the flap of a retina tear is always directed anteriorly and it is the anterior flap of the retinal tear, which is lifted up into the vitreous as a consequence of the vitreous traction.

The situation in a giant retinal tear is quite different. As a consequence of its huge size, the small anterior retinal flap with vitreous attached to it become quite redundant. The posterior flap, which in a small horseshoe tear has a passive role, becomes the dominant factor. This is because this flap has no support and consequently has a tendency to fall back on the posterior retina (Fig.15.1).

Furthermore, the residual vitreous fibrils attached to this flap become involved in the process of proliferative vitreoretinopathy and contract. This contraction results in the posterior retinal flap of a giant retinal tear initially getting displaced from its position; subsequently the flap appears to be standing up right; and finally it begins to roll up and get inverted. Once the retina flap is positioned up right in the vitreous cavity without a tendency to fall back with ocular movements, one can be sure that its mobility is significantly restricted.

The concept of the mobility of the posterior retinal flap is the pivot around which the surgical management of a giant retinal tear is planned. In the initial stages of its occurrence, when the tear exists without displacement of the retinal flap from its normal position or is still mobile, permitting the retina to fall back in to its normal position, its management by laser/ cryo and conventional scleral buckling procedures is still possible.[4] However, once significant restriction of mobility of the posterior retina flap occurs, one has to resort to complex vitreoretinal procedures for successful reattachment of the retina.[5]

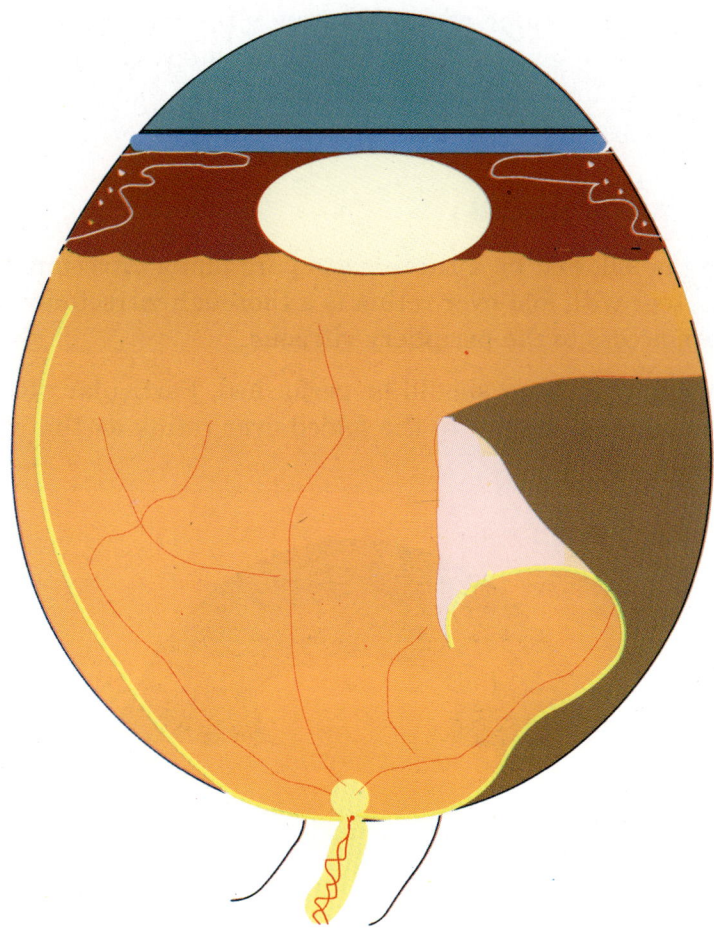

Fig. 15.1 *Giant retinal tear*

EXTENT OF PROLIFERATIVE VITREORETINOPATHY (PVR)

The presence of a giant retinal tear results in the exposure of a large area of bare retinal pigment epithelium. These eyes are therefore at high risk for development of proliferative vitreoretinopathy.[6] Furthermore, proliferative vitreoretinopathy develops very rapidly in these eyes. Proliferative vitreoretinopathy (PVR) could take the form of star folds in various parts of the retinal surface and especially in the quadrants involved by the giant retinal tear. These could be a consequence of preretinal and subretinal membranes. Epiretinal membrane at the edge of the giant retinal tear could results in a rolling (scrolling up) of the tear edge.[4] Circumferential contraction of the vitreous fibrils attached to the torn retinal edge could cause it to contract in a purse-string fashion, and occasionally even to adhere here to the opposite retinal surface. In the macular area, the presence of a pre-retinal membrane may induce a macular pucker. These proliferative changes ultimately results in the torn retina completely folding over and becoming immobile and crumpled up. The onset and progression of proliferative vitreoretinopathy makes the surgical procedure more difficult and could make the anatomic and visual result much worse.

Accurate assessment of the degree of proliferative vitreoretinopathy is therefore essential not only in order to be able to give the prognosis to the steps of the surgical procedure. It is especially important for the surgeon to assess the feasibility of complete removal of vitreoretinal traction due to preretinal proliferation in the area of the retina, which is not torn.

PROCEDURE (SURGICAL TECHNIQUE)

Conjunctival peritomy is followed by a three ports pars plana vitrectomy. The initial step for repairing of any giant tear with fold-over retina is a thorough vitrectomy. Lensectomy is sometimes indicated to gain access to the periphery vitreous.

A complete as possible vitrectomy should be performed. Particular attention is given to ensuring that no gel is present posterior to the folded-over retina as this will prevent the later unfolding of the break (Fig.15.2).

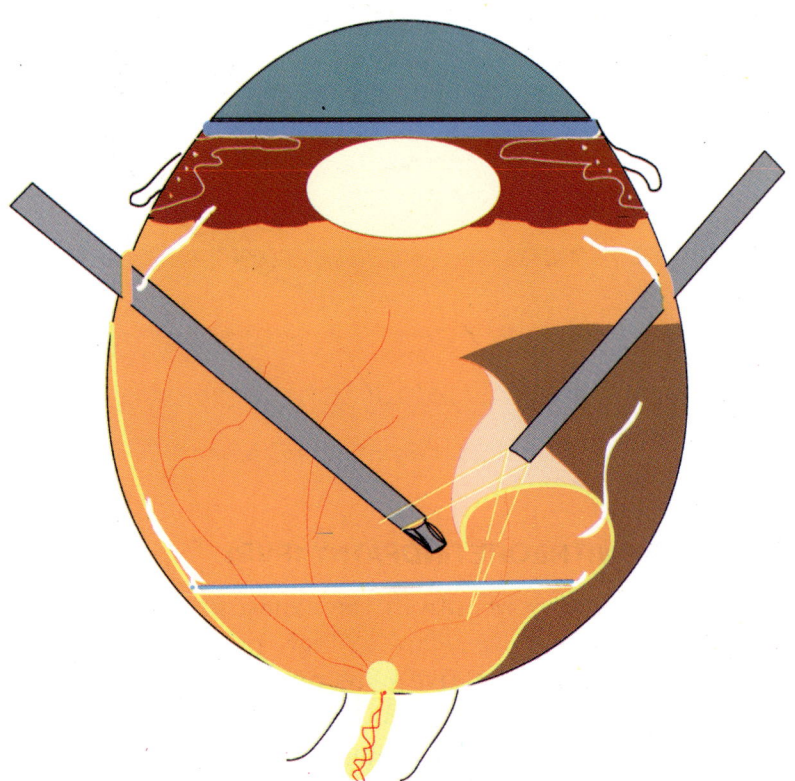

Fig. 15.2 *Thorough vitrectomy with unfolding the retina*

Vitreous base is shaved by the help of vitreous shaver using scleral depressor (Fig.15.3).

If anterior flap is produced it should be ampulated because contraction within this flap can also re-open the break. The posterior flap must be repositioned which can be grasped with gentle suction using a silicone cannula and carefully rotated anteriorly (Figs.15.4 and 15.5).

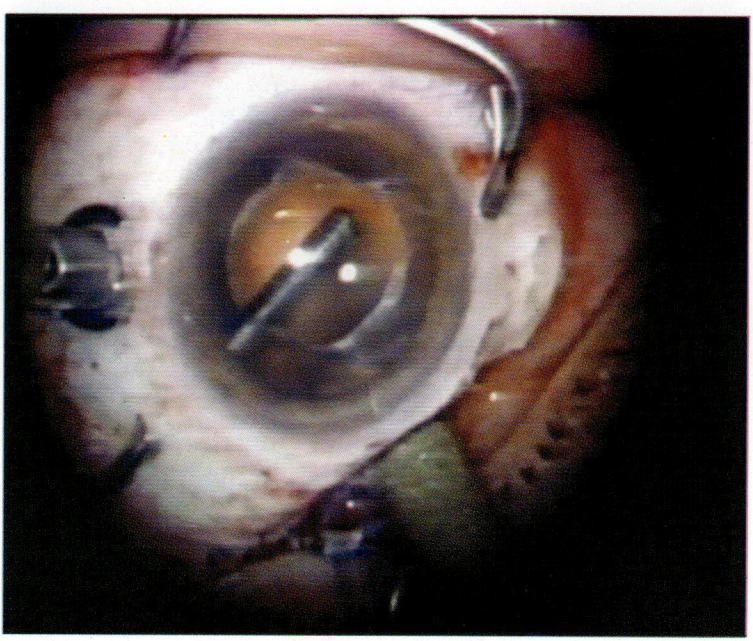

Fig. 15.3 *Vitreous base is removed by depressing the sclera by scleral depressor*

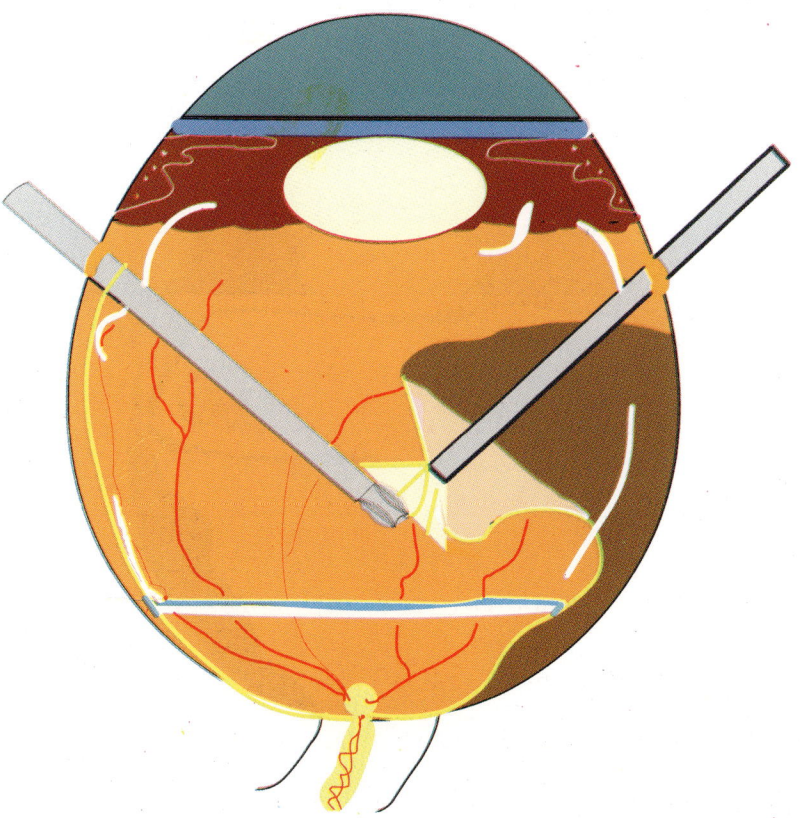

Fig. 15.4 *Rotation of flap with silicone cannula*

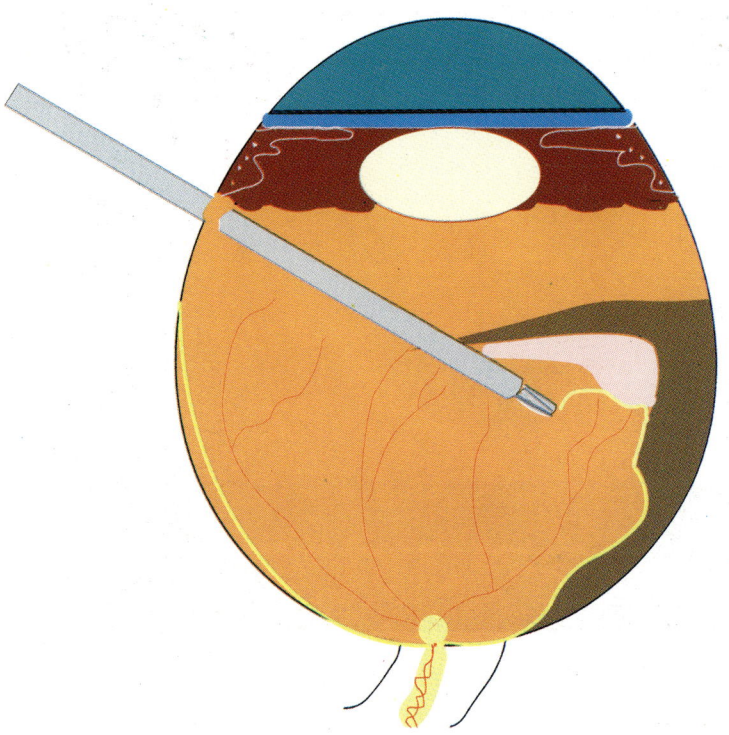

Fig. 15.5 *Flap anteriorly rotated*

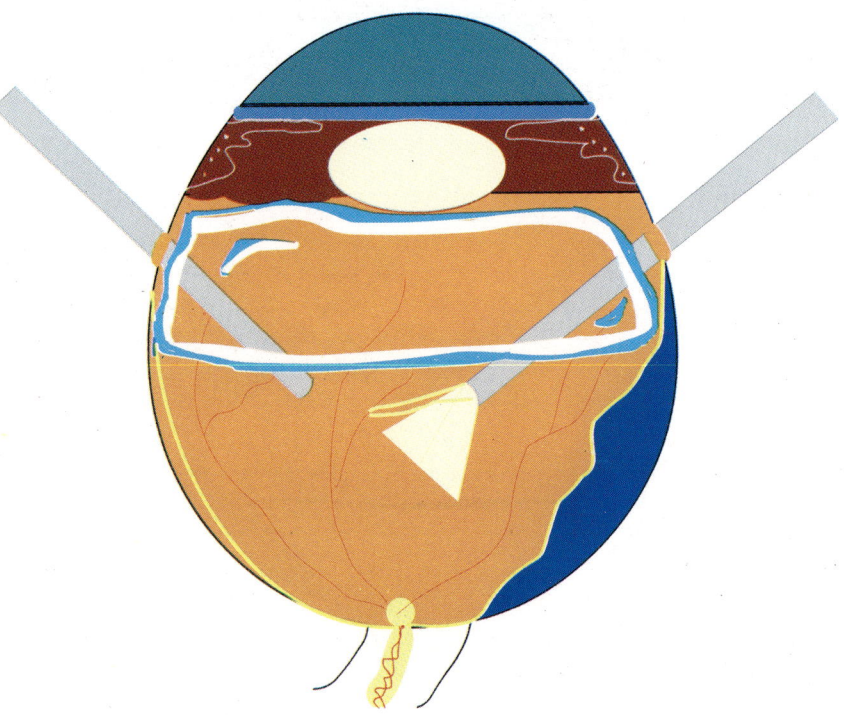

Fig. 15.6 *Trapping subretinal fluid under the retina.*

After air – fluid exchange, subretinal fluid trapped under the retina (Fig.15.6).

To drain the subretinal fluid the eye is tipped in the direction of tear and drainage is performed from the edge (Fig.15.7).

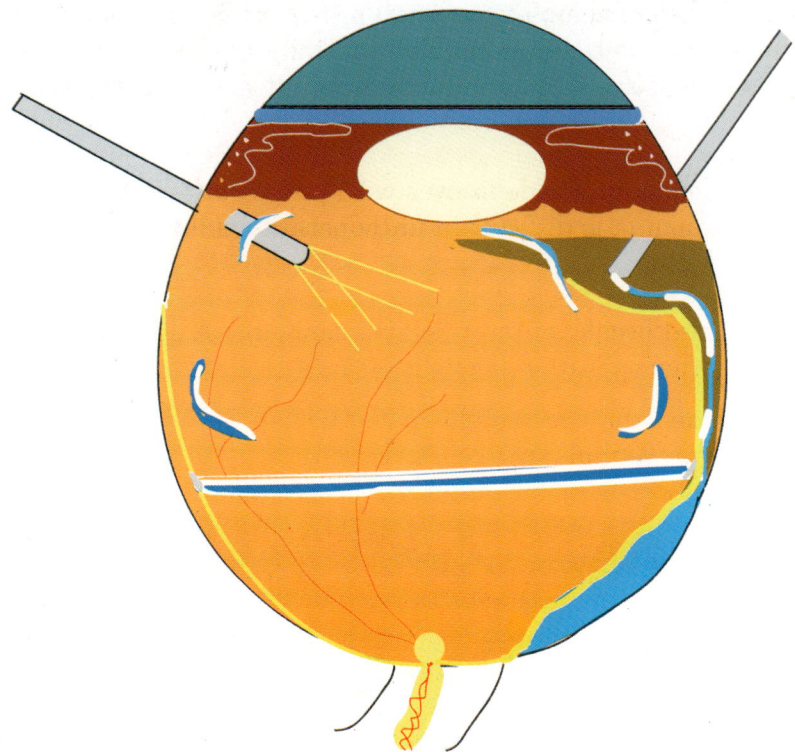

Fig. 15.7 *Drainage of subretinal fluid*

This technique works much better and tear that extend very posteriorly then on anteriorly place tear. To drain posteriorly fluid from anterior tear the cannulated extrusion needle can be placed beneath the tear and position posteriorly.

SILICONE OIL TECHNIQUE IN GIANT RETINAL TEAR

Paul Cibis, of St. Louis, was responsible for the early popularity of intraocular silicone oil.[7] John Scott used silicone oil as an instrument to separate membranes and push the retina back, without vitrectomy. It was Haut who first combined use of silicone oils as internal tamponade after vitrectomy.[8] Zivojnovic popularized their technique and contributed immensely to its successful usage by defining its role clearly.[9] A standard three-port vitrectomy is done with the goal of removing all formed vitreous. It is of extreme importance that all retinal traction is released and the retina is completely reattached before the use of silicone oil. The per fluorocarbon (PFCL) can be useful in producing traction in the posterior pole and stabilizing the anterior retina, to facilitate dissection of membrane. Perflurocarbon may be removed before the gas exchange or during fluid air exchange. An inferior iridectomy is performed in aphakic eyes, which may also be beneficial in eyes with a posterior chamber intraocular lens if zonular rupture is suspected (Fig.15.8).

The decision regarding the need for a scleral buckle is made preoperatively based on the assessment of the feasibility of complete removal of the preretinal membranes in the area of the retina which is not torn. The use of buckle especially important in patients in whom the giant retinal tear is situated superiorly and extensive vitreoretinal traction is present in the inferior quadrant.

Silicone oil is an excellent tamponade in eyes with proliferation vitreoretinopathy or eyes in which postoperative positioning is difficult in uncooperative adults, debilitated individual and children.

The posterior flap of giant break is first unfolded, using direct intraocular manipulation with the endoilluminator and the aspiration needle (Fig.15.9).

Once the flap is unfolded the eye is held with the flap dependent and silicone oil slowly exchange for fluid in the preretinal surface (Fig.15.10).

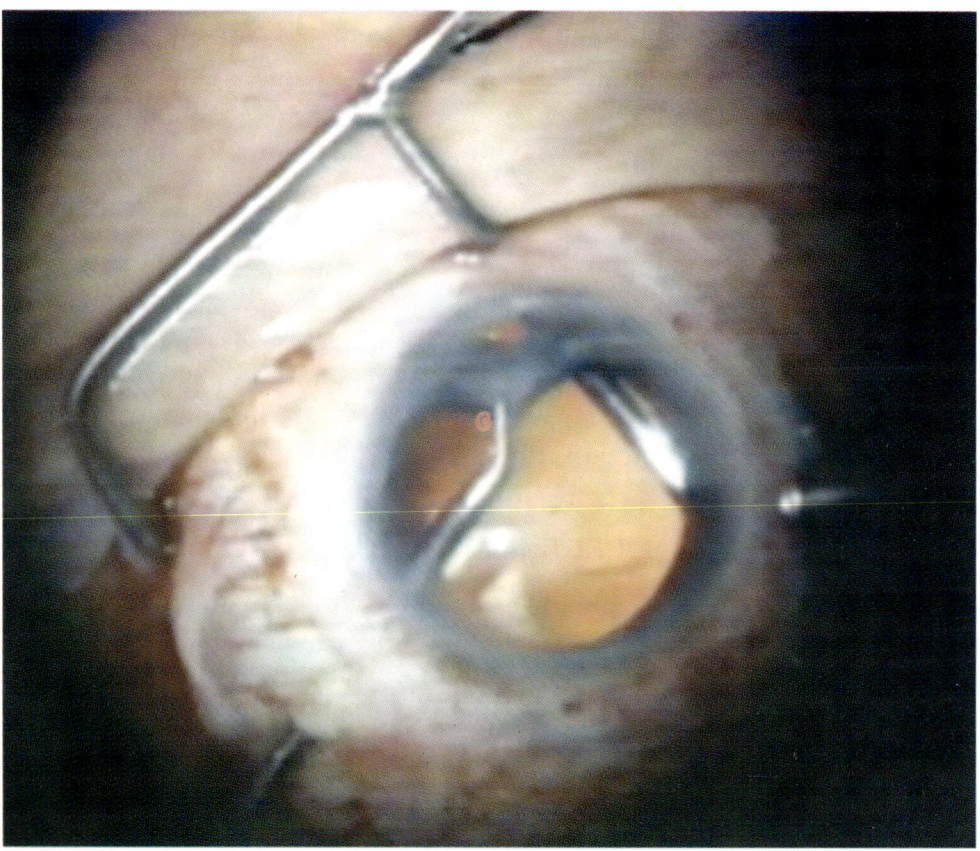

Fig. 15.8 *Inferior iridectomy*

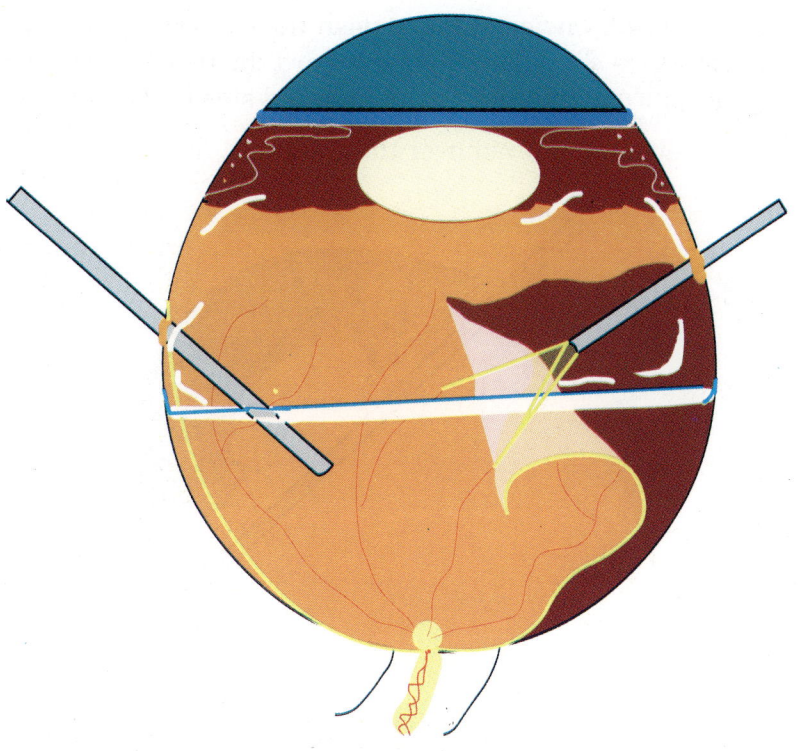

Fig. 15.9 *Following vitrectomy, silicone oil is infused in the eye*

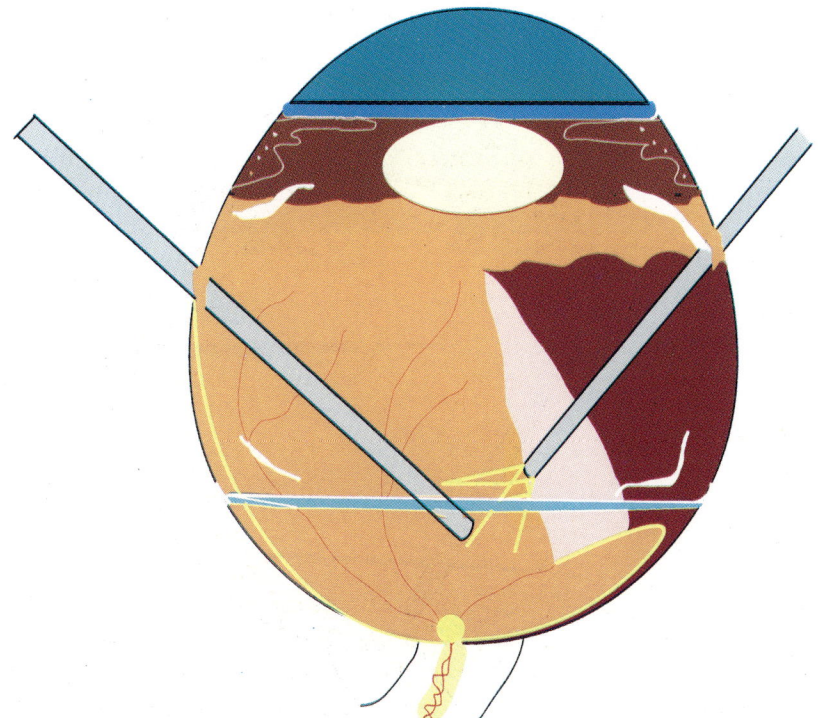

Fig. 15.10 *Fluid is drained as silicone oil floats above the balanced salt solution*

The slow expansion of the silicone oil tends to push the sub-retinal fluid in to the pre-retinal space where it can be aspirated. The eye is tipped toward the tear to vacuum of the last amount of subretinal fluid as the silicone continued to be injected slowly (Fig.15.11).

Any residual posterior fluid is removed over the optic disc (Fig.15.12).

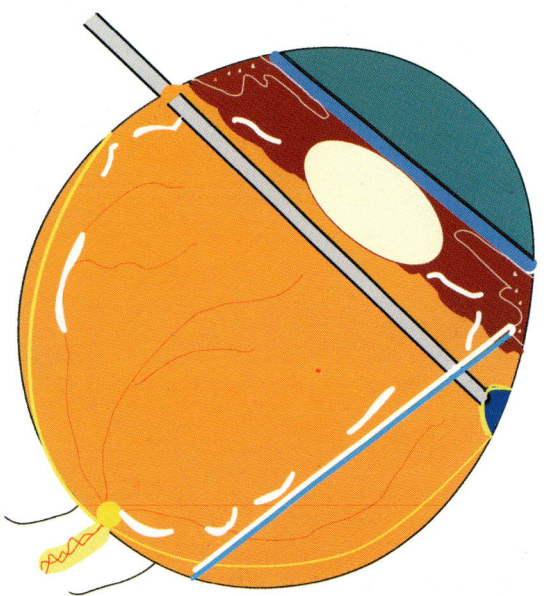

Fig. 15.11 *Last amount of subretinal fluid is drained out*

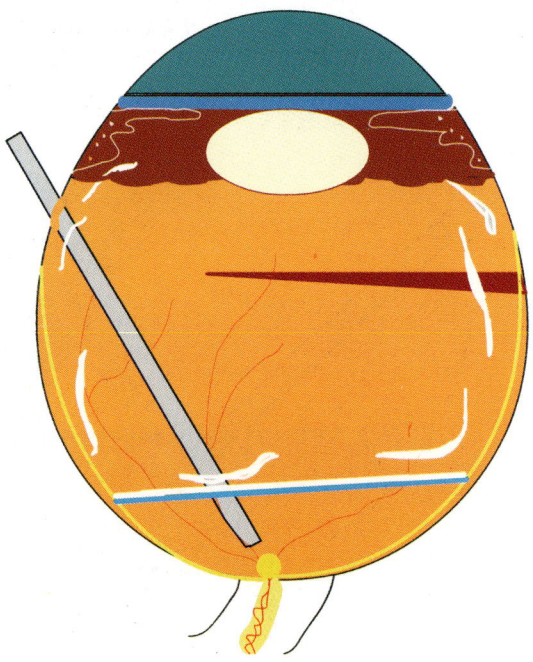

Fig. 15.12 *Subretinal fluid is completely removed*

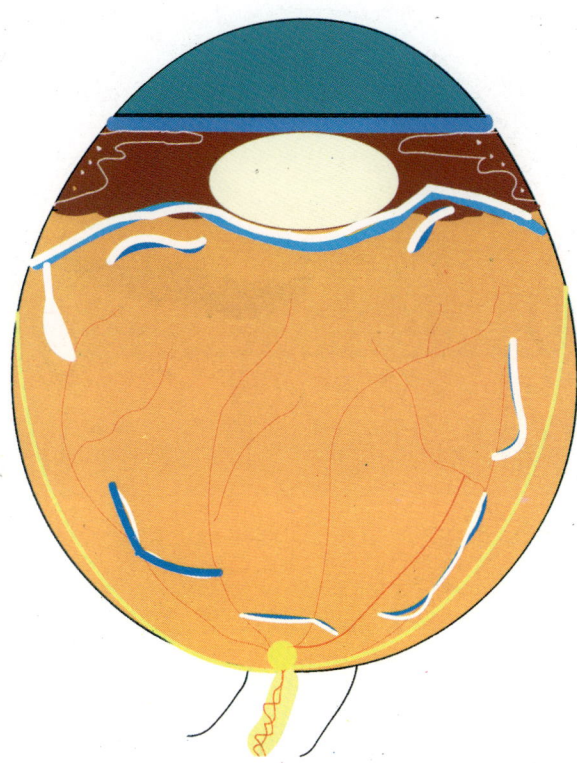

Fig. 15.13 *Silicone oil is filled completely and retina attached*

The silicone oil is filled completely leaving the retina attached (Fig.15.13).

In certain cases, a deliberated posterior retinotomy is required to internally drain subretinal fluid trapped posteriorly after the giant break is closed. The silicone oil provides a good tamponade postoperative period. The anterior end of the break treated with cryopexy, the remainder of break is treated with confluent endophotocoagulation. Every effort is made to avoid treating bare retinal pigment epithelium (RPE).

In spite of proper vitreous-base shaving, and through vitrectomy majority of cases re-detachment occurs from re-opening of one or the other ends of the break or from new break formation caused by vitreous base contraction in area of previously uniform retina, circumferential buckle is used in uniform equatorial retina. Closer of the giant break is maintained by silicone tamponade. Although a scleral buckle usually is applied for giant tears with proliferative vitreo retinopathy, it is not needed for all giant tear repairs.

If buckle to be performed, it is often best to apply the buckle before repositioning the tear to reduce the likelihood of dislodging the retina during the positioning and suturing of the buckle (Fig.15.14).

At the end of the surgery, last drop of perfluorocarbon must be removed with great care to avoid dislodging the retina (Fig.15.15).

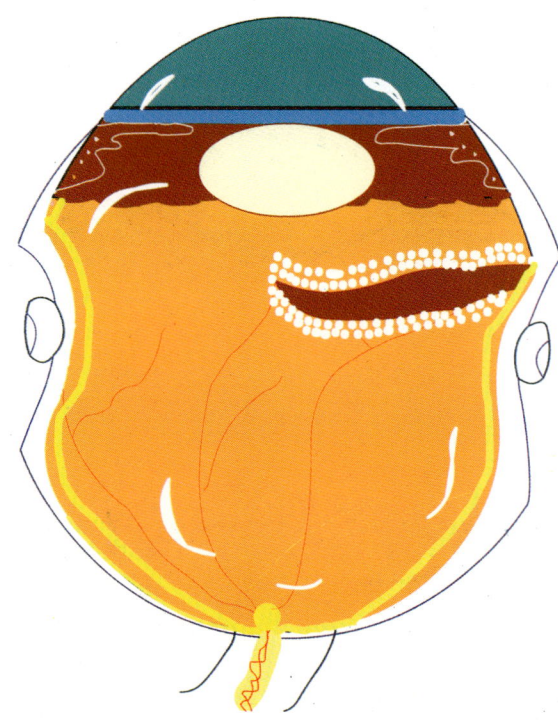

Fig. 15.14 *Scleral buckle with laser photocoagulation*

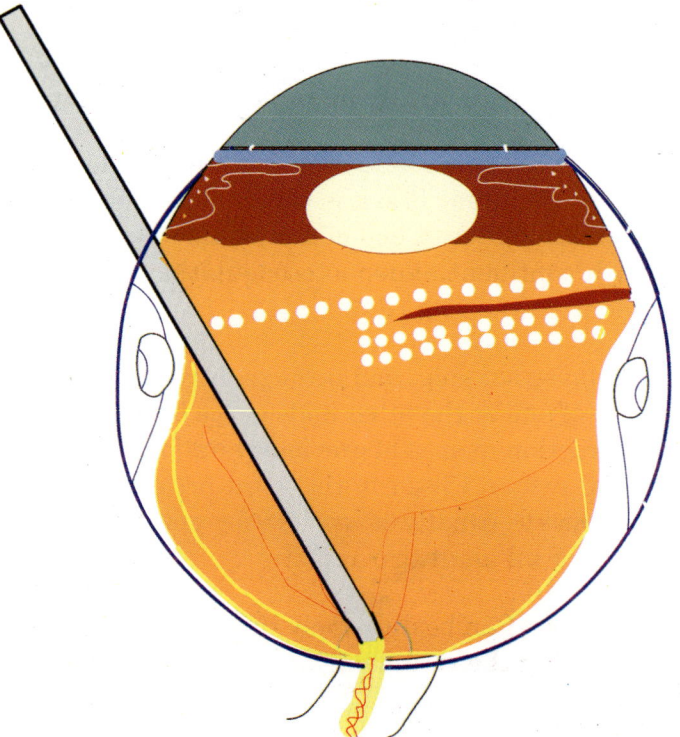

Fig. 15.15 *Last drop of perfluorocarbon is removed.*

SILICONE OIL REMOVAL

The technique of silicone oil removal is relatively simple. A formal three-port vitrectomy is favourable as any residual or recurrent preretinal membranes or other media opacities can be removed. Balanced salt solution is infused through the parsplana using the infusion cannula. In aphakic patients, where additional surgery is not required a small corneal incision made by the MVR-blade is sufficient to allow the engross of the silicone oil. An 18 or 19-gauge thin-walled needle inserted through the pars-plana and attached by a small piece of tubing to a 60 ml syringe allows generating sufficient suction force to evacuate oil in phakic or psudophakic eyes. Mechanical viscous fluid extractors, which are attached to the main console, can also be used. Silicone oil, sometimes tend to be tapped in the vitreous base and under the iris and in membranes. Hidden small silicone bubble may be removing with the help of flute needle. However, total removal of oil traces is never possible.

The minimal time after which silicone oil can be removed is considered to be three weeks. In general it is preferred that the silicone oil to be removed by three to six months postoperatively.[10] and even earlier. There are, however, several cases in which silicone oil has remained in eyes for several year.[9]

LIQUID PERFLUOROCARBON IN GAINT RETINAL TEAR

Perfluorocarbon liquids were rapidly recognized as being a very useful tool in the treatment of giant retinal tear. It is an excellent intraocular tool for reattaching the retina. The liquid is heavier than water or saline and displaces subretinal fluid forward. Following vitrectomy, the perflurocarbon is injected slowly over the optic disc and care should be taken to inject directly into the bubble to avoid creating multiple bubbles (Fig.15.16).

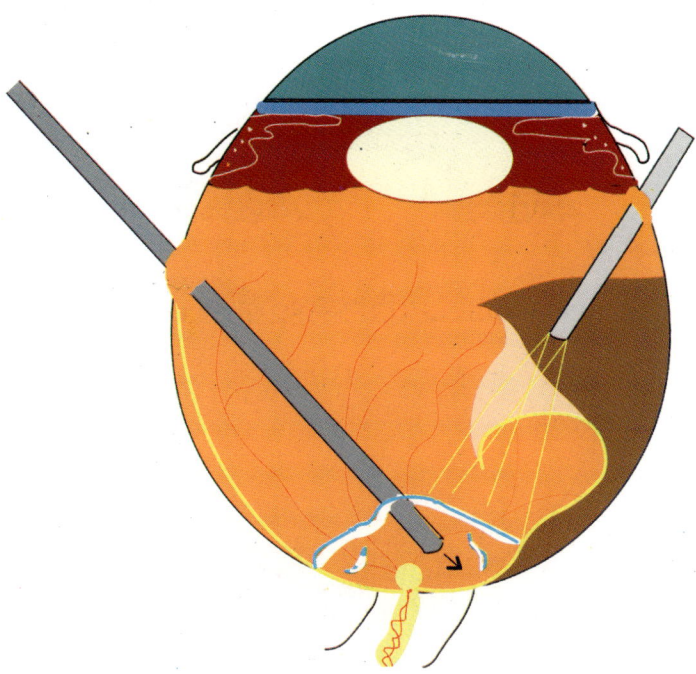

Fig. 15.16 *Slow injection of PFCL over optic nerve*

As soon as the bubble enlarges, the retina is pushed anteriorly and the fluid is extruded from under the retina (Fig. 15.17).

This process is best monitored through a wide angle viewing system. While injecting perfluorocarbon, care is taken not to allow the perfluorocarbon to go beneath the retina (Fig.15.18).

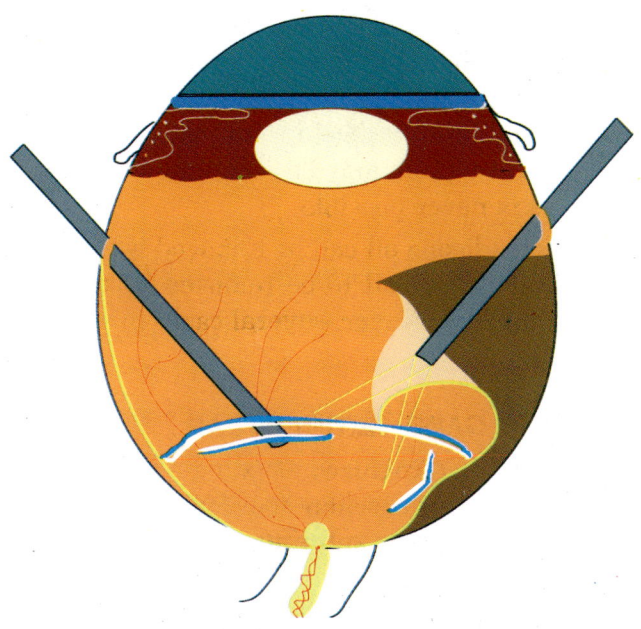

Fig. 15.17 *Retina pushed anteriorly as PFCL bubble enlarges*

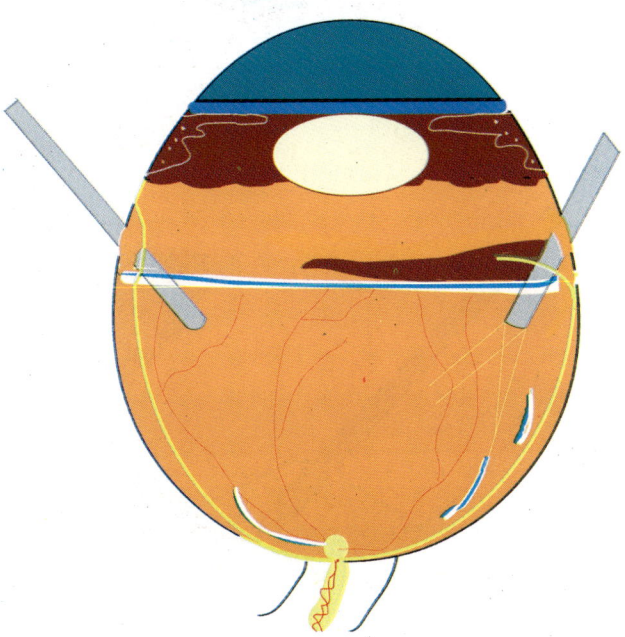

Fig. 15.18 *PFCL brought of to posterior edge of tear*

An air–fluid exchange is now performed, and the edge of the tear treated either by cryo-therapy or laser while the perflurocarbon maintains the retinal position.

The basic technique for managing rhegmatogenous retinal tears with or without prolifera-tive vitreoretinopathy is similar for most of the eyes. Scleral sutures are placed for a circumfer-ential scleral buckle before vitrectomy is performed. The narrow buckle is used is the giant retinal tear is less than 180° break and if it is more than 180° broad buckle may be used. The crystalline lens has to be scarified which allows removing complete anterior vitreous at the edge of the giant tear. It also improves access to the edge of the giant tear to prevent inversion of the tear when the fluid–gas exchange is performed. Aggressive removal of vitreous base is done because the vitreous base is unstable in many eyes with giant retinal tears and may cause extension of the tear postoperatively with recurrent retinal detachment.

The goal is to make the retina mobile so it will repose to the eyewall after the perfluorocarbon liquid–gas exchange. The perfluorocarbon liquid is injected in a 3 to 5 ml syringes through 25 or 27 gauge blunt needle over the optic disc. Once the vitreous has been removed and the retina is mobile, the intravitreal saline-infusion solution will be displaced out of the eye around the sides of the 25-gauge blunt needle in the 20-gauge sclerotomy as the perflurocarbon liquid is injected. It is important to inject the perflurocarbon liquid slowly to allow the subretinal fluid to pass from the vitreous cavity and out of the eye.

It is important that the tip of the edge of the giant retinal tear must be perilously dried so the retina does not slip posteriorly or invert during removal of the more posterior perfluorocarbon liquid (Fig.15.19).

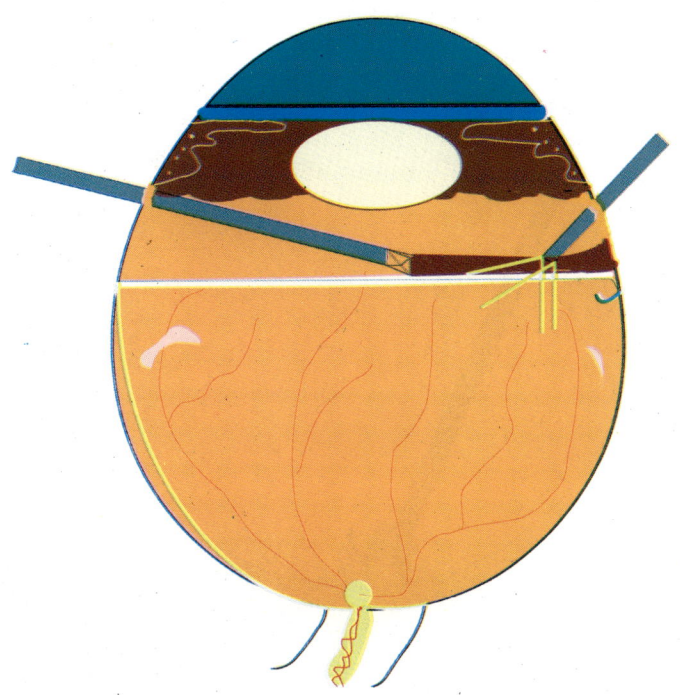

Fig. 15.19 *Air–fluid exchange and edge of tear is drained for laser photocoagulation.*

It is mandatory to decrease the suction to 25 to 50 mm of Hg while drying the edge of the retina. Removal of saline from the anterior vitreous is also slow and careful. The capillary attraction between retina and retinal pigment epithelium will hold the retina in position once the retinal pigment epithelium (RPE) is dried at the edge of the retinal tear and all the subretinal fluid has been removed using flexible tip cannula. However, care must to be taken to remove all of the perflurocarbon liquid from the vitreous cavity as it accumulate over the optic disc during fluid–gas exchange Laser endophotocoagulation is then placed around the edge of the tear and 360° buckle applied once the eye is filled with gas. The suture around the buckle is tightened to create a moderate to high buckle effect. After the laser photocoagulation completed gas is injected into the vitreous cavity and sclerotomy incision are closed. The patient is instructed to maintain face down position postoperatively to provide intraocular tamponade and maintain the position of the edge the giant tear against the retinal pigment epithelium.

TREATMENT OF GIANT TEAR

After attachment of the giant tear, both the anterior and posterior edge of the tear should be treated by endo laser photocoagulation (Fig. 15.20). Treatment is carried out 360° to guard against subsequent extension of the tear. PFCL is removed by either passive or active suction replacing the liquid with air or silicone oil. After the last drop of PFCL are remove over the disc the retina is examine care fully if any residual liquid, which could be removed. Performing cryotherapy before vitrectomy has been advocated because cells liberated from the pigment epithelium during surgery will be removed by vitrectomy, theoretically reducing the risk of

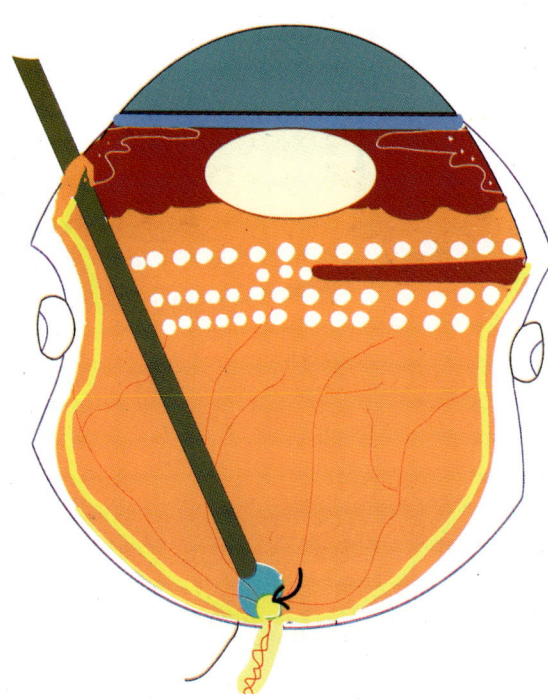

Fig. 15.20 *Endolaser photocoagulation done both anterior and posterior edge of tears with passive removal of PFCL*

postoperative proliferative vitreoretinopathy. Endolaser is superior to cryotherapy as there is less chance of release of pigments. This can be done to treat any posterior iatrogenic breaks as well as the giant tear. Treatment in phakic eyes may be difficult with endophotocoagulation, particularly in the superior quadrants.

Photocoagulation applied through the indirect ophthalmoscope with scleral depressor is helpful in these cases.

POSTOPERATIVE COMPLICATIONS

Complications following surgery for a giant retinal tear includes severe fibrinus anterior segment reaction, glaucoma, hyphaema, and slippage of the retinal tear, pre-retinal membrane formation and redetachment due to proliferative vitreoretinopathy. Slippage almost always implies that there is at least a minute amount of residual sub-retinal fluid remaining, which can be drained by doing posterior retinotomy (Fig. 15.21). Applying intense diathermy to a small area of the retina creates this.

Through the posterior retinotomy (Fig.15.22), fluid may be drained and the retina is repositioned by gently brushing it in to place with silicone tipped cannula. Endolaser is applied to the retinotomy and to the edges of the giant break (Fig.15.23).

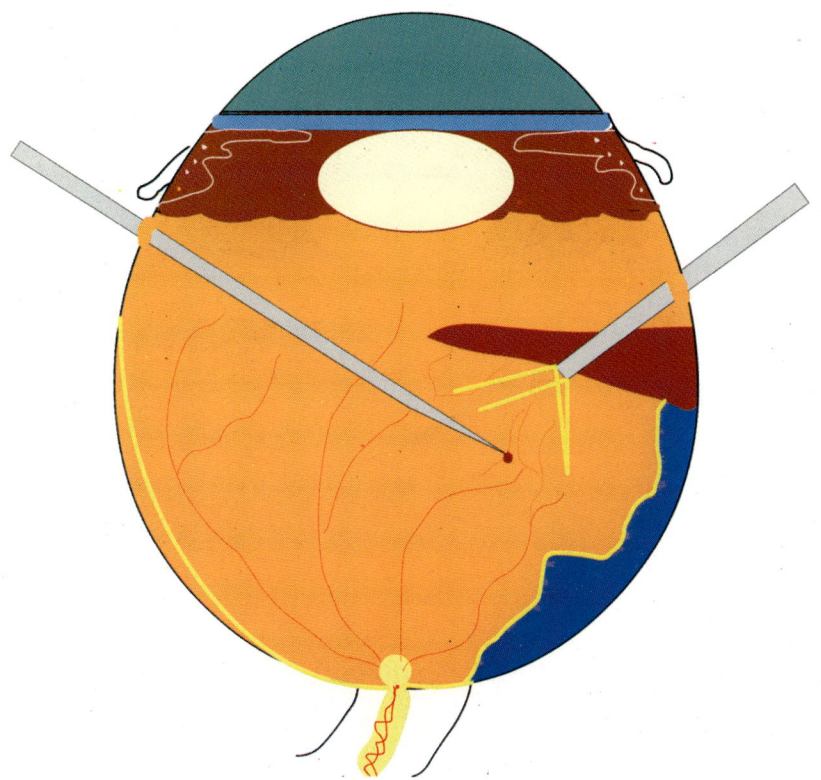

Fig. 15.21 *Posterior retinotomy is created*

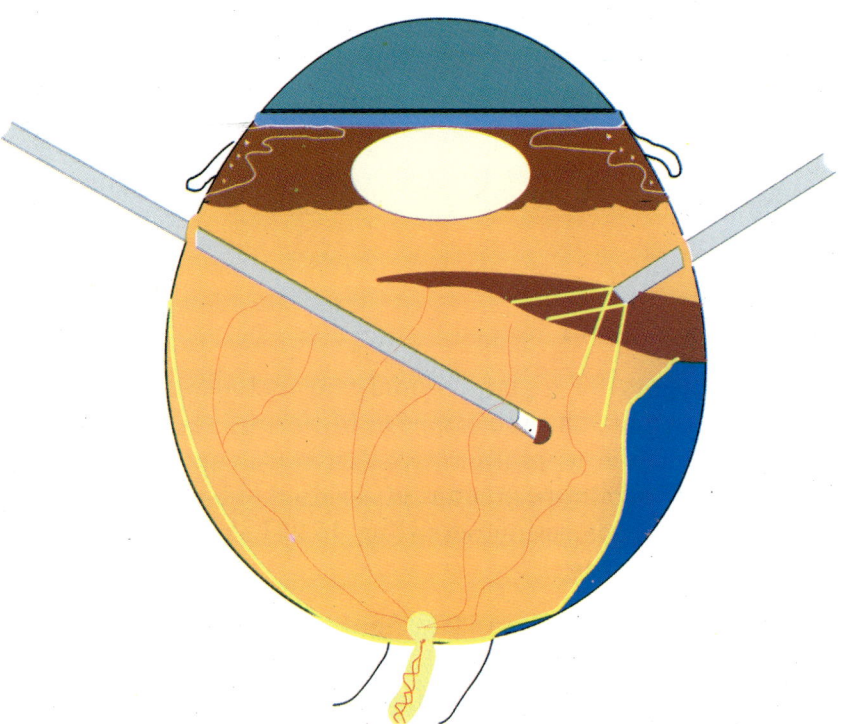

Fig. 15.22 *Fluid is drained through posterior retinotomy by silicone-tipped cannula.*

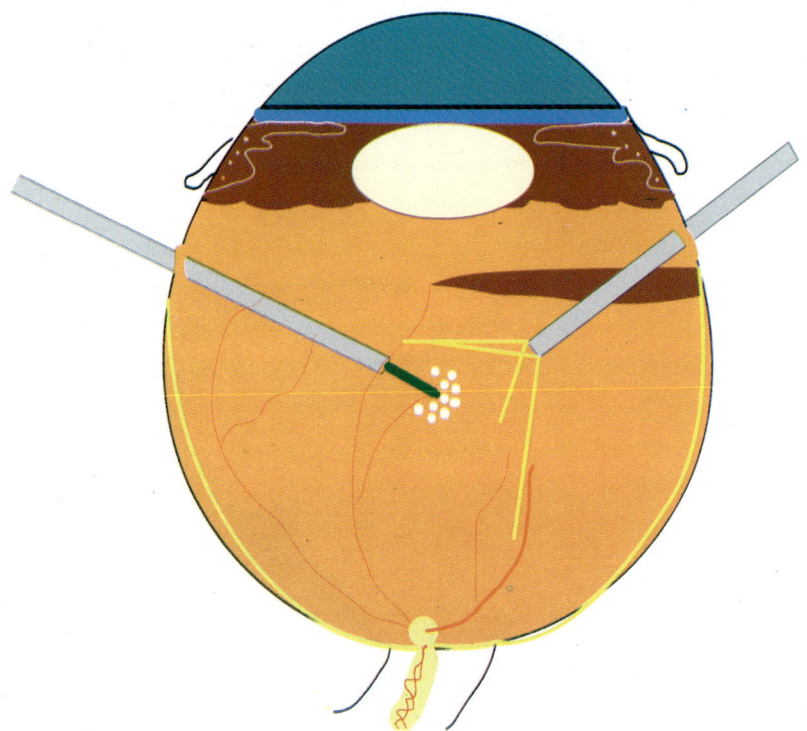

Fig. 15.23 *Laser is applied to the retinotomy and to the edge of giant retinal tear.*

The most important and common complication following an initially successful vitreoretinal surgery for a giant retinal tear is the formation of an epiretinal membrane Removal of the epiretinal membrane under silicone oil can be done as second sitting later on.

MANAGEMENT OF FELLOW EYE

Fellow eyes of patients with a nontraumatic (idiopathic) giant retinal tear are at risk for development of retinal detachment. Finding that have been reported in these fellow eyes at presentation include giant retinal breaks, retinal detachment or even retinal dialysis in 31.1% of patients. A further 23.7% developed one or more of these finding over a follow up period, which ranged from 1 to 29 years. The commonest ophthalmoscopic finding in fellow eyes which developed a giant retinal break was extensive white with pressure. Eyes with myopia greater than 10.00 Diopter's, increase area of white with pressure, and increasing condensation of the vitreous base show a high incidence of giant retinal breaks.[13, 12]

It is, therefore, recommended that the fellow eyes of patients with a non-traumatic giant retinal tear having theses features should be treated by an encircling band with 360° cryopexy or laser photocoagulation.

Today patients with giant retinal tears can expect final reattachment rates of 90% (with multiple surgical procedure).[13]

These rates are lower for patients with giant retinal tear (GRT) associated with penetrating trauma. Long-term anatomic re-attachment rates vary from 86%, 6 months postoperatively to 73%, 5 years following surgery are quite favourable with 66% of patients achieving a visual acuity of 6/6 and 32% achieving a visual acuity 6/18 or more[14]. While there is no significant effect of the size of the giant retinal tear (GRT) on visual prognosis, the degree of proliferative vitreoretinopathy could affect the visual outcome following surgery.

REFERENCES

1. Freeman HM, Cox MS and Schepens CL: Traumatic retinal detachments. Int. *Ophthalmol*. Clin; 14 (4): 151, 1974.

2. Freeman, H.M : Current management of giant retinal breaks and fellow eyes. In: Ryan SJ (Ed.) *Retina*, Vol 3, St. Louis, CV Mosby Co, pp. 2313-2328, 1994.

3. McLeod O: Giant retinal tear after central vitrectomy. *Br. J. Ophthalmol*, 69: 96, 1985.

4. Freeman HM: Fellow eyes of giant retinal breaks. *Trans. Am. Ophthalmol. Soc.*; 76: 343-382, 1978.

5. Michels RG: Complicated types of retina detachment. In: Michels RG Ed. *Retinal Detachment,* St. Louis, CV Mosby Co., pp 638-669, 1990.

6. Sipplerley JO, Machemer R: Histologic evaluation of adhesive properties of early lesions in diathermy and cryopexy. *Int. Ophthalmol*; 2 : 107, 1981.

7. Clibis PA, Becker B, Okun E, et. al. The use of liquid silicone in retinal detachment surgery. *Arch Ophthalmol*, 68 : 590, 1962.

8. Haut J Ulleren M, Boulard ML, et. al: Utilisation du silicone intraocular après vitrecomic comme troitement des restrictions massive in vitreo. *Bull Soc. Ophthalmol Fr* 78; 361, 1978.

9. MC Cuen BW 2nd, De Juan E Jr, Machemer R : silicone oil in vitreoretinal surgery Part 1st. Surgical techniques, *Retina* 5: 189, 1985.

10. Chang S: Giant retinal tears : Surgical management with perflurocarbon liquids. In Ryan SJ (Ed.) : *Medical and Surgical Retina*, St. Louis. The C.V. Mosby Co., pp 199-207, 1994.

11. Zivojnovic R : *Silicone oil in vitreo retinal surgery*. Dordrecht, The Nether lands, Martinus Nilhoff/ Dr. W Junk, 1987.

12. Leaver : Management of giant retinal tears with silicone oil. In Ryan SJ (Ed) : *Medical and Surgical Retina*, St. Louis, C.V. Mosby Co., pp 208-221, 1994.

Role of Vitrectomy in Endophthalmitis

Introduction

Endophthalmitis is defined as an inflammation of the inner coats of the eye associated with exudates in the vitreous which may be infectious or noninfectious in origin (Fig. 16.1). It is no doubt that it is catastrophic complication of intraocular surgery, penetrating injury, and endogenous infection. The most frequent pathogens causing acute bacterial endophthalmitis are gram positive cocci, i.e. *Staphylococcus albus* and *Staphylococcus aureus*, followed by the gram-negative organisms, especially *Pseudomonas aerugenosa*, *Streptococcus* and fungi.[1] In recent years attention has been directed to late onset endophthalmitis caused by *Propionibacterium acnes*.

DIAGNOSIS OF ENDOPHTHALMITIS

The ophthalmologist must maintain a high indent of suspicion for endophthalmitis; in patients with inflammation above the expected level, because early treatment is critical in achieving a good outcome (Fig 16.1) .

In addition to the clinical findings, the treatment can be made essentially by means of an anterior chamber and vitreous tap, so that fluid can be sent for culture. Anterior tap is not sufficient because up to 40% of cases in which the vitreous tap is positive, the anterior tap is negative. The vitreous tap should be obtained before antibiotics are administered.[2]

INTRAVITREAL INJECTION OF ANTIBIOTICS

The mainstay of treatment for postoperative endophthalmitis is intravitreal injection of antibiotics. Usually a combination of two antibiotics is chosen, which are selected based on their

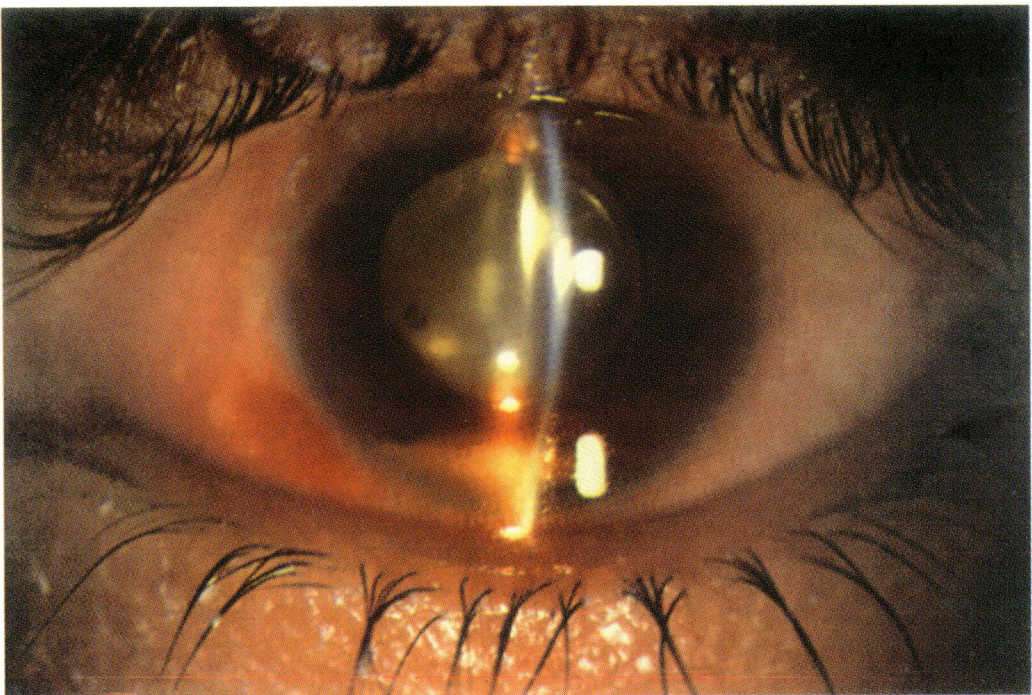

Fig. 16.1 *Postoperative endophthalmitis*

activity against coagulase negative staphylococci (the most common bacterial cause of endophthalmitis), and gram negative bacilli. The most commonly used and effective combination for their purpose at present is vancomycin (1 mg/0.1 ml) and ceftazidime (2.25 mg in 0.1 ml). While amikacin (400 µg/0.1 ml) could be used in place of ceftazidime, it possesses a higher risk of macular toxicity and should be avoided if possible. To limit the postoperative inflammation dexamethasone 400 µg/0.1 ml may be used.[3]

TECHNIQUES OF INTRAVITREAL INJECTION

Intravitreal injection of antibiotics should be given in the operation theatre under proper aseptic precautions. It is usually performed under topical anaesthesia. However, peribulbar anaesthesia could be administered if the patient is uncooperative.

The most common site for administering intravitreal injection is inferotemporally 3 mm from the limbus in aphakic and 3.5 mm in phakic eyes (Fig .16.2).

Initially around 0.5 cc vitreous should be aspirated with a 21 guage needle for making smears as well as for culture sensitivity; then antibiotics are injected in to the vitreous cavity with a 26 gauge needle. In case of a dry tap, aqueous paracentesis could be done to obtain material for smear and culture sensitivity and even more importantly, for bringing down the intraocular pressure prior to the intravitreal injection. It is not necessary to use two different needles for injecting the two antibiotics through different syringes is mandatory. The needle should be kept facing towards the center of the globe. The bevel of the needle should be dented upward, to-

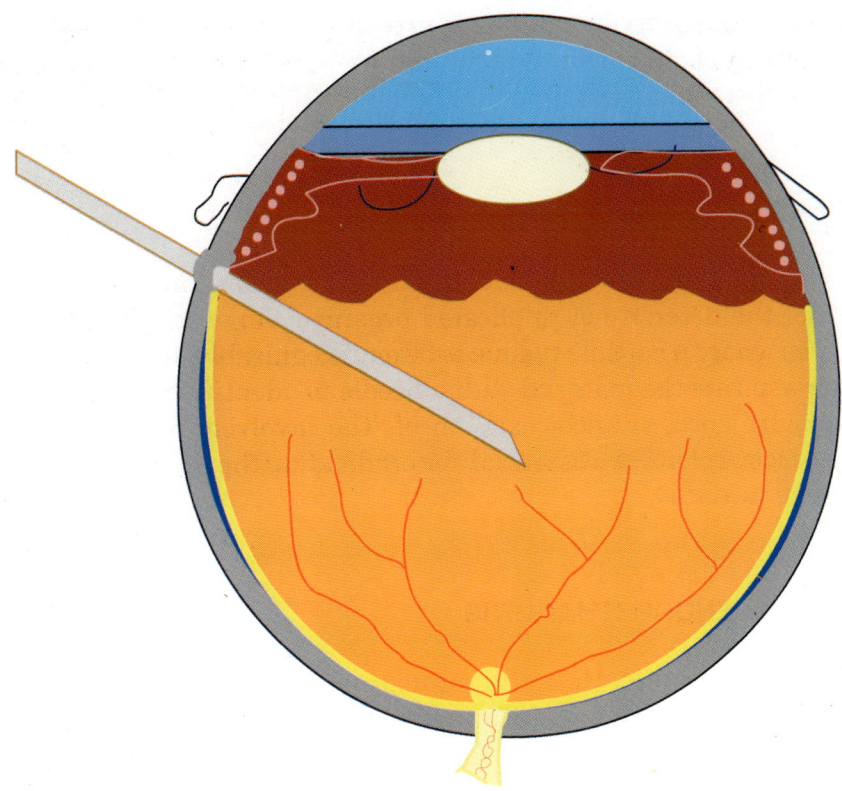

Fig. 16.2 *Intravitreal administration of antibiotic*

wards the cornea. The antibiotics should be taken in two separate glass tuberculin syringes. Disposable tuberculin syringes should be avoided. This is so because it is possible to inject the antibiotic slowly drop by drop with a glass tuberculin syringe by rotating the plunger while pushing it forward. This motion is not possible with disposable syringe. Thus, a jet of fluid is more likely to be injected with a disposable syringe.

ROLE OF VITRECTOMY IN ENDOPHTHALMITIS

The exact role of vitrectomy in the initial management of endophthalmitis is at present controversial. Vitrectomy is probably unnecessary in mild cases but may be beneficial in severe or resistant cases. The theoretical advantages include removal of the offending organism and toxins, enhanced distribution of antibiotics, removal of vitreous membrane which could lead to tractional retinal detachment and clearing of vitreous opacities. In cases of moderate or severe vitreous opacification one can do pars plana vitrectomy. Extensive therapeutic vitrectomy is not performed in mild cases of endophthalmitis. In those cases a vitreous tap (diagnostic vitrectomy) for culture and intravitreal injection of antibiotics is usually adequate.

In case of severe infection, vitrectomy is ideal as removing the vitreous will remove many of the toxins that damage the retina as well as allowing the antibiotics better access to the retina.

In many of these cases, a pupillary membrane is present which obstructs visualization of the vitreous cavity. The surgeon should remove the pupillary membrane by entering the anterior chamber through a limbal stab incision.

REMOVAL OF THE LENS CAPSULE

The management of chronic postoperative endophthalmitis is more controversial and difficult to generalize because of the diversity of implicated organism. In endophthalmitis caused by propionibacterium acnes where a capsule plaque is often recognizable, it is advisable to remove the involved capsule or aspirate the material with a needle to identify the organism on a grams stain. Despite the low virulence, surgical excision of the involved area of posterior capsule containing the plaque or focus of may be essential for eradicating the infection. Then intravitreal antibiotic therapy can be initiated.

TIPS FOR VITRECTOMY IN ENDOPHTHALMITIS

In modern area, there is no doubt that the mainstay of management for postoperative endophthalmitis is intravitreal antibiotics. However, there are certain situations in which vitrectomy may result not only in salvaging a favourable outcome in patients with this devastating disease process. Some of the practical tips regarding successful use of this very effective tool in the ophthalmologists armamentarium are as follows.

1. Inaccurate projection of light is not a contraindication for vitrectomy. In fact, it probably has almost no prognostic role at all.

2. Patients who have not responded to their first intravitreal injection of antibiotics given 48 hours earlier are candidates for an immediate vitrectomy.

3. Patients with a retinal detachment on B-scan ultrasonography; have a poor prognosis following vitrectomy, when there is dense exudates extending up to the posterior one-third of the vitreous cavity on ultrasonography.

4. Surgery is easier in patients with partial or total posterior vitreous detachment.

5. The decision regarding when to undertake vitrectomy is, however, based on clinical finding but not by ultrasonography.

SURGICAL TECHNIQUE

Surgery under general anesthesia is preferable for uncooperative patients as a rule, however, peribulbar anesthesia is adequate for vitrectomy. The wound margin must be inspected and strengthened by placing additional sutures before starting vitrectomy. Three port pars plana vitrectomy is usually under taken and 6 mm infusion cannula must be used. This can be inspected by depressing the cannula towards the pupillary area and should be sure of its presence inside the vitreous cavity. The infusion bottle must be kept higher around 20 inches from the patient's eye. In pseudophakic endophthalmitis, there is almost always a fibrin membrane covering the iris and the pupillary area. It can be removed through pars plana route by making an iridectomy next to the temporal port with the vitrectomy cutter with the help of MVR blade which is passed through the iridectomy to engage the fibrin membrane and dislodge it from its adhesion to the iris and the intraocular lens (IOL) surface. The membrane is then dissected away in the anterior chamber by introducing the vitrectomy probe through the iridectomy.

For vitrectomy cutter (800 to 1500 cuts per minutes) and low suction (50 to 100 mm of Hg) should be used in case of endophthalmitis. This will ensure that no under traction is put on the vitreous gel during the vitrectomy.

In some cases cornea is oedematous during operation, also poor pupillary dilatation, and haze on the intraocular lens, a complete vitrectomy may not be possible. In some cases a very clear view of the posterior retina is noticed. Some times there is accumulation of white inflammatory debris on the posterior retina which may be vaccumed with the same technique as used for removing blood. However, if there are inflammatory membranes attached to the retina, no attempt should be made to remove them because of the risk of tearing the retina. Most of this inflammation will resolve during the first few days of the postoperative period if the infecting bacteria are not highly virulent. Core vitrectomy is sufficient in majority cases. Lavage of the vitreous cavity can be carried out with vitreous cutter by continuing to use the vitreous cutter (in cutting mode) placed in the central vitreous cavity for at least (5–10 minutes) after the infected gel has been removed. This is possible to carry out the lavage without causing any turbulence within the vitreous cavity. Corneal epithelium debridement can be carried out at any time during vitrectomy if epithelial oedema is preventing adequate visualization, without any risk of causing a corneal ulcer.

After as much vitreous is removed, required doses of antibiotics intravitreal of are injected slowly through the sclerotomy. The eye should be tipped inferiorly and rocked slightly to create fluid currents because the antibiotics tend to sink posteriorly and may give dangerous concentration to the macula.

After closing of the sclerotomies, sclerocorneal wound should be checked once more since the corneal sutures could become loose due to maneuver. The results of vitrectomy are excellent if timely diagnosis and intervention are done in time. However, poor results may be seen is cases who have history of diabetes, corneal infiltration, ring-ulcer, abnormal intraocular pressure, rubeosis, absent of red-reflex or a ruptured posterior capsule. Today, however, with appropriate management, it is possible not only to salvage many of the cases of this devastating condition, but it is also possible to help them to retain some useful vision also.[4]

REFERENCES

1. Johnson MV et al : The endophthalmitis vitrectomy study relationship between clinical presentation and microbiologic spectrum. *Ophthalmology* 104: 261, 1997.

2. Meredith TA : Vitrectomy for injections endophthalmitis. In Ryan S (Ed.) *Retina* 3 edn; Vol. 3, St. Louis, Mosby Year Book, 1998.

3. Endophthalmitis : Vitrectomy study group. Results of the endophthalmitis vitrectomy study; a randomized intravenous antibiotics for the treatment of postoperative bacterial endophthalmitis. *Arch Ophthalmol* 113: 1479, 1995.

4. Endophthalmitis vitrectomy study group; microbiologic factors and visual out come in the endophthalmitis vitrectomy group. *Am J Ophthalmol* 122; 834, 1996.

Complications of Operative Vitreous Surgery

Introduction

Intraoperative complications in vitreous surgery have tremendously reduced due to advancement in technology and as well as expertise the whole procedure. Most of these complications are intraoperative, caused mainly by either pharmacobiological or mechanical insult to ocular structure and tissues. Some of these complications also occur in postoperative period, mainly as an extension of intraoperative complications.

COMPLICATIONS FOLLOWING SCLEROTOMY

The site of incision of sclerotomies should be within 3 to 4.5 mm from the limbus. Anterior incision can damage the lens or ciliary body and a posterior opening can evulse the vitreous base causing retina dialysis and sometimes also lead to retinal detachment (Fig. 17.1).

Many a times due to low tension the infusion cannula dose not enter the vitreous cavity and suprachoroid infusion may occur (Fig.17.2).

This happens with detachment of choroids. In cases of low tension, a long 6 mm cannula is helpful so that it passes through the coats of vitreous to prevent this complication. When there is incarceration of peripheral retina into the sclerotomy site, the infusion bottle can be lowered and retina should be milked inside, if there is no success, a forceps from the opposite sclerotomy can be introduced to pull the incarcerated retina out from the other sclerotomy. However, in case this also fails, fluid–gas exchange and removal of incarcerated tissue should be done. Some times bleeding from sclerotomy site is very annoying and happens in case of resurgery.

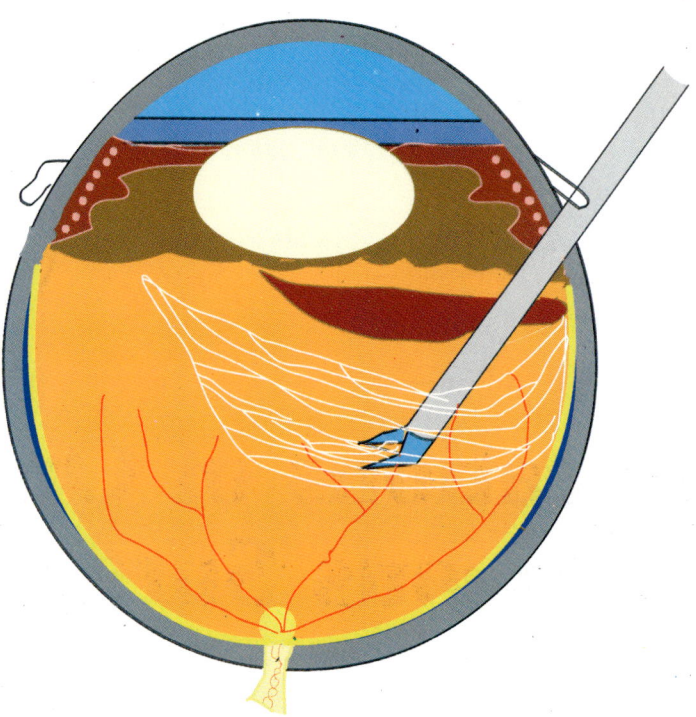

Fig 17.1 Tearing of the retina at the entry site

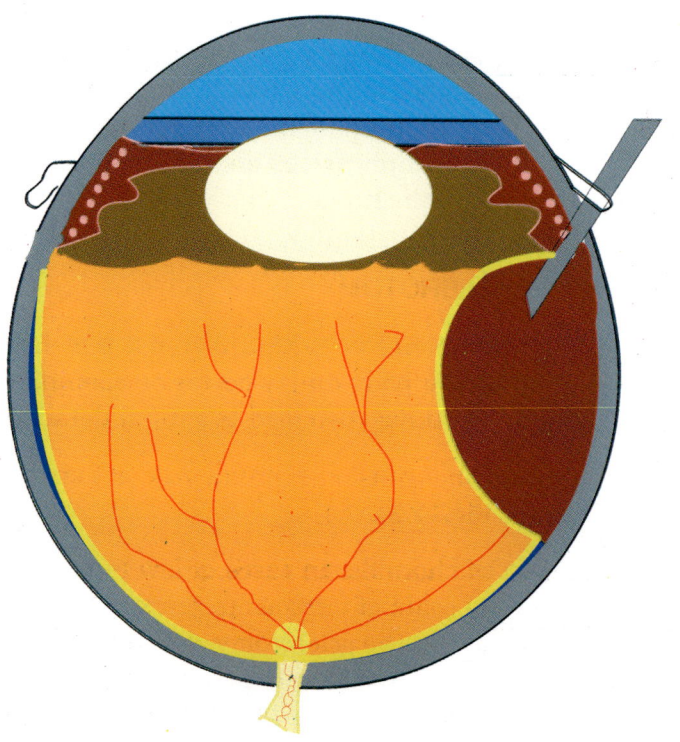

Fig 17.2 *If infusion at the choroid results in choroidal effusion, procedure must be stopped*

Application of surface diathermy suffices the bleeding vessels at the edge of the sclerotomy site. However, in the event of continuous bleeding possibility of changing sclerotomy site should be kept in mind.

CORNEAL COMPLICATIONS

Cornea is the window of the eye and it allows viewing of the posterior segment. Therefore, its clarity is essential during surgery. The most common complication is corneal odema, which occurs mainly due to raised intra ocular pressure and sometimes due to corneal epithelium oedema. In both the instances viewing of posterior segment are difficult and often frustrating. When corneal epithelium is the cause of corneal oedema, epithelium can be removed, thus improving the clarity. Any blunt instrument can be used to scrape the superficial layers of cornea till the epithelium comes off. Use of sharp instrument sometime can lead to damage of the basement membrane. Persistence of postoperative corneal oedema is mainly due to endothelial damage, which may be due to either direct mechanical insult to corneal endothelium during surgery, or due to prolonged usage of irrigating solution. One should avoid putting phenylephrine eye drop as it sometimes produces persistent corneal oedema. All these cases present with descemets fold and improve with healing of corneal endothelium. Hypertonic saline drops take care to reduce corneal oedema. Postoperative epithelial defects may require cessation of topical medication and keeping the lid patched with pad and bandage for 24 to 48 hrs. Occasionally a therapeutic contact lens may be required in non-healing defects.

RETINAL COMPLICATIONS

Retina tears occur during vitrectomy at entry site which is usually 2 to 3% of vitrectomies even when extensive manipulations are not required.[1] This occurs secondary to direct retinal trauma by the instruments or it may secondary to vitreous traction. Instruments entering the eye may catch on the vitreous base to create these tears. The entire periphery should be examined at the end of each procedure including sclerotomy sites. Peripheral tears are caused when vitreous is pulled interiorly as instruments are removed. At time due to high suction, sucking of the retina occurs into the vitrectomy probe. Sometime, while using a flush flute needle, tear occurs while lifting the membrane or sucking. Retina tears may occur at sites where membrane is being stripped from the retina when the adhesion is extraordinarily tight. The cutting probe may create retina holes. When the retina is very mobile, it may be pulled unexpected by the cutting port by the normal levels of suction even from distances of 2 to 3 mm. Sometimes, cutting with scissor blades horizontal to the retina tends to cause oval defects when a piece of retina is inadvertently included in the scissor bite. Vertical scissors tends to cause linear cuts in the retina beneath the membrane either because of pressure from the lower scissors blade or from passing the lower tip through the retina and then cutting it.

Prevention of these mishaps can be done immediately. When the retina gets engaged in vitrectomy probe, the machine should be stopped and suction should be replaced by gentle injection. This frees the retina, and iatrogenic small retina breaks if occurs require endo laser of the whole area around it. However, in the event of a large tear, a fluid/gas exchange is required depending upon the types of a cases and application endolaser around the tear is desirable. All attempts should be made to drain the subretinal fluid internally.

CHOROIDAL HAEMORRHAGE

During vitrectomy sudden appearance of a dark cone in the periphery of the field of view suggests a choroidal haemorrhage or effusion. The position of the irrigation cannula must always be checked to ensure that it remains in the vitreous cavity and not infusing into the choroids when there is inadvertent infusion into the choroids, the procedure must be stopped. One can choose a new sclerotomy site with longer cannula to continue the procedure.

VITREOUS HAEMORRHAGE

Vitreous hemorrhage occurs while handling neovascular membrane; neo-vascularisation of retina, iatrogenic tears formation and from the sclerotomy wound during surgery. Once the haemorrhage occurs, the infusion bottle should be immediately raised to maximum height for the haemorrhage to stop. Once the haemorrhage stops, a search should be made to find the source of bleeding accordingly, this should be diathermized. When there is bleeding due to epiretinal membrane after it stops and the retinal hemorrhage can be cleared by vacuum needle or large flute needle also. However, in the event of continued bleeding from new vessels, diathermy can be applied. Focal endophotocoagulation over the bleeder is also recommended as an alternative procedure.

LENS COMPLICATION

When working in the periphery, the light pipe may accidentally touch the back of the lens, leaving a linear defect. Mechanical damage to the lens can occur during sclerotomy or during introduction of infusion cannula or other intraocular instruments. During sclerotomy, if the incision is too anterior, damage to the lens is always a possibility. Mechanical injury to lens is always avoidable and careful entry into the vitreous cavity obviates such mishap. Care should be taken to use reflected light from the posterior segment or light from the operating microscope to reduce the risk of this complication.

However, once such a damage occurs, one should assess the extent of damage and if it is obstructing view of surgery, damaged lens may be removed either by vitreous cutter or fragmentome if nucleus is sclerotic.

MIOSIS DURING VITREOUS SURGERY

Miosis can produce problems during surgery. Intracameral diluted adrenaline (1:10000) gives via the limbus may help in dilatation of pupil as a considerable number of patients have small pupils preoperatively. The pupil can be mechanically stretched by temporary sutures (10-0) proline (Eckhardts technique). Eckhardt used this technique for making a quadrangular/triangular dilatation of pupil. This provides adequate visibility during surgery.

COMPLICATIONS OF SILICONE OIL

Emulsification. Emulsification probably occurs because of the shearing effect created by the difference between the velocities of movement of the silicone bubble and that of the eye and the fluid concentrated in the vitreous fluid may contribute to the shearing effect. It occurs invariably in all cases.

Keratopathy. Band-shaped keratopathy or stromal opacification may occur in 30% cases. Band keratopathy responds well to debridement of the cornea with diluted disodium ethylene diamine tetraacetic acid (EDTA), with application of a bandage lens postoperatively. Stromal opacification is treated by corneal transplant, in eyes with visual potential. Corneal transplant is usually carried out at the time of silicone oil removal.

Cataract. All phakic eyes containing intravitreal silicone oil develop cataracts. This is related to contact between the silicone globule and the posterior lens capsule and the resulting mechanical obstruction to diffusion of nutrients. The incidence of cataract is most pronounced between 6 and 18 months after surgery and opacification can develop or progress even after silicone withdrawl.

Pupillary Block. The inferior iridectomy by Ando has reduced the incidence of pupillary block considerably. Postoperative closure of peripheral iridectomy is highly correlated with forward oil migration and occurs most frequently in eyes with proliferative diabetic retinopathy. Silicone oil can migrate into the anterior chamber even in phakic eyes. This occurs through unsuspected zonular dehiscences. If small, this can be ignored and be removed along with the main bubble.

Hypotony. Hypotony has been reported in 16% cases. This has been attributed to the extensive anterior proliferation seen in most cases of complicated proliferative vitreo retinopathy (PVR). The anterior membranes, surgical attempts to remove them and extensive laser contribute towards lowering of intraocular pressure. Silicone oil removal should be avoided in cases with hypotony.

Peri silicone Proliferative Macular Pucker. Macular pucker has been reported to occur in approximately 30% cases. Membranes should be removed at the time of oil removal.

Recurrent Retinal Detachments. Recurrence of retinal detachment has been reported to occur in 25-40% cases. Reoperation should be done if the eye has visual potential. The recurrences in most cases are not attributable to silicone oil but to the primary disease process. The use of liquid vitreous substitutes have revolutionized vitreoretinal surgery. As new indications for these liquids continue to evolve, and their use becomes more widespread, their many benefits will be appreciated by the vitreoretinal surgeons. Most complications with silicone oil can be avoided if one is aware that silicone oil is not a permanent tamponading agent but should be removed as soon as possible. The twin objective of retinal reattachment surgery is possible in a majority of cases by meticulous initial surgery while injecting silicone oil, and by careful evaluation at time of oil removal.

During injection of silicone oil if excessive force exerted it pushes the retina and causes tear formation . This happens when there is a incomplete relief of retina traction from proliferative tissue or due to pre existing retinal traction, the silicone oil is pushed behind the retina. When it happens, a glossy retinal reflex from choroids is visible. Removal of silicone oil should be done immediately after stopping the injection.

Small amount of silicone oil may be squeezed out of retina by blunt instrument but for large amount either suction underneath the retina is applied and large retinotomy is performed to release the silicone oil. While injecting silicone oil, care should be taken so that it does not touch the corneal endothelium directly. Once silicone oil fills up vitreous cavity and it reaches the infusion tube or pupillary plane, ringer lactate or balance salt solution (BSS) is injected using a bent cannula directed into the anterior chamber via sclerotomy. This ensures that the silicone oil is pushed back into the vitreous cavity and the anterior chamber is filled with ringers lactate solution or balance salt solution (BSS).

GLAUCOMA IN VITREOUS SURGERY

Glaucoma is one of the serious complications, which are usually seen after vitreous surgery.[2] Different types of glaucoma are encountered postoperatively.

Pupillary block Glaucoma. Air or gas can block the pupil postoperatively and can be effectively prevented by proper positioning, i.e. facedown position.

Silicone oil Glaucoma. This is a common postoperative complication following silicone oil injection. Pupillary block glaucoma, which often occurs is prevented by an inferior iridectomy (Ando) performed at 6 O' clock position. Silicone oil, being lighter than water, rises up and aqueous can percolate through the inferior peripheral iridectomy. Constant monitoring of IOP after ejecting silicone oil is, however, mandatory, as the cause of glaucoma is often multifactorial. Emulsification of oil, formation of peripheral anterior synechia, etc. contributes to this glaucoma.

Erythroclastic Glaucoma. This is a form of hemolytic glaucoma often occurring due to incomplete vacuum cleaning. The phenomenon is transient and self limited, treatable conservatively with antic glaucoma medication.

Neo-vascular Glaucoma. Rise of intraocular pressure has been seen in certain cases after surgery, which is mainly due to neovascularisation at the trabecular meshwork. It occurs 2 to 12 weeks after operation. It is a recalcitrant type of glaucoma and lowering of intraocular pressure by conventional therapy is often a problem. Cyclocryocoagulation and cyclophotocoagulation are usually beneficial.

Steroid Glaucoma. Postoperative excessive use of steroid may sometimes lead to steroid-induced glaucoma. Discontinuation of steroid completely and use of conservative anti-glaucoma medication helps in controlling the intraocular pressure.

Open angle Glaucoma. This usually occurs secondary to the metabolic trauma to trabeculer meshwork occurring from the infusion fluid, treatment is conservative.

RETINAL BURN

Light burns may be created when the media is clear and there is prolonged macular surgery or prolonged opening and closing allowing concentrated light on one area of the retina. Pale swelling of the retina is seen and later this burn may lead to an oval appearance with patchy coarse pigmentation of retinal pigment epithelium .[3,4]

ENDOPHTHALMITIS

Postoperative endophthalmitis incidence is reduced due to better care and improved sterilization technique. Prevention is key and proper instrument sterilization, shorter operating time and better preparation of irrigating solution, all reduce the risk of infection. Antibiotic regimens which cover both gram-positive and gram-negative organisms are administered sub-conjunctively after surgery. Postvitreal injection of combination antibiotic covering both gram-positive and gram negative, e.g. Amikacin 400 mg + 2.25mg cephazolin can be administered. If no improvement occurs within 48-72 hrs, a repeat vitrectomy can then be performed with guarded prognosis.

REFERENCES

1. Charles S: *Vitreous Microsurgery*, 2nd edn, Baltimore, Williams & Wilkins 1987.

2. Faulborn J, Conway BP, Machermer R: Surgical complication of pars plana vitreous surgery, *Ophthalmology* 85:116,1978.

3. Fuller D, Machemer R, Knighton RW: Retina damage produced by intra-ocular fiber optic light *Am J Ophthalmol* 85: 519, 1978.

4. Robertson DM, Feldman RB: Photic retinopathy from the operating room microscope. *Am J Ophthalmol* 101:561,1986.

5. The silicone study group: Vitrectomy with silicone oil or sulphur hexafluoride gas in eyes with severe proliferative vitreoretinopathy silicone study report. *Arch Ophthalmol* 110:770, 1992.

Index

Advantages of EIBOS 24
Anatomic considerations 99
Anterior hyaloidal proliferation 115
Basic diabetic vitrectomy 104
Basic working principle of vitrectomy equipment 27
Binocular indirect ophthalmo microscope (BIOM) 24
Care of instruments 43
   cleaning 43
   disinfections and sterilisation 43
   instruments sets 43
   storage 43
Cataract 217
Choroidal haemorrhage 216
Classification 119
Closure, fluid-air exchange 70
Coaxial and oblique zoom illumination 19
Coaxial zoom illumination 19
Complications of silicone oil
   recurrent retinal detachments 217
   emulsification 217
   hypotony 217
   keratopathy 217
Corneal clouding 168
Cortical vitreous 2
Delamination of diabetic membrane 107
Diabetic membrane delamination 113
   bimanual dissection technique 113
Diabetic vitrectomy 99
   en bloc techniques in diabetic membrane 111
   indication of diabetic vitrectomy 103
   intraoperative complications of diabetic membrane dissection 116
   introduction to 99
   segmentation on fibrovascular proliferation 107
   surgical objectives 104
Drainage complications 168
EBIOS
   advantages of 24
   cleaning and sterilization 26
   description of functions 26
   diagrammatic representation of parts 25

erected image binocular ophthalmoscopic system 24
   how to use 26
Endophthalmitis 219
Erected image binocular ophthalmoscopic system (EIBOS) 24
Failure of primary retinal detachment pitfalls 172
Fluid-air exchange 62
   after retinal reapplication using a liquid perfluorocarbon 68
   associated with drainage of subretinal fluid 68
   combined with drainage of subretinal fluid though a posterior dehiscence 68
Fluorescein angiography unit 11
Foot switch, an overview 22
Fundus contact lenses for vitreoretinal surgery 23
Giant retinal tear 187
   diagnosis and preoperative evaluation 187
   introduction 187
   location 188
   management of 187
      extent of proliferative vitreoretinopathy (PVR) 189
      fellow eye 205
      mobility of posterior retinal flap 188
      postoperative complications 203
      procedure (surgical technique) 190
      silicone oil removal 199
      silicone oil technique in giant retinal tear 193
      treatment of giant tear 202
Glaucoma in vitreous surgery 218
   neo-vascular glaucoma 218
   open angle glaucoma 218
   pupillary block glaucoma 218
   silicone oil glaucoma 218
   steroid glaucoma 218
   erythroclastic glaucoma 218
Indication for vitrectomy in rhegmatogenous retinal detachment 180
Infrastructure 10

Intraoperative complications of scleral
   buckling 168
IR-PFCL exchange 68
Large retinal intraocular foreign body 138
Laser photocoagulation unit 12
Laser photocoagulation 69
Liquid perfluorocarbon in giant retinal tear 199
Locations and extent of penetrating injuries
   related to prognosis 139
Loss of lens fragments into the vitreous 74
Macular hole surgery 83
   removal of ilm 88
   surgical technique 84
   when to perform surgery in macular hole 84
Macular hole 81
   clinical features 81
   diagnosis 83
   introduction 81
Macular pucker (macular distortion) 90
Main cause of failure of retina detachment (rd)
   surgery 172
Management of ocular trauma and retained
   intraocular foreign bodies 131
Miosis 168
   during vitreous surgery 216
Ocular trauma 138
   encapsulated RIOFB 138
   glass and other foreign bodies 139
   introduction to 131
   repair of scleral laceration, ruptures and
      prognosis 139
   retained IOFB - in the vitreous cavity 138
   risk of intraoperative haemorrhage 133
   role of infection in timing of surgery 132
   role of vitrectomy 133
   subretinal intraocular foreign body 138
   surgery of pvr in penetrating trauma 140
   timing of surgery 132
   vitrectomy endolaser silicone oil
      tamponade 133
   wound closure 132
Operating microscope and wide angle fundus
   observation system 17
Operating microscope 17
   beam splitter and eyepiece head 18
   care, sterilization and maintenance 20
   checking after surgery 20
   filter and protection for eyes 19
   foot switch 21
   illumination 19
   introduction to 17
objective lens assembly 18
   trouble-shooting and remedies of 21
   zoom device 18
Operative vitreous surgery, Complications of
   213
Pars plana lensectomy 53
Pars plana vitrectomy 45
   basic Technique 45
   for retinal detachments 181
   conjunctival incisions 47
   infusion cannula 49
   instrument handling 51
   introduction to 45
   irrigation fluids 46
   making the entry sites 47
   management of small pupil 54
   mid-peripheral iridectomy 55
   multiple sphincterotomies 55
   mydriasis 45
   nonsurgical treatment of small pupils 54
   patient preparation 45
   preparation of the surgical field 46
   radial iridectomy for miotic pupil 55
   sphincterotomy or pupilloplasty 55
   steps for removal of lens 53
   surgical treatment of small pupil 54
   vacuum technique 61
   basic technique 45
Patient preparation 42
Patient preparation for vitreous surgery and
   care of instruments 37
   anaesthesia 39
   check lists for vitrectomy and fragmatome
      units 39
   checking the microscope 39
   checking the microsurgical equipment 39
   checklist of instruments in ot 39
   dilatation of pupils 38
   introduction to 37
   irrigation fluid 42
   patient preparation 37
   preparation for surgery 38
   preparation of eye 38
Pneumatic retinoplexy 174
   introduction to 174
   preoperative evaluation 174
   procedure 175
Postoperative complications 169
   anterior segment ischemia 170
   changes in refractive error after scleral
      buckling 171

choroidal detachment   170
cystoid macular oedema   171
extrusions and buckle infection   170
glaucoma   169
macular pucker   171
postoperative diplopia   171
Precaution with
    cryotherapy   173
    scleral buckling   173
Preparing vitrectomy unit for use   30
Preventive steps to avoid primary failure   173
Primary vitrectomy in retinal detachment
        caused by macular hole   182
Primary vitrectomy in retinal detachment
        caused by peripheral breaks 185
Primary vitrectomy in retinal detachment
        caused by posterior breaks 183
Proliferative vitreoretinopathy (PVR) 140
    in ocular trauma 140
    anatomic presentation in 120
    membrane removal 123
    membrane removal with perflurocarbon
        technique in 128
    optimal time for operation in 122
    principles of treatment of, to close all retinal
        breaks   122
    vitrectomy technique in 122
Pupillary block   217
Removal of foreign bodies   133
Retained intraocular foreign bodies 138
    encapsulated RIOFB   138
    glass and other foreign bodies   139
    in the vitreous cavity   138
    introduction to   131
    removal of foreign bodies   133
    repair of scleral laceration, ruptures and
        prognosis   139
    risk of intraoperative haemorrhage   133
    role of
        infection in timing of surgery   132
        vitrectomy   133
    surgery of pvr in penetrating trauma   140
    timing of surgery   132
    vitrectomy endolaser silicone oil
        tamponade   133
    wound closure   132
Retained lens fragments and intraocular lens
        dislocation 73
    emphasized during cataract surgery   74
    identification of risk factors   73
    introduction to   73

time of removal of retained lens fragments
        and dislocated lens   74
Retinal burn   218
Retinal detachment 79
Retinopathy of prematurity (ROP) 141
    classification   141
    complications   150
    introduction   141
    laser/cryo treatment in retinopathy of
        prematurity   146
    management of pupil   147
    pathogenesis   141
    peripheral traction problems   149
    plus disease   145
    posterior tractional problems   148
    screening   145
        stage 1: demarcation line   142
        stage 2: ridge   143
        stage 3: ridge with extra-retinal
        fibrovascular   proliferation   144
        stage 4: partial retinal development   144
        stage 5: total retinal detachment   145
    staging   142
    surgical management of retinopathy of
        prematurity   146
    surgical options   148
    threshold disease   145
Rhegmatogenous retinal detachment 151
    basic requirement of retinal detachment
        surgery   156
    basic surgical technique   155
    buckle position, suture finalisation and
        adjustments   161
    Custodis technique   167
    diagnosis   151
    drainage of subretinal fluid   160
    introduction to   151
    localisation and treatment of retinal
        breaks   154
    management of subretinal fluid
        drainage   159
    methods of buckling   156
    securing the ends of the band   159
    surgical anatomy of conjunctiva, tenon's
        capsule and muscles isolation   152
Role of vitreous surgery in primary
        rhegmatogenous retinal detachment 179
    introduction to 179
Scleral perforations   168
Setting up the vitreoretinal unit 9
Subfoveal choroidal neovascularization   93

Subretinal intraocular foreign body   138
Subretinal neovascularization   93
   complications   97
   instrumentation   94
   postoperative management   97
   surgical technique   95
Surgery for proliferative vitreoretinopathy   119
   introduction to   119
Surgical anatomy and its importance in
      vitreoretinal surgery   1
Surgical anatomy
   introduction to   1
Surgical landmarks, important   4
Surgical treatment of macular surface disorder
   81
Techniques of intraocular foreign body
      removal   134
Ultrasonography unit   11
Vitrectomy accessories   13
Vitrectomy equipment   32
   air-module   32
   aspiration   35
   back-flush features   29
   cleaning and sterilizing instruction for
      accessories   35
   cleaning instructions   36
   compressed air inlet   34
   diathermy module   31
   dual illumination module   31
   foot switch functions   28
   irrigation   35
   irrigation/aspiration (I/A) and viscus fluid
      extraction module   34
   preoperating procedure   30
   recommendation guidelines for ethylene oxide
      sterilization parameters   35
   recommendation guidelines for steam
      sterilization   35

vitrectomy/VFI module   33
Vitrectomy in endophthalmitis   210
   surgical technique   210
Vitrectomy in simple vitreous haemorrhage   122
   technique in proliferative vitreoretinopathy
      122
Vitrectomy, role of, in endophthalmitis   207
   diagnosis of endophthalmitis   207
   intravitreal injection of antibiotics   207
   introduction   207
   removal of the lens capsule   210
   role of vitrectomy in endophthalmitis   209
   techniques of intravitreal injection   208
   tips for vitrectomy in endophthalmitis   210
Vitreoretinal tray   13
Vitreoretinal unit
   consumable items   14
   duty of responsible staff   14
   introduction to   9
   operating room assistants   16
   operating room   12
   standby anaesthesiologist   15
   sterilization   14
   supportive service   15
   surgeon and trained assistant   15
Vitreous anatomy   2
Vitreous body, main   3
Vitreous haemorrhage flow chart   59
Vitreous humour   2
Vitreous surgery complications   213
   complications following sclerotomy   213
   complications of silicone oil   217
   corneal complications   215
   introduction to   213
   lens complication   216
   retinal complications   215
   vitreous haemorrhage   216
Wide angle fundus observation system   23